# Developmental Toxicology
*Target Organ Toxicology Series*

# Target Organ Toxicology Series

Editor-in-Chief: Robert L. Dixon
*National Institute of Environmental Health Sciences*
*Research Triangle Park, North Carolina*

**Blood Toxicology**
*Richard D. Irons and James E. Gibson, editors*

**Cardiovascular Toxicology**
*Ethard W. Van Stee, editor*

**Developmental Toxicology**
*Carole A. Kimmel and Judy Buelke-Sam, editors, 352 pp., 1981*

**Immune Toxicology**
*Jack H. Dean and Albert E. Munson, editors*

**Liver Toxicology**
*Gabriel L. Plaa and William R. Hewitt, editors*

**Lung Toxicology**
*Gary E. R. Hook, editor*

**Nervous System Toxicology**
*Clifford L. Mitchell, editor*

**Toxicology of the Endocrine System**
*John A. Thomas, Kenneth S. Korach, and John A. McLachlan, editors*

**Toxicology of the Eye, Ear, and Other Special Senses**
*A. Wallace Hayes, Reginald Cook, and David Eckerman, editors*

**Toxicology of the Gonads**
*Robert L. Dixon and Raymond D. Harbison, editors*

**Toxicology of the Intestines**
*Carol M. Schiller, editor*

**Toxicology of the Kidney**
*Jerry B. Hook, editor, 288 pp., 1981*

*Target Organ Toxicology Series*

# Developmental Toxicology

## Editors

### Carole A. Kimmel, Ph.D., and Judy Buelke-Sam, M.A.

*Perinatal and Postnatal Evaluation Branch*
*Division of Teratogenesis Research*
*National Center for Toxicological Research*
*Food and Drug Administration/DHHS*
*Jefferson, Arkansas*

Raven Press ■ New York

Raven Press, 1140 Avenue of the Americas, New York, New York 10036

**Library of Congress Cataloging in Publication Data**
Main entry under title:

Developmental toxicology

(Target organ toxicology series)
Incluces bibliographical references and
index.
1. Fetus—Effect of drugs on.
2. Teratogenic agents.   I. Kimmel, Carole A.
II. Buelke-Sam, Judy.   III. Series.
RG627.6.D79D48        618.3'2        79-5302
ISBN 0-89004-542-9

*To*
*James G. Wilson*
*Mentor and Friend*

# Foreword

The *Target Organ Toxicology* monographs have evolved from the need for periodic review of the methods used to assess chemically induced toxicity. In each monograph, experts focus upon the following areas of a particular organ system: (1) a review of the morphology, physiology, biochemistry, cellular biology, and developmental aspects of the system; (2) a description of the means routinely used to assess toxicity; (3) an evaluation of the feasibility of tests used in the assessment of hazards; (4) proposals for applying recent advances in the basic sciences to the development and validation of new test procedures; (5) a description of the incidence of chemically induced human disease; and (6) an assessment of the reliability of laboratory test data extrapolation to humans and of the methods currently used to estimate human risk.

Thus, these monographs should be useful to both students and professionals of toxicology. Each provides a concise description of organ toxicity, including an up-to-date review of the biological processes represented by the target organ, a summary of how chemicals perturb these processes and alter function, and a description of methods by which such toxicity is detected in laboratory animals and humans. Attention is also directed to the identification of probable toxic chemicals and the establishment of exposure standards which are both economically and scientifically feasible, while adequately protecting human health and the environment.

Robert L. Dixon
*Editor-in-Chief*

# Preface

Developmental toxicology involves the consolidation of a diverse range of disciplines, which is exemplified by the chapters in this volume. This specialty within toxicology encompasses many of the areas covered by the larger field, but is even more complex because of the ever-changing nature of the developing organism. Indeed, the susceptibility of an organism to insult is influenced by continual changes in the state of differentiation, organization, and growth. In addition, the expression of toxicity following such insult may be dependent on a chain of morphological, physiological, or chemical events (pathogenesis) that occur before the "final" defect is manifest. Thus, the timing of agent exposure and of endpoint evaluation must be considered carefully in the design and interpretation of developmental toxicity studies.

The link between thalidomide exposure and limb malformations in the early 1960s forced expansion of the field of teratology and resulted in numerous studies of structural malformations. Over the past 10 years, newer aspects of developmental toxicology have been explored and recognized as important in evaluating risk following developmental exposure. This volume is intended to provide essential basic information in the field and to indicate the current state of the art, in many cases describing newer methods applicable to the study of developmental toxicology. The subject areas covered are: development and differentiation, including discussion of the morphological and biochemical bases and the role played by the placenta; developmental determinants of toxicity, including genetic and metabolic factors and cellular receptors; perinatal and postnatal functional evaluations; and assessment of test methods, including current and future procedures and the use of developmental toxicity data for risk assessment.

An important task now at hand is to integrate information from thorough studies on the manifestations of developmental insult, the pharmacodynamics of an agent, and the potential mechanisms of action into an overall profile of developmental toxicity. This type of approach, which is discussed in the last chapter, requires careful planning and cooperation as well as a large commitment of time and resources. However, the integrated study of a full range of endpoints, potential mechanisms, and comparative pharmacodynamics should lead to more precise determination of hazard and subsequent extrapolation to man. The information contained in this volume will point out the achievements as well as the complexities of this field and the many areas which need further study. We hope that more integrated approaches to developmental toxicology will be pursued to provide a better basis for predicting, and thus minimizing, human developmental toxicities.

This volume will be of interest to toxicologists, developmental biologists, pharmacologists, teratologists, pediatricians, and other scientists and clinicians studying prenatal exposure to natural and man-made substances.

Jefferson, Arkansas                                                      Carole A. Kimmel
                                                                          Judy Buelke-Sam

# Acknowledgments

We are indebted to the National Institute of Environmental Health Sciences, the Society of Toxicology, and the community of academic and federal scientists for the symposia upon which this set of monographs is based. The successful efforts of Joseph R. Borzelleca and Perry J. Gehring in initiating and coordinating the symposia are greatly appreciated.

Robert L. Dixon
Editor-in-Chief

We are very grateful for the cooperation of the distinguished group of contributors to this volume. The research efforts they collectively report provide an optimistic outlook for the future of developmental toxicology. We also thank Ms. Rose Huber, Mrs. Cindy Hartwick, the NCTR General Services Branch, and especially Mrs. Ruth York for their invaluable assistance in compiling this volume.

Carole A. Kimmel
Judy Buelke-Sam

# Contents

# Contributors

**Jane Adams, Ph.D.**
*Perinatal and Postnatal Evaluation Branch*
*Division of Teratogenesis Research*
*National Center for Toxicological Re-*
*search*
*Food and Drug Administration*
*Jefferson, Arkansas 72079*

**F. D. Andrew, Ph.D.**
*Biology Department*
*Pacific Northwest Laboratory*
*Richland, Washington 99352*

**A. Barth, Dr. Med.**
*Institute of Pharmacology and Toxicology*
*Friedrich Schiller University of Jena*
*Löbderstrasse 1*
*DDR-69 Jena*
*German Democratic Republic*

**F. Beck, M.D., Ch.B., D.Sc.**
*Department of Anatomy*
*The Medical School*
*University of Leicester*
*Leicester LE1 7RH, England*

**Fred G. Biddle, Ph.D.**
*Kinsmen Pediatric Research Centre*
*Alberta Children's Hospital*
*1820 Richmond Road S.W.; and*
*Departments of Pediatrics and Medical*
*    Biochemistry*
*Faculty of Medicine*
*University of Calgary*
*Calgary, Alberta, Canada T2N 1N4*

**Judy Buelke-Sam, M.A.**
*Perinatal and Postnatal Evaluation Branch*
*Division of Teratogenesis Research*
*National Center for Toxicological Re-*
*search*
*Food and Drug Administration*
*Jefferson, Arkansas 72079*

**John R. Chapman, B.S.**
*Immunotoxicology Branch*
*Division of Molecular Biology*
*National Center for Toxicological Re-*
*search*

*Food and Drug Administration*
*Jefferson, Arkansas 72079*

**J. David Erickson, D.D.S., Ph.D.**
*Bureau of Epidemiology*
*U.S. Public Health Service*
*Department of Health and Human Services*
*Center for Disease Control*
*Atlanta, Georgia 30333*

**Sergio E. Fabro, M.D., Ph.D.**
*Department of Obstetrics and Gynecology*
*The George Washington University*
*Washington, D.C. 20037*

**Richard M. Hoar, Ph.D.**
*Toxicology Division*
*Hoffmann-LaRoche, Inc.*
*Nutley, New Jersey 07110*

**Carole A. Kimmel, Ph.D.**
*Perinatal and Postnatal Evaluation Branch*
*Division of Teratogenesis Research*
*National Center for Toxicological Re-*
*search*
*Food and Drug Administration*
*Jefferson, Arkansas 72079*

**G. L. Kimmel, Ph.D.**
*Developmental Mechanisms Branch*
*Division of Teratogenesis Research*
*National Center for Toxicological Re-*
*search*
*Food and Drug Administration*
*Jefferson, Arkansas 72079*

**U. Kleeberg, Dr. med.**
*Institute of Pharmacology and Toxicology*
*Friedrich Schiller University of Jena*
*Löbderstrasse 1*
*DDR-69 Jena*
*German Democratic Republic*

**W. Klinger, Prof. Dr. sc. med.**
*Institute of Pharmacology and Toxicology*
*Friedrich Schiller University of Jena*
*Löbderstrasse 1*
*DDR-69 Jena*
*German Democratic Republic*

**D. M. Kochhar, Ph.D.**
*Department of Anatomy*
*Jefferson Medical College*
*Thomas Jefferson University*
*Philadelphia, Pennsylvania 19107*

**K. S. Korach, Ph.D.**
*Transplacental Toxicology Group*
*Laboratory of Reproductive and Develop-*
*  mental Toxicology*
*National Institute of Environmental Health*
*  Sciences*
*P.O. Box 12233*
*Research Triangle Park, North Carolina*
*  27709*

**J. C. Lamb IV, Ph.D.**
*National Toxicology Program*
*P.O. Box 12233*
*Research Triangle Park, North Carolina*
*  27709*

**George W. Lucier, Ph.D.**
*Laboratory of Organ Function and Toxi-*
*  cology*
*National Institute of Environmental Health*
*  Sciences*
*P.O. Box 12233*
*Research Triangle Park, North Carolina*
*  27709*

**P. S. Lytz, B.S.**
*Biology Department*
*Pacific Northwest Laboratory*
*Richland, Washington 99352*

**J. A. McLachlan, Ph.D.**
*Transplacental Toxicology Group*
*Laboratory of Reproductive and Develop-*
*  mental Toxicology*
*National Institute of Environmental Health*
*  Sciences*
*P.O. Box 12233*
*Research Triangle Park, North Carolina*
*  27709*

**Ian W. Monie, M.D.**
*Department of Anatomy*
*University of California*
*San Francisco, California 94143*

**D. Müller, Dr. sc. med.**
*Institute of Pharmacology and Toxicology*
*Friedrich Schiller University of Jena*
*Löbderstrasse 1*
*DDR-69 Jena*
*German Democratic Republic*

**R. R. Newbold, C.T. (A.S.C.P.)**
*Transplacental Toxicology Group*
*Laboratory of Reproductive and Develop-*
*  mental Toxicology*
*National Institute of Environmental Health*
*  Sciences*
*P.O. Box 12233*
*Research Triangle Park, North Carolina*
*  27709*

**A. K. Palmer, B.Sc.**
*Huntingdon Research Centre*
*Huntingdon*
*Cambridgeshire PE18 6ES, England*

**Jerry M. Rice, Ph.D.**
*Perinatal Carcinogenesis Section*
*Laboratory of Experimental Pathology*
*National Cancer Institute*
*Bethesda, Maryland 20205*

**Dean W. Roberts, Ph.D.**
*Immunotoxicology Branch*
*Division of Molecular Biology*
*National Center for Toxicological*
*  Research*
*Food and Drug Administration*
*Jefferson, Arkansas 72079*

**Anthony R. Scialli, M.D.**
*Columbia Hospital for Women*
*2435 L Street, N.W.*
*Washington, D.C. 20037*

**Richard G. Skalko, Ph.D.**
*Department of Anatomy*
*College of Medicine*
*East Tennessee State University*
*Johnson City, Tennessee 37614*

**Y. Suzuki, Ph.D.**
*Asia University*
*24-10, 5-Chome Sakai*
*Musashino-shi*
*Tokyo 180, Japan*

*Developmental Toxicology*, edited by
C. A. Kimmel and J. Buelke-Sam. Raven Press,
New York © 1981.

# Biochemical Mechanisms in Developmental Toxicology

### Richard G. Skalko

*Department of Anatomy, College of Medicine, East Tennessee State University, Johnson City, Tennessee 37614*

## TERMS AND CONCEPTS

The study of developmental events entails an analysis of the progressive change in the potential of cells. This progression is orderly, reproducible, and follows a distinct relationship to time. It is well known that certain environmental agents and drugs have the ability to interfere with this progression and, in so doing, to produce an embryotoxic effect. The study of the normal sequence of developmental processes *(developmental biology)* and the analysis of chemically induced alterations in this sequence *(developmental toxicology)* are intimately related. However, the difficulties associated with understanding basic problems in development, such as cellular differentiation, are magnified considerably when biologically significant exogenous influences are introduced. Thus, if one examines some of the more recent theories of cellular differentiation, the difficulty in understanding the restriction of developmental potential becomes apparent. These theories include changes in cyclic nucleotides and inorganic ions within developing cells as a function of time (32), the response of the cell membrane and its receptors to changes in the microenvironment of the cell and the transfer of this information to the genome (6), and the temporal restriction of gene activity within a cell leading to the expression of a single phenotype (7).

All of these theories represent solid attempts to define, in temporal terms, the underlying cellular and biochemical mechanisms by which developing cells normally respond to their environment in a specific and reproducible manner. The basic challenge that confronts developmental toxicologists, then, is not only the practical definition of those agents that are capable of eliciting a toxic response but the analysis of those normal developmental mechanisms that are altered and lead to subsequent abnormal development.

The scientific origins of the study of abnormal morphogenesis *(teratology)* in classical descriptive and experimental embryology have been documented and extensively reviewed by Zwilling (68) and Corner (8). As the study of environmentally induced teratogenesis progressed, it became obvious that the expressivity of a toxic effect by the conceptus was both highly reproducible and specific (42). Thus, in both practical and

*1*

theoretical terms, the demonstration of specific responses by the embryo to exogenous agents would suggest that those methods and concepts that are useful to the analysis of normal development could also be applied to abnormal development. The converse should also be true, and indeed, it has been possible to utilize the procedures of experimental teratogenesis to explore basic problems in cell lineage (19) and in the elaboration of extracellular matrices (24). In both developmental biology and developmental toxicology, it is also essential to define events in cellular terms and, in the study of the response of embryos to abnormal environmental cues, to define those susceptible cell populations that are influenced by a particular treatment. It is in this regard that the tools and concepts of the science of toxicology are invaluable.

If a chemical *(toxin)* produces an adverse effect in any biological system, there is a basic assumption that it affects some cells and does not affect others, that is, that its action is selective to some degree (1). Authors have referred to those cells that are particularly affected by exogenous chemicals as "uneconomic" (1), "sensitive" (51), or "target" cells (38). Those cells that appear to be unaffected by such exposure are described as being either "economic" (1) or "tolerant" (51). Such a toxin would produce its selective effects according to two broad principles: (a) the agent is equally toxic to both "sensitive" and "tolerant" cells, but, due to discrete metabolic differences between the two cell types, it is accumulated (or retained) by the "sensitive" cells at a distinctly higher level; (b) the agent reacts fairly specifically with a cytological or biochemical feature of the "sensitive" cells which may either be absent from or play a less important role in the biology of the "tolerant" cells (1). These two principles quite obviously are not mutually exclusive, and it is possible that both mechanisms could be responsible for a single toxic response to any specific agent.

The application of these principles in the study of developmental toxicology is a complex undertaking. Because of the central role that time plays in development, the embryo is in constant change and is a different organism at any two points in time no matter how small the interval between them (59). However, developmental events are so regular that, even with inherent and well-documented alterations of form and function, they are amenable to analysis. Because of this, it is possible to employ these principles and, in doing so, develop testable models of chemically induced embryotoxicity (38,66). If these principles are to have broad applicability, however, it is necessary to modify some concepts that are still used, specifically the long-held view that teratological and toxicological responses are the manifestation of two distinct biological processes (4). In view of the many recent attempts to explain abnormal development in toxicological terms, it is more reasonable to accept the view expressed by Neubert et al. (37) that teratogenesis represents a special form of embryotoxicity.

## BIOCHEMICAL ONTOGENY IN ANIMAL DEVELOPMENT

Although the study of biochemical ontogeny in nonmammalian vertebrate embryos has had a long and productive history (41,61), similar analyses of mammalian development have been fairly recent (26,49). It is the purpose of this selective review to survey elements of biochemical ontogeny that appear, at the present time, to have particular relevance to the study of chemically induced embryotoxicity.

## Early Development

Mammalian development begins with a unique membrane event, the fusion of the surface membranes of a mature spermatozoon and a recently ovulated secondary oocyte. The successful completion of this event provides a "trigger" for a whole series of programmed cellular events that lead to the formation of a complex structure, the blastocyst (11). Interest in this period of development from the perspective of toxicology has been slow but grew out of the demonstration that, rather than being resistant to toxic influences, the preimplantation embryo can respond to teratogenic agents both *in vitro* (34,50) and *in vivo* (54). Coincident advances in cell biology, particularly the demonstration of cell surface heterogeneity and the importance of this phenomenon in programmed developmental events (6,9), have led to a more systematic analysis of early development and, in particular, alterations in the cell membrane.

Two principal approaches have been used to study cell surface changes during mammalian development. These are: (a) the ontogeny of cell-surface antigens (53,60) and (b) the ontogeny of lectin-binding sites (15,65) (see also G. L. Kimmel, *this volume*). These studies have, for the most part, shown that the surface of embryonic cells is more closely related to that of tumor cells than to the surface of normal adult tissues (60). Attempts to define distinctive and stage-specific embryonic antigens (SSEA) have met with only moderate success. Some degree of specificity has been obtained in the binding of immune sera against fertilized ova, mature sperm, and ectoplacental cone tissue to the cell surfaces of mouse embryos at various stages in development (53). One specific antigen, F9, is expressed on embryonal carcinoma cells, cells of cleavage-stage embryos and sperm surfaces (5,15). The study of this antigen has been extensive because it represents an "immature" gene product that is not expressed on adult cells. It is related to the expressivity of a specific mutation at the complex T locus in the mouse. This mutation ($t_{12}$) is lethal during the preimplantation period of development in the homozygous condition and is considered allelic for the gene coding for F9. The amount of F9 occurring on $t_{12}/t_{12}$ homozygotes is less than on their heterozygous littermates (28). These findings have a corollary in the expressivity of another mutant, staggerer, which affects cerebellar development in the homozygous state. In this latter mutant, there are defects in synapse formation between the granule cells and Purkinje cells. This effect is associated with an inability of the homozygous cell types to express the antigenic characteristics of a mature cell (57).

Another useful marker for studying alterations in the cell surface in development is the binding of plant lectins, such as concanavalin A, in order to demonstrate changes in distribution of cell surface sugars ($\alpha$-D-mannose and $\alpha$-D-glucose). In a recent study, Wu (65) has shown that concanavalin A binding sites increase in number throughout preimplantation development, being lowest in two-cell embryos and highest in the late blastocyst. This increase is thought to reflect changes that are essential for the cell-cell interaction that occurs between the trophoblast and endometrium during the implantation process.

Extracellular matrices also demonstrate specific biochemical alterations during early mammalian development, particularly the distribution of the various subclasses of collagen (58). Basement membrane collagen (type IV) first appears at the late, or compacted, morula stage and is localized around cells of the inner cell mass. As development proceeds, the distribution of type IV collagen also changes, it being localized first in the embryonic basement membrane and Reichert's membrane and only later in all basement membranes including those of the ectoderm, chorion, amnion, and visceral yolk sac. By day 8 of development (four somites), collagens I and III, referred to as "interstitial" collagens, appear simultaneously and are detectable in the somites, the head and heart mesenchymes and in their basement membranes.

While many other biochemical parameters are also known to change during early mammalian development (26,46), two specific ones deserve mention since their activities reflect specific developmental events, and, as such, they are convenient markers for early morphogenesis. These are: the activity of the X-linked enzyme, hypoxanthine–guanine phosphoribosyl transferase (HGPRT), and the isozymes of lactate dehydrogenase (LDH). In the former instance, the enzyme activity associated with both paternal and maternal X-chromosomes persists through the eight-cell stage with inactivation of one of the chromosomes (a random event) occurring at the late morula–early blastocyst stage of development (21). In the latter instance, only the maternal isozyme (LDH-1; B-subunits) is active in oocytes and preimplantation embryos. The A subunit (LDH-5) is an expression of the embryonic genome, and its activity appears to occur coincident with implantation. Spielmann et al. (55) have shown that implantation, per se, is not essential for expression of the embryonic genome. By utilizing culture conditions that prevent blastocyst hatching but allow trophoblastic giant cell transformation, these authors have shown that LDH-5 activity begins at a time in development when it can be demonstrated *in vivo*.

## The Developmental Biology of Model Systems

In all areas of toxicology and, indeed, of experimental medicine, the definition of "model systems" for the purpose of analyzing complex disease processes has had a long and productive history. The problem of extrapolation of the results obtained by the use of either *in vitro* assays or a different but susceptible species has been discussed by many (62), but these systems are of value in permitting an analysis of the component parts in cellular and biochemical terms. In mammalian development, there are two *in vitro* systems deserving of interest, since they are amenable to the influence of exogenous agents on their progression in culture. While not absolutely identical to the situation *in vivo*, they are analogous to a remarkable degree. These are the rat pancreas (43) and the mouse limb bud (18,36; see also D. M. Kochhar, *this volume*).

The development of the pancreas, *in vivo* and *in vitro*, encompasses the complete range of epithelio–mesenchymal interactions as they are manifest in glandular organs. The pancreas begins as a diverticulum of the foregut that soon becomes capped by mesenchyme. This event is crucial to further development and leads to proliferation and morphogenesis of the epithelium into islet tissue and the excretory ducts and acini of the exocrine pancreas. The mesenchyme produces a factor that is required for the normal production of epithelial cells in the pancreas, and, in its absence, the epithelium stays constant in size and produces exclusively endocrine tissue (44). The accumulation of insulin and of the exocrine enzymes (specifically pancreatic amylase) has been shown to be biphasic. The primary transition leads to the formation of typical pancreatic morphology and a low level of production of the various exocrine enzymes and of insulin. This level of cell-specific products remains constant for several days, a period of development called the *protodifferentiated state*. A secondary transition occurs between days 16 and 19 of gestation in which the cells of the pancreatic rudiment undergo frank cytodifferentiation and morphogenesis with the appearance of greatly enhanced levels of the specific proteins. This occurs coincident with the development of zymogen granules in the acinar cells and $\beta$-granules in the beta cells. The differentiation of cell surface glycoconjugates in all cell types occurs in parallel (29).

The development of the limb also involves a form of epithelio–mesenchymal interaction. There is a reciprocal relationship between the apical ectodermal ridge (AER) and the subridge mesenchyme which is essential for normal growth and morphogenesis of the extremity (69). With growth, the mesoderm of the limb becomes segregated with the inner core being the presumptive skeleton and the peripheral cells giving rise to the muscles, tendons, and connective tissue (33). In addition to these elements, the peripheral nervous system is intimately involved in limb morphogenesis. It has been suggested that during nerve–muscle interaction, inductive influences, which are as yet undefined, are operative (31).

The complexity of limb development is apparent when morphogenesis is studied *in vitro*. In contrast to the case of the pancreas, current methods do not permit an analysis of all factors that are involved in normal limb development. They do, however, provide a convenient means of studying chondrogenesis. This is achieved by the use of culture conditions that suppress growth (as measured by DNA content) but enhance the expression of the chondrogenic phenotype. This results in a net increase in total RNA, total protein, and content of the collagen-specific amino acid, hydroxyproline (39). It is possible, however, to utilize the biochemical methods similar to those developed for limbs *in vitro* to monitor other elements of the developing limb *in vivo*. This has been accomplished successfully by Kwasigroch and Neubert (22) who have shown that the activity of the muscle-specific enzyme creatine phosphokinase (CPK) increases dramatically between days 11 and 16 of gestation, coincident with myoblast fusion.

## CHEMICALLY INDUCED BIOCHEMICAL ALTERATIONS

A basic and all-pervasive problem in developmental toxicology is the lack of a precise definition of those biochemical pathways that are absolutely critical for normal development. As has been emphasized by many authors (63), embryotoxic agents may influence multiple pathways and many cellular activities simultaneously. Our inability to define a discrete and unequivocal site of action for a single one of the many toxins to which embryos are exposed represents a serious obstacle to our collective ability to develop biologically valid models of embryotoxicity. The cumulative body of evidence strongly suggests, however, that under well-defined experimental conditions, it is possible to produce fairly specific biochemical effects. As an example, the central role of DNA synthesis and cell proliferation in development has been repeatedly confirmed by observations on the teratogenicity of cytotoxic agents (23,45,46,49).

The normal developmental program of differentiating cells can be modulated by exogenous chemicals, and this effect can be monitored by studying the synthesis of the terminal components of cytodifferentiation, the cell-specific products. In the developing pancreas, the exposure of pancreatic rudiments to the glucocorticoid dexamethasone results in an intensive increase in the synthesis of pancreatic amylase (44). This effect is highly specific and affects the expressivity of some pancreatic genes while those coding for other exocrine proteins remain unaffected. If the thymidine analog 5-bromodeoxyuridine (BrdU) is used, a completely opposite sequence of events occurs. This compound blocks the synthesis of cell-specific products without adversely affecting growth. When pancreatic rudiments from 14-day embryos are cultured in the presence of BrdU, the development of the exocrine components is suppressed with a dose-dependent decrease in the activity of pancreatic amylase (12,44).

The use of the mouse limb bud, both *in vitro* and *in vivo*, has provided much useful information about the influence of teratogens on the synthesis of cell-specific products. Long and Johnson (25) demonstrated that the ontogeny of a series of isozyme patterns in the hindlimbs of mice was altered with the production of tibial hemimelia. Kochhar and his co-workers (2,14,18) have shown that a wide spectrum of teratogens, e.g., 6-diazo-5-oxo-L-norleucine (DON), retinoic acid, BrdU, and thalidomide, inhibit expressivity of the chondrogenic phenotype in mouse limb buds after *in vitro* exposure. This effect also occurs if the anlagen are exposed *in utero* and are then cultured (20). Similar observations by other laboratories (27,40) have confirmed the validity of combining *in vivo* and *in vitro* methods to monitor the effects of teratogens on limb development. The use of these techniques to analyze underlying biochemical mechanisms is just beginning (see D. M. Kochhar, *this volume*). It is of interest to note that Kwasigroch and Neubert (22) have confirmed that the effect of retinoic acid on chondrogenesis is highly specific as measured by decreased content of hydroxyproline in 14-day limbs (after day-10 exposure *in vivo*).

## OVERVIEW

Developmental toxicology currently has two distinct roles. The first is to provide a sound biological basis for risk assessment and for the safety evaluation of known and suspected teratogenic agents. The second is to utilize the methodology of both developmental biology and toxicology to contribute to our understanding of the basic biology of abnormal development. It is quite clear that to fulfill the first role, major progress must be achieved in accomplishing the second. Indeed, it can be argued that our major responsibility is to provide more meaningful basic information in order to modify current testing procedures and that failure to do so will increase rather than decrease the risk of exposing the human conceptus to potential toxins.

In his classic review, Karnofsky (17) outlined the basic problems that are associated with the use of multiple species and multiple agents in developmental toxicology. In the aftermath of the thalidomide tragedy, he stated that our research emphasis should be directed to the accomplishment of two practical objectives: the definition of the mechanism of action of thalidomide, and the development of reliable test methodologies. In spite of extensive progress, the charge to accomplish these goals is still with us. We do not, as yet, have a firm and unequivocal definition of the mechanism of action of any teratogenic agent, and current test methodologies are based on the developmental biology of 20 years ago. With time, these methods have become less relevant, and while we need to modify them, any alteration must be based on sound scientific information. Zbinden (67) has made a strong case for the absolute need to apply the explosive advances in basic science to analyze mechanisms of toxicity in general. He points out quite succinctly, however, that toxicology is a regulated science, so that the application of newer methods is dependent on the needs of the regulatory agencies. Since it is often difficult to assess the true relevance of an observation achieved with a newer and more sophisticated technique, the practical application of recent findings is quite slow.

However, the development of concise experimental protocols will supply us with the necessary scientific base to provide meaningful biological information and improve our currently mandated testing procedures. To provide a proper toxicological base, three types of data should be obtained (3). These are: (a) information on pharmacokinetics (48,64,66); (b) information on pharmacodynamics, the interaction of the reacting chemical species with target tissue/cell (16,35); and (c) dose–response relationships (47,52). To provide a firm developmental base is a formidable task, since many complex processes are essential for normal differentiation, and many of these tend to occur in parallel. These include, but are not restricted to, cell–cell interaction, cytodifferentiation, morphogenesis, growth, and expressivity of the embryonic genome. The central role of the cell surface cannot be underestimated in all of these developmental events. It plays an obligatory role in cell–cell interaction (13), expresses modulations that reflect cytodifferentiation (9,29,60), and directs the interaction between the cell and its microenvironment (6).

Two recent studies that utilize the techniques and concepts of modern developmental biology have made major contributions to our understanding of how embryotoxic agents exert their effect. In the first of these, Ekblom et al. (10) have analyzed the effect of DON (a glutamine analog known to interfere with the synthesis of glycosaminoglycans and glycoproteins) on kidney tubule induction *in vitro*. When metanephrogenic mesenchyme is cultured with spinal cord (separated by a millipore filter), the inductive influence of spinal cord lasts for 24 hr and results in normal kidney tubule formation. If these components are cultured in the presence of DON during the inductive period, there is a dose-dependent decrease in the number of tubules formed per explant. If, however, the analog is not present during the inductive period but is present during the period of differentiation (24–72 hr after explantation), it is without effect. The analog has no demonstrable effect on the formation of cell–cell contacts between the two tissue elements, and the authors conclude that DON interferes with tubule induction by decreasing the synthesis of glycosaminoglycans and reducing the number of lectin-binding sites on the cell surface. This produces an inability to transmit the inductive signal and results in the absence of kidney tubule formation.

The second experiment (30,31) represents an excellent attempt to apply the methods and concepts of developmental biology to the resolution of an enigmatic problem, the mechanism of action of thalidomide (17). After reviewing many theories proposed over the past two decades, McBride (30) suggested that another form of cell–cell interaction, that between the peripheral nervous system and the developing components of the limb bud, is important in the genesis of thalidomide embryopathy. He suggested that the outgrowth of neurites derived from the neural crest (sensory neurons) act as primary inducers for normal limb development. The absence or reduction of the level of this influence produced the panorama of limb defects that have been observed in humans. He supported this hypothesis in a series of experiments in which he showed that removal of the lumbar neural tube resulted in a high level of amelia on the operated side. These observations support prior studies in rabbits that showed that one consistent effect of thalidomide treatment was its association with varying degrees of pathology in the dorsal root ganglia (56). Whereas it is true that the biochemical alterations associated with these experiments are unknown, they form a framework within which it may be possible to analyze inductive influences and their effects on normal and abnormal limb morphogenesis.

In conclusion, it is hoped that this selective review of some of the biochemical factors that are manifest in studies of both normal and abnormal development will serve as a stimulus for future efforts. Although development is the result of a complex series of biological events, the judicious use of modern biochemical and cytochemical techniques should continue to yield useful insights into those steps that are critical for normal cytodifferentiation and morphogenesis. The application of the results obtained and the concepts they represent is essential for an understanding of those discrete mechanisms by which embryotoxic agents exert their effects.

# REFERENCES

1. Albert, A. (1965): Fundamental aspects of selective toxicity. *Ann. N. Y. Acad. Sci.*, 123:5–18.
2. Aydelotte, M. B., and Kochhar, D. M. (1975): Influence of 6-diazo-5-oxo-L-norleucine (DON), a glutamine analogue, on cartilaginous differentiation in mouse limb buds *in vitro*. *Differentiation*, 4:73–80.
3. Bass, R., Bochert, G., Merker, H.-J., and Neubert, D. (1977): Some aspects of teratogenesis and mutagenesis in mammalian embryos. *J. Toxicol. Environ. Health*, 2:1353–1374.
4. Becker, B. A. (1975): Teratogens. In: *Toxicology, The Basic Science of Poisons*, edited by L. J. Casarette and J. Doull, pp. 313–332. Macmillan, New York.
5. Bennett, D. (1975): The T locus of the mouse. *Cell*, 6:441–454.
6. Brunner, G. (1977): Membrane impression and gene expression. Towards a theory of cytodifferentiation. *Differentiation*, 8:123–132.
7. Caplan, A. I., and Ordahl, C. P. (1978): Irreversible gene repression model for control of development. *Science*, 201:120–130.
8. Corner, G. W. (1961): Congenital malformations: The problem and the task. In: *First International Conference on Congenital Malformations*, pp. 7–17. J. B. Lippincott, Philadelphia.
9. Edelman, G. M. (1976): Surface modulation in cell recognition and cell growth. *Science*, 192:218–226.
10. Ekblom, P., Lash, J. W., Lehtonen, E., Nordling, S., and Saxen, L. (1979): Inhibition of morphogenetic cell interactions by 6-diazo-5-oxo-norleucine (DON). *Exp. Cell Res.*, 121:121–126.
11. Gardner, R. L. (1975): Analysis of determination and differentiation in the early mammalian embryo using intra- and interspecific chimeras. In: *The Developmental Biology of Reproduction*, edited by C. L. Markert and J. Papaconstantinou, pp. 207–236. Academic Press, New York.
12. Githens, S., Pictet, R., Phelps, P., and Rutter, W. J. (1976): 5-Bromodeoxyuridine may alter the differentiative program of the pancreas. *J. Cell Biol.*, 71:341–356.
13. Glaser, L. (1980): From cell adhesion to growth control. In: *The Cell Surface: Mediator of Developmental Processes*, edited by S. Subtelny and N. K. Wessells, pp. 79–97. Academic Press, New York.
14. Greene, R. M., and Kochhar D. M. (1975): Limb development in mouse embryos: Protection against teratogenic effects of 6-diazo-5-oxo-norleucine (DON) *in vivo* and *in vitro*. *J. Embryol. Exp. Morphol.*, 33:355–370.
15. Jacob, F. (1979): Cell surface and early stages of mouse embryogenesis. In: *Current Topics in Developmental Biology, Vol. 13, Part 1*, edited by A. A. Moscona and A. Monroy, pp. 117–137. Academic Press, New York.
16. Jusko, W. J. (1972): Pharmacodynamic principles in chemical teratology: Dose–effect relationships. *J. Pharmacol. Exp. Ther.*, 183:469–480.
17. Karnofsky, D. A. (1965): Drugs as teratogens in animals and man. *Annu. Rev. Pharmacol.*, 5:447–472.
18. Kochhar, D. M. (1975): The use of *in vitro* procedures in teratology. *Teratology*, 11:273–288.
19. Kochhar, D. M., and Agnish, N. D. (1977): "Chemical surgery" as an approach to study morphogenetic events in embryonic mouse limb. *Dev. Biol.*, 61:388–394.
20. Kochhar, D. M., and Aydelotte, M. B. (1974): Susceptible stages and abnormal morphogenesis in the developing mouse limb analysed in organ culture after transplacental exposure to vitamin A (retinoic acid). *J. Embryol. Exp. Morphol.*, 31:721–734.
21. Kratzer, P. G., and Gartler, S. M. (1978): HGPRT activity changes in pre-implantation mouse embryos. *Nature*, 274:503–504.
22. Kwasigroch, T. E., and Neubert, D. (1978): A simple method to test chondrogenic and myogenic tissues for differential effects of drugs. In: *Role of Pharmacokinetics in Prenatal and Perinatal Toxicology*, edited by D. Neubert, H. -J. Merker, H. Nau, and J. Langman, pp. 621–630. Georg Thieme Verlag, Stuttgart.
23. Langman, J., Rodier, P., Webster, W., Crowley, K., Cardell, E. L., and Pool, R. (1975): The influence of teratogens on cellular and tissue behavior during the second half of pregnancy and their effect on postnatal behavior. In: *New Approaches to the Evaluation of Abnormal Embryonic Development*, edited by D. Neubert and H.-J. Merker, pp. 439–467. Georg Thieme Verlag, Stuttgart.
24. Linsenmayer, T. F., and Kochhar, D. M. (1979): *In vitro* cartilage formation: Effects of 6-diazo-5-oxo-norleucine (DON) on glycosaminoglycan and collagen synthesis. *Dev. Biol.*, 69:517–528.

25. Long, S. Y., and Johnson, E. M. (1968): Enzyme ontogeny in normal and hemimelic limbs of mice. *J.Embryol. Exp. Morphol.*, 20:415–430.
26. Manes, C. (1975): Genetic and biochemical activities in preimplantation embryos. In: *The Developmental Biology of Reproduction*, edited by C. L. Markert and J. Papaconstantinou, pp. 133–163. Academic Press, New York.
27. Manson, J. M., Dourson, M. L., and Smith, C. C. (1977): Effects of cytosine arabinoside on *in vivo* and *in vitro* mouse limb development. *In Vitro*, 13:434–442.
28. Marticorena, P., Artzt, K., and Bennett, D. (1978): Relationship of F9 antigen and genes of the T/t complex. *Immunogenetics*, 7:337–347.
29. Maylié-Pfenninger, M. F., and Jamieson, J. D. (1980): Development of cell surface saccharides on embryonic pancreatic cells. *J. Cell Biol.*, 86:96–103.
30. McBride, W. G. (1979): The pathogenesis of thalidomide embryopathy. In: *Advances in the Study of Birth Defects, Vol. 1*, edited by T. V. N. Persaud, pp. 113–127. University Park Press, Baltimore.
31. McBride, W. G. (1979): The inductive influence of neurons in limb development. In: *Advances in the Study of Birth Defects, Vol. 1*, edited by T. V. N. Persaud, pp. 129–139. University Park Press, Baltimore.
32. McMahon, D. (1974): Chemical messengers in development: A hypothesis. *Science*, 185:1012–1021.
33. Milaire, J. (1965): Aspects of limb morphogenesis in mammals. In: *Organogenesis*, edited by R. L. DeHaan and H. Ursprung, pp. 283–300. Holt, Rinehart and Winston, New York.
34. Monesi, V., and Molinaro, M. (1970): Macromolecular synthesis and effect of metabolic inhibitors during preimplantation development in the mouse. In: *Advances in the Biosciences, Vol. 6*, edited by G. Raspé, pp. 101–117. Pergamon Press, Oxford.
35. Nau, H., and Neubert, D. (1978): Development of drug-metabolizing monooxygenase systems in various mammalian species including man. Its significance for transplacental toxicity. In: *Role of Pharmacokinetics in Prenatal and Perinatal Toxicology*, edited by D. Neubert, H.-J. Merker, H. Nau, and J. Langman, pp. 13–44. Georg Thieme Verlag, Stuttgart.
36. Neubert, D., and Barrach, H.-J. (1977): Techniques applicable to study morphogenetic differentiation of limb buds in organ culture. In: *Methods in Prenatal Toxicology*, edited by D. Neubert, H.-J. Merker, and T. E. Kwasigroch, pp. 241–251. Georg Thieme Verlag, Stuttgart.
37. Neubert, D., Merker, H.-J., Kohler, E., Krowke, R., and Barrach, H.-J. (1970): Biochemical aspects of teratology. In: *Advances in the Biosciences, Vol. 6*, edited by G. Raspé, pp. 575–622. Pergamon Press, Oxford.
38. Neubert, D., Merker, H.-J., Nau, H., and Langman J. (1978): *Role of Pharmacokinetics in Prenatal and Perinatal Toxicology*. Georg Thieme Verlag, Stuttgart.
39. Neubert, D., Merker, H. -J., and Tapken, S. (1974): Comparative studies on the prenatal development of mouse extremities *in vivo* and in organ culture. *Naunyn Schmiedebergs Arch. Pharmacol.*, 286:251–270.
40. Neubert, D., Tapken, S. and Merker, H.-J. (1974): Induction of skeletal malformations in organ cultures of mammalian embryonic tissues. *Naunyn Schmiedebergs Arch. Pharmacol.*, 286:271–282.
41. Papaconstantinou, J. (1967): Metabolic control of growth and differentiation in vertebrate embryos. In: *The Biochemistry of Animal Development, Vol. 2*, edited by R. Weber, pp. 57–113. Academic Press, New York.
42. Runner, M. N. (1965): General mechanisms of teratogenesis. In: *Teratology: Principles and Techniques*, edited by J. G. Wilson and J. Warkany, pp. 95–103. University of Chicago Press, Chicago.
43. Rutter, W. J., Pictet, R. L., Harding, J. D., Chirgwin, J. M., MacDonald, R. J., and Przybyla, A. E. (1978): An analysis of pancreatic development: Role of mesenchymal factor and other extracellular factors. In: *Molecular Control of Proliferation and Differentiation*, edited by J. Papaconstantinou and W. J. Rutter, pp. 205–227. Academic Press, New York.
44. Rutter, W. J., MacDonald, R. J., Van Nest, G., Harding, J. N., Przybyla, A. E., Chirgwin, J. C., and Pictet, R. L. (1978): Pancreas-specific genes and their expression during differentiation. In: *Differentiation and Development*, edited by F. Ahmad, J.Schultz, T. R. Russell, and R. Werner, pp. 65–90. Academic Press, New York.
45. Scott, W. J., Jr. (1977): Cell death and reduced proliferative rate. In: *Handbook of Teratology, Vol. 2*, edited by J. G. Wilson and F. C. Fraser, pp. 81–98. Plenum Press, New York.
46. Sherman, M. I. (1979): Developmental biochemistry of pre-implantation mammalian embryos. *Annu. Rev. Biochem.*, 48:443–470.

47. Skalko, R. G. (1965): The effect of $Co^{60}$-radiation on development and DNA synthesis in the 11-day rat embryo. *J. Exp. Zool.*, 160:171–182.
48. Skalko, R. G. (1975): Kinetic aspects of the placental transport of drugs. In: *New Approaches to the Evaluation of Abnormal Embryonic Development*, edited by D. Neubert and H.-J. Merker, pp. 326–352. Georg Thieme Verlag, Stuttgart.
49. Skalko, R. G., and Jacobs, D. M. (1978): The effect of 5-fluorouracil on [³H] nucleoside incorporation into the DNA of mouse embryos and maternal tissues. *Exp. Mol. Pathol.*, 29:303–315.
50. Skalko, R. G., and Morse, J. M. D. (1969): The response of the early mouse embryo to actinomycin D treatment *in vitro*. *Teratology*, 2:47–54.
51. Skalko, R. G., Packard, D. S., Jr., Schwendimann, R. N., and Raggio, J. F. (1971): The teratogenic response of mouse embryos to 5-bromodeoxyuridine. *Teratology*, 4:87–94.
52. Skalko, R. G., Tucci, S. M., and Dropkin, R. H. (1979): The influence of teratogens on mouse embryo chromosome structure. In: *Advances in the Study of Birth Defects, Vol. 3*, edited by T. V. N. Persaud, pp. 15–27. University Park Press, Baltimore.
53. Soltor, D., and Knowles, B. B. (1979): Developmental stage-specific antigens during mouse embryogenesis. In: *Current Topics in Developmental Biology, Vol. 13, Part 1*, edited by A. A. Moscona and A. Monroy, pp. 139–165. Academic Press, New York.
54. Spielmann, H., and Eibs, H. -G. (1978): Recent progress in teratology: A survey of methods for the study of drug actions during the preimplantation period. *Arzneim. Forsch.*, 28:1733–1742.
55. Spielmann, H., Eibs, H.-G., Jacob-Muller, U., and Bischóff, R. (1978): Expression of lactate dehydrogenase isozyme 5 (LDH-5) in cultured mouse blastocysts in the absence of implantation and outgrowth. *Biochem. Genet.*, 16:191–202.
56. Stokes, P. A., Lykke, A. W. J., and McBride, W. G. (1976): Ultrastructural changes in the dorsal root ganglia evoked by thalidomide preceding limb development. *Experientia*, 32:597.
57. Trenkner, E. (1979): Postnatal cerebellar cells of *staggerer* mutant mice express immature components on their surface. *Nature*, 277:566–567.
58. Wartiovaara, J., Leivo, I., and Vaheri, A. (1980): Matrix glycoproteins in early mouse development and in differentiation of teratocarcinoma cells. In: *The Cell Surface: Mediator of Developmental Processes*, edited by S. Subtelny and N. K. Wessells, pp. 305–324. Academic Press, New York.
59. Wilde, C. E., Jr. (1974): Time flow in differentiation and morphogenesis. In: *Concepts of Development*, edited by J. Lash and J. R. Whitaker, pp. 241–260. Sinauer Associates, Stamford, Connecticut.
60. Wiley, L. M. (1979): Early embryonic cell surface antigens as developmental probes. In: *Current Topics in Developmental Biology, Vol. 13, Part 1*, edited by A. A. Moscona and A. Monroy, pp. 167–197. Academic Press, New York.
61. Williams, J. (1965): Chemical constitution and metabolic activities of animal eggs. In: *The Biochemistry of Animal Development, Vol. 1*, edited by R. Weber, pp. 13–71. Academic Press, New York.
62. Wilson, J. G. (1978): Survey of *in vitro* systems: Their potential use in teratogenicity screening. In: *Handbook of Teratology, Vol. 4*, edited by J. G. Wilson and F. C. Fraser, pp. 135–153. Plenum Press, New York.
63. Wilson, J. G., and Fraser, F. C. (1977): *Handbook of Teratology, Vol. 2, Mechanisms and Pathogenesis*. Plenum Press, New York.
64. Wilson, J. G., Ritter, E. J., Scott, W. J., and Fradkin, R. (1977): Comparative distribution and embryotoxicity of acetylsalicylic acid in pregnant rats and rhesus monkeys. *Toxicol. Appl. Pharmacol.*, 41:67–78.
65. Wu, J. T. (1980): Concanavalin A binding capacity of preimplantation mouse embryos. *J. Reprod. Fertil.*, 58:455–461.
66. Young, J. F., and Holson, J. F. (1978): Utility of pharmacokinetics in designing toxicological protocols and improving interspecies extrapolation. *J. Environ. Pathol. Toxicol.*, 2:169–186.
67. Zbinden, G. (1979): Application of basic concepts to research in toxicology. In: *Workshop on Cellular and Molecular Toxicology*, edited by D. W. Fawcett and J. W. Newberne, pp. 605–616. Williams & Wilkins, Baltimore.
68. Zwilling, E. (1955): Teratogenesis. In: *Analysis of Development*, edited by B. H. Willier, P. Weiss, and V. Hamburger, pp. 699–719. W. B. Saunders, Philadelphia.
69. Zwilling, E. (1961): Limb morphogenesis. In: *Advances in Morphogenesis, Vol. 1*, edited by M. A. Abercrombie and J. Brachet, pp. 301–330. Academic Press, New York.

*Developmental Toxicology*, edited by
C. A. Kimmel and J. Buelke-Sam. Raven Press,
New York © 1981.

# Comparative Development of Specific Organ Systems

*Richard M. Hoar and **Ian W. Monie

*Toxicology Division, Hoffmann-LaRoche, Inc., Nutley, New Jersey 07110; and
**Department of Anatomy, University of California, San Francisco, California 94143

In studying the toxic effects of agents on the developing embryo or fetus, it is sometimes desirable to compare the pattern of development of a particular organ system in animals of different species. This chapter provides such information for some key developmental events in man, the macaque, guinea pig, rabbit, rat, mouse, hamster, and a few other mammals. Corresponding data are also provided for the chick in view of its long-standing use in embryological studies.

It will be appreciated that restrictions of space and, at times, the lack of data limit the amount of information presented. Those interested in fuller details should consult the references.

## GENERAL CONSIDERATIONS

Since precise time of fertilization is not determinable, when calculating the length of gestation or the time that elapses before a particular developmental event occurs, it is customary in man and in the macaque to refer to ovulation age and to ovulation or copulation age in the case of other mammals. Menstrual age, also used in the timing of human pregnancies, is about 14 days longer than ovulation age. Incubation age is employed for the chick, and it should be remembered that by the time the egg is laid, development has been proceeding for 24 to 36 hr. For a discussion on the timing of developmental events consult Kalter (28).

It must be emphasized that the times given herein are approximations, since rate of development is influenced by both genetic and environmental factors. In addition, investigators may differ in their methods of calculating gestational age and the time when an organ is actually established. Thus, in regard to the former, the day of finding sperm in the rat vagina or of a "plug" in the mouse vagina may be considered by some investigators as "day zero" and by others as "day one" of pregnancy. In birds, the temperature of incubation has a marked influence on the rate of embryonic growth.

Embryos and fetuses are usually classified according to age, length, weight, or, in the case of the very young, by the number of somites present. However, because embryos of the same chronological age can develop at different rates, tables have

*13*

been prepared that classify stage according to the extent of development achieved. Those most in use are the "Carnegie Stages" (43) and the "Horizons" (56–58) for human embryos, the "Standard Stages" (65) for a variety of animals, and the "Chick Stages" (20). A comparison of those developmental stages used in the classification of human embryos is given in Table 1.

Average gestation periods and the times at which some important developmental events occur in man and common laboratory animals are shown in Table 2. The approximate lengths of gestation in days for some other animals used at times in research are: opossum, 13; ferret, 42; dog, 61; cat, 63; pig, 115; sheep, 150; and baboon, 180. Usually, when gestation is short, development is rapid, and litter size is large. In the latter case, the littermates in the early stages of development often vary considerably in size, but differences tend to diminish as gestation advances.

The fertilized ovum, lying within an envelope called the zona pellucida, undergoes repeated division as it moves along the uterine tube. By the time it reaches the uterus, it is a hollow ball of cells (blastocyst) which, on dissolution of the zona pellucida, attaches to the endometrium and commences implantation (Table 2). The trophoblast cells comprising the outer shell of the blastocyst now invade the endometrium and gradually facilitate the transfer of substances between mother and embryo. Within the blastocyst, the inner cell mass gives rise to the embryonic disk, the yolk sac, and the amniotic sac, the mode of development of the last mentioned varying somewhat according to the species.

When fully established, the embryonic disk consists of three "germ layers" known as the ectoderm, the endoderm, and the intraembryonic mesoderm. Ectoderm gives rise to skin, hair, tooth enamel, nails, and the nervous system; endoderm to the respiratory and alimentary tracts; and mesoderm to bones, ligaments, muscles, the cardiovascular system, and most of the urogenital system.

TABLE 1. *Developmental classification of human embryos*

| Developmental Stage | Witschi Standard Stages | Streeter Horizons | Carnegie Stages |
|---|---|---|---|
| Cleavage and blastula | 1-7 | I-III | 1-3 |
| Gastrula | 8-11 | IV-VII | 4-6 |
| Primitive Streak | 12 | VIII | 6-7 |
| Neurula | 13-17 | IX-XII | 7-12 |
| Tailbud Embryo | 18-24 | XII-XIII | 12-13 |
| Complete Embryo | 25 | XIV | 14 |
| Metamorphosing Embryo | 26-33 | XV-XXII | 15-22 |
| Fetus | 34 | XXIII | 23 |
| | 34-36 | | Fetal Period |

References: 43, 56-58, 65

TABLE 2. *Times of some key developmental events in days*

| | Implanta-tion | Primitive Streak | 10-somite Stage | Lower Limb Buds | Hand (Forepaw) Rays | Palatal Folds Uniting* | Gestation Period |
|---|---|---|---|---|---|---|---|
| Man | 7.5 | 17 | 25 | 32 | 37 | 57 | 267 |
| Macaque | 9 | 17 | 23 | 28 | 35 | 46 | 167 |
| Guinea Pig | 6.5 | 13 | 15 | 18.5 | 22 | 26 | 67 |
| Rabbit | 7.5 | 7.25 | 8.5 | 11 | 14.5 | 19.5 | 32 |
| Rat | 6 | 9 | 10.5 | 12 | 14 | 17 | 22 |
| Mouse | 5 | 8 | 8.5 | 10.3 | 12.3 | 15 | 19 |
| Hamster | 5 | 7 | 8 | 9.75 | 11 | 12 | 16 |
| Chick | - | 0.5 | 1.5 | 3 | 4.75 | ** | 21 |

|———————————Embryonic Period————————————|

References: Man: 1, 21, 37, 44, 53, 56-58; Macaque: 23, 24, 53;
Guinea Pig: 19, 52, 53, and personal observations of R.M. Hoar;
Rabbit: 15, 34, 35, 53, 63; Rat: 1, 15, 16, 37, 53; Mouse: 37, 42, 45, 53, 55;
Hamster: 10, 11, 53; Chick: 1, 20 31, 37, 42, 46, 53.

*Not all at the same stage of union.
**In the chick palatal folds do not fuse.

At about day 17 in man, the primitive streak appears in the ectoderm of the caudal end of the embryonic disk and gives origin to the intraembryonic mesoderm. At its rostral end lies the primitive (Hensen's) node from which the notochord, precursor of the vertebral column, grows cranially. Gestation periods, embryonic periods, and the times of various developmental events in man and animals under consideration are given in Table 2. Organ systems are established during the embryonic period, and it is during this time that the conceptus is usually most sensitive to teratogenic insult.

The human embryo serves as the model in the account of the formation of systems discussed below, and comments on time and patterns of development in other animals are made only where they differ significantly from those of man. Structures referred to in the tables are illustrated by simple diagrams.

## NERVOUS SYSTEM

The nervous system begins as the neural plate which is formed from the ectoderm of the embryonic disk (Table 3) at about day 19 in man. The plate quickly becomes a groove, the lateral margins of which gradually approach and fuse to form the

TABLE 3. *Development of the nervous system/time in days*

| | Neural Plate | Neuropores Closed* | Three Brain Vesicles | Cerebral Hemispheres | Cerebellum | Olfactory Bulbs |
|---|---|---|---|---|---|---|
| Man | 19 | 25-27 | 26 | 30 | 37 | 37 |
| Macaque | 20 | 25-27 | 25 | 29 | 36 | 38 |
| Guinea Pig | 13.5 | 15.25-15.5 | 15.3 | 17 | 19 | 23 |
| Rabbit | 8 | 9.5-10.5 | 9.5 | 11 | 15 | 14 |
| Rat | 9.5 | 10.5-11 | 10.5 | 12 | 14 | 13.5 |
| Mouse | 7 | 9.0-9.5 | 8 | 10 | 12 | 11 |
| Hamster | 7.5 | 8.5-9.0 | 8.5 | 9 | 11 | 11 |
| Chick | 1 | 2.3-2.75 | 1.5 | 3 | 4.5 | 7 |

References: As in previous Tables
Abbreviations: AN - anterior neuropore; D - diencephalon; L - myelencephalon;
M - mesencephalon; N - metencephalon; NT - notochord; P - prosencephalon;
PN - posterior neuropore; R - rhombencephalon; T - telencephalon
*Anterior neuropore first; posterior neuropore second

neural tube. Union begins in its midportion at about day 22 and proceeds cranially and caudally. For a short time the tube has openings at either end, the anterior and posterior neuropores, but these close at about 25 and 27 days, respectively.

As the cranial end of the neural tube is closing, three brain vesicles form rostrally, the prosencephalon, the mesencephalon, and the rhombencephalon. The fate of each of these is as follows: the prosencephalon divides into the telencephalon (cerebral hemispheres) and the diencephalon (thalami, posterior lobe of the pituitary gland, pineal body, and optic vesicles); the mesencephalon (midbrain); and the rhombencephalon which divides into the metencephalon (pons and cerebellum) and the myelencephalon (medulla oblongata). The remainder of the neural tube forms the spinal cord.

By the end of the fourth week, the brain, when viewed laterally, presents cephalic and cervical flexures, and during the sixth week another, the pontine flexure, forms between them and flexes in the opposite direction. This last flexure causes attenuation of the roof of the rhombencephalon in which the foramen of Magendie appears in man. The existence of this foramen in many animals is said to be questionable (66). Clusters of blood vessels push the roof inwards and become associated with the choroid plexus of the fourth ventricle.

Cerebral hemispheres are apparent in human embryos by day 30, and olfactory bulbs grow forward from the telencephalon at about day 37. At the same time, the cerebellum is becoming distinguishable. Each cerebral hemisphere grows in the form of a horseshoe, and its cavity, the lateral ventricle, remains in communication with the third ventricle in the diencephalon. The corpus callosum appears during the 12th week and resembles the adult structure by the 20th week. Sulci are present in the human cerebral hemispheres by the fifth fetal month and are well in evidence by birth. In all other animals except primates, the hemispheres remain smooth. In the chick, the cerebral hemispheres are small, but the optic bulbs, midbrain, and the cerebellum are well developed.

As the neural folds unite to form the neural tube, neural crest cells migrate from their margins and become widely dispersed within the embryo. They form dorsal root, cranial nerve, and possibly sympathetic ganglia, as well as chromaffin tissue, and the adrenal medulla. In addition, they contribute to branchial arch cartilages, the leptomeninges, and the facial mesenchyme.

Neuroblast formation continues in man until about 7.5 months prenatally and in the cat until birth. In man, their subsequent growth and development occurs mainly during the last 2.5 months of gestation and, in the cat, through the first 8 weeks postnatally (59).

Neurons form in the fetal rat brain principally between days 13 and 20, except in the cerebellum where they do not appear until about day 19, and continue to form during the early postnatal weeks. In the fetal mouse, neurons form between days 10 and 20, but in the hippocampus, cerebellum, and olfactory bulb, they continue forming throughout the first 2 or 3 weeks after birth. In both mouse and rat, two peak periods of active neuronal growth are distinguishable. For details of these various features see Rodier (49).

Myelination commences between the fifth and sixth months in the cervical portion of the human spinal cord in the segmental and intersegmental pathways and a little later in the vestibulospinal and spinocerebellar tracts. Corticospinal tracts, such as the pyramidal tract, begin to myelinate just before birth and are not fully myelinated until the second or third year. The human brain is largely unmyelinated at birth and myelinates slowly until adolescence or later. Visual, auditory, olfactory, motor, and sensory fibers myelinate prior to commissural and association fibers. The reticular formation is not fully myelinated until the second decade.

There is little myelin in the rat nervous system at birth, but it forms rapidly between the 10th and 20th days postnatally and continues to form at a slower rate up to about 3 months. In the cat, myelination is occurring actively during the last 3 weeks of gestation and the first month postnatally, then forms at a slower rate until the 12th month (59). In the chick, myelination commences about day 15 of incubation (27).

Stimulation of the neck region elicits movement in the human fetus about the seventh or eighth week, in the rat fetus at day 16, and in the chick on day 3 of incubation (26).

## SPECIAL SENSES

### Eye

Eye formation begins with the outgrowth from the diencephalon of the optic vesicle which invaginates to form the optic cup (Table 4). The latter induces the lens plate in the overlying ectoderm which then sinks below the surface to become the lens vesicle. The inner layer of the optic cup forms the sensory part of the retina, and the outer layer forms the pigmented part of the retina. Optic nerve fibers arise from cells in the sensory layer of the retina and extend along the optic stalk to the brain.

Rods and cones develop in the sensory layer of the retina in both man and chick, but in the rat and mouse, only rods are formed. In the newborn rat, the retina is immature, and rods do not appear until the fifth day postnatally at which time ganglion cells are actively differentiating; the latter arrange themselves in a single layer a few days later (4,12). Details of the development of the mouse eye have been provided by Rugh (51) and by Pei and Rhodin (48).

In many animals, the eyelids fuse during fetal life and separate before or after birth. In the human fetus, the period of closure is from about 60 to 175 days and in the rat, from day 18 prenatally to 16 days postnatally. In the chick, the eyelids approximate at day 13 of incubation but never actually unite.

Other components of the eye such as the choroid, cornea, sclera, and the extraocular muscles arise from condensation of the surrounding mesenchyme. The musculature of the iris, however, is said to arise from ectoderm in man and possibly in other animals as well (21).

TABLE 4. *Development of eye and ear/time in days*

|  | Optic Vesicle Forming | Lens Separated | Optic Nerve Fibers Present | Otic Vesicle Forming | Cochlea Appearing | Otic Capsule Cartilaginous |
|---|---|---|---|---|---|---|
| Man | 24 | 35 | 48 | 25 | 44 | 56 |
| Macaque | 23 | 32 | 39 | 25 | 37 | 42 |
| Guinea Pig | 15.5 | 18 | 21.5 | 15.5 | 20.5 | 22 |
| Rabbit | 9 | 11.5 | 15 | 9 | 13 | 20 |
| Rat | 10.5 | 12.5 | 14 | 11.5 | 13.5 | 15 |
| Mouse | 9.5 | 11.5 | 13 | 8.5 | 12 | 14.5 |
| Hamster | 8 | 10 | 11 | 8.5 | 10 | 11 |
| Chick | 1.3 | 2.5 | 4 | 2.3 | 7 | 8 |

References: 48, and in previous Tables.

The human eye is sensitive to light about the seventh month prenatally, and at birth, light is distinguishable from dark. Eye movements become coordinated about 3 months after birth. Color perception is probably not established until the second year (29).

### Ear

The ear commences as the otic placode, a thickened portion of the cephalic ectoderm, at about day 22 in man (Table 4). It sinks inwards to form the otic vesicle and becomes the membranous labyrinth of the inner ear. Outpouchings from the latter produce, in turn, the ductus endolymphaticus, the semicircular canals, and the cochlea. The craniodorsal extension of the first branchial arch pouch establishes the pharyngotympanic tube, the middle ear, and the mastoid antrum.

The three ear ossicles, malleus, incus, and stapes, are derived mostly from the dorsal portion of the first and second branchial arch cartilages. In man, they ossify and attain adult structure and proportions during fetal life (2). In birds, they are represented by one bone, the columella, which is homologous with the stapes.

The external auditory meatus is a remnant of the craniodorsal end of the first external branchial cleft. Tubercles fuse around it to form the pinna of animals. During fetal life, the inner ear is surrounded by the cartilaginous otic capsule which gradually ossifies to become the petrous temporal bone. Cochlear and vestibular mechanisms are functional in the human newborn, but hearing is impaired for several days by fluid and debris in the middle ear and in the external auditory meatus.

Details of the antenatal development of the nonhuman inner ear will be found in the following references: rat (5,32); mouse (50); and macaque (64). For a detailed account of the postnatal development of the inner ear of the rat, consult Wada (62).

### RESPIRATORY SYSTEM

The respiratory diverticulum grows out from the ventral part of the foregut of the human embryo at about day 28 and shortly divides into two asymmetrical lung buds (Table 5). The latter then each divide, and the process is repeated until, by birth, some 18 generations of these buds are established. After birth, more divisions occur, and by the eighth year, there are around 23 generations (14) terminating in alveoli.

The human right lung has three lobes, and the left lung two lobes. In the macaque, the right lung has four lobes, and the left lung three lobes (9). In the rat, the right lung has four lobes, and the left lung one lobe. The major bronchial divisions appear in man at about day 46, in the macaque at about day 38, and in the rat at about day 15.5.

The human lung is at first a compact "glandular" structure in which most of the future air ducts are closed until the 17th week when they begin to canalize. A few weeks later, active vascularization of lung tissue commences, and by the 24th week, alveoli are recognizable (13). In the macaque, canalization commences at about the

TABLE 5. *Development of respiratory system/time in days*

| | Respiratory Diverticulum | Asymmetric Lung Buds | Major Bronchial Divisions | Surfactant Appears |
|---|---|---|---|---|
| Man | 28 | 32 | 46 | 170 |
| Macaque | 27 | 29 | 36 | 140 |
| Guinea Pig | 16 | 18.5 | 21.5 | - |
| Rabbit | 10.5 | 12 | 15 | 27 |
| Rat | 12 | 13 | 15.5 | 19 |
| Mouse | 9.5 | 10.5 | 13 | 18 |
| Hamster | 9 | 9.5 | 10.5 | - |
| Chick | 3 | * | * | 17 |

References: 9, 33 and in previous Tables
Abbreviations: I - type I cell; II - type II cell
*Pattern of avian lung development different from that of mammal.

12th week of gestation. An interesting feature of this animal is the eventual conversion of many of the pseudobronchioles into prealveolar ducts between birth and adulthood, a change that markedly increases the amount of air space within the lung (9).

Surfactant, a complex substance containing phospholipid, is secreted by Type II cells in the walls of the alveoli and facilitates the expansion of the collapsed alveoli once respiration commences. In man, it appears at about the 24th week and is usually sufficient in amount by the 35th week to permit normal respiration. Stress and cortisol (6) accelerate its rate of formation. In the lamb, surfactant appears at about day 120 (33). The times at which it is detectable in some other animals are shown in Table 5.

The avian lung differs from that of the mammal in that alveoli and air sacs are replaced by air capillaries that form loops arising from and terminating in ducts called parabronchi. Surfactant is present in the air capillaries at about day 17 (33).

The pulmonary arteries in mammals arise from the medial portions of the sixth branchial arch arteries, and during fetal life their intrapulmonary branches have narrow lumens that are highly resistant to blood flow. At birth, with the commencement of breathing and the increased oxygen tension of the blood, these vessels dilate, and pulmonary blood flow increases. The muscle content of the pulmonary arteries ramifying within the lungs decreases during the first few months after birth (22,41). In birds, the pulmonary arteries also arise from the sixth branchial arch arteries.

The design of the pulmonary arterial tree in the postnatal mammal differs according to the species. In man, the macaque, and the mouse, the transition from large to small arteries (i.e., from elastic to transitional, muscular, and endothelial arteries) occurs gradually, but in the rat, rabbit, and guinea pig, the change is sudden, and each type of artery is sharply defined (18).

Although rapid shallow respiratory-type movements occur in the human fetus after the first trimester (8) and in the lamb at about day 40 of gestation, inhalation of significant amounts of amniotic fluid does not seem to occur unless under stress. In the chick, the onset of respiratory movements occurs a few days prior to hatching.

## CARDIOVASCULAR SYSTEM

Two heart tubes form in the cephalic part of the human embryonic disk towards the end of the third week of gestation and begin fusing into a single heart tube at about day 21 (Table 6). During the fourth week, the single heart tube undergoes segmentation into four chambers: the sinus venosus which receives blood from the major veins; the primitive atrium; the primitive ventricle; and the bulbus cordis or conus arteriosus. From the last chamber, the blood enters the truncus arteriosus which communicates with the paired ventral aortae. The heart tube becomes S-shaped at about day 25, and septation soon follows within the atrium and the ventricle. The former divides into the definitive right and left atria, and the sinus venosus gradually becomes incorporated into the right atrium. The primitive ventricle gives rise to the definitive left ventricle, and the bulbus cordis to most of the

TABLE 6. *Development of heart and great arteries/time in days*

|  | Fusing Heart Tubes | S-shaped Heart | Septation Occurring | Foramen Ovale Present | Truncal Septation Complete | Aortic Arch Arteries Forming |
|---|---|---|---|---|---|---|
| Man | 21 | 25 | 28 | 44 | 46 | 22-32 |
| Macaque | 22 | 25 | 28 | 34 | 36 | 22-30 |
| Guinea Pig | 15 | 16 | 19.5 | 21 | 22 | 15.5-21.5 |
| Rabbit | 8.5 | 9.5 | 13 | 14 | 16.5 | 9-11 |
| Rat | 9.5 | 10 | 11.5 | 13 | 15.5 | 10-12 |
| Mouse | 7 | 8.5 | 10.5 | 12 | 14 | 8.5-11 |
| Hamster | 8 | 8.5 | 9.25 | 13 | 15 | 8-9.5 |
| Chick | 1.2 | 2 | 2.3 | 5 | 7 | 1.5-4.5 |

References: 54, and in previous Tables
Abbreviations: A - primitive atrium; B - bulbus cordis;
IF - interventricular foramen; LA - left atrium; LV - left ventricle;
RA - right atrium; RV - right ventricle; T - truncus arteriousus;
V - primitive ventricle

right ventricle. In mammals, an opening in the interatrial septum, the foramen ovale, permits part of the bloodstream entering the right atrium from the inferior (posterior) vena cava to pass to the left atrium. In the chick, the foramen ovale is represented by multiple perforations in the interatrial septum (31).

The interventricular foramen that temporarily connects the right and left ventricles is eventually closed by the encroachment of the truncobulbar septum which also divides the truncus arteriosus into the ascending aorta and the pulmonary trunk. These two events are completed in man at about the end of the seventh week.

The heart begins beating on the following days: man, 22 (probably); hamster, 8; rat, 10; guinea pig, 16.5; and chick, 1.5. The paired aortae arising from the truncus arteriosus sweep cranially, then caudally as the first aortic (branchial, pharyngeal) arch arteries. Between days 22 and 32 in man, additional aortic arch arteries appear on either side of the developing pharynx until a total of six pairs has been formed; however, the fifth of these is very transient. All vessels are not present at the same time. Only the third, fourth, and sixth pairs of arteries persist to give rise to the carotids, aortic arch, brachiocephalic and pulmonary arteries, and the ductus arteriosus. The last mentioned is the lateral portion of the sixth left arch artery and serves as a bypass for blood from the pulmonary trunk to the descending aorta, the former left dorsal aorta. In the chick, there is both a right and left ductus arteriosus, and the descending aorta is formed from the former right dorsal aorta.

At birth, respiration results in increased blood flow within the lungs, and the pressure of blood in the left atrium consequently rises to equal that of the right atrium. This results in the functional closure of the foramen ovale in mammals. In the chick, the same mechanism causes relaxation of the interatrial septum, and its perforations gradually close during the 2 or 3 days prior to hatching.

Closure of the ductus arteriosus takes place in two steps: primary closure caused by the contraction of muscle within its walls, and secondary closure resulting from a combination of subintimal proliferation, necrosis, and fibrosis. In the guinea pig and rabbit, primary closure occurs within a few minutes of birth, whereas in man, the process takes about 10 to 15 hr. Secondary closure in the rat, guinea pig, rabbit, and lamb occurs after 3 to 5 days, whereas in man, it takes about 2 to 3 weeks. Where primary closure occurs slowly, as in man, blood may flow temporarily through the ductus arteriosus from the aorta to the pulmonary arteries (25). Coronary arteries extend from the ascending aorta into the myocardium during the sixth week of gestation in man, in the rat on day 15.5, and in the chick on day 14.5 (54).

In addition to the foramen ovale and the ductus arteriosus, other structures peculiar to the fetal circulation are the umbilical vessels and the ductus venosus. The latter connects the umbilical vein with the inferior (posterior) vena cava and closes within a few days of birth in man and many mammals, but in the pig and horse, it disappears some weeks before birth (7).

Two umbilical veins form in young mammalian embryos and are retained in the lamb, but in man and the rat, the right umbilical vein disappears during the sixth week and on day 13, respectively (39). In the chick, both the right umbilical vein and the subintestinal vein atrophy at about day 4 of incubation. After birth, the umbilical vein in man closes at the umbilicus, but proximally, it may retain its lumen.

Two umbilical arteries develop both in mammals and birds. In man, during the fourth week, they unite in the body stalk to form a single vessel, but in the following week, this shortens, and the two umbilical arteries that joined to form it gradually extend the full length of the cord (36). Most mammals have two umbilical arteries within the cord, but in the rat, there is only one throughout gestation, and of the two intraabdominal umbilical arteries that unite to form it, one disappears at about day 17. In the chick, the right umbilical artery begins to atrophy at about day 8 of incubation. Whereas in man and the rat the umbilical arteries arise from the internal iliac arteries, in the lamb, they spring from a single vessel arising from the distal aorta.

Vitelline arteries form early in development in mammals and birds, and where there is both an allantoic and a yolk-sac placenta, as in the rat, they persist until birth; where only an allantoic placenta is formed, as in man, they disappear early in gestation. In the young rat embryo, there is a communication between the vitelline and umbilical arteries until day 11 of gestation; should it persist, abnormal vascular patterns result (38).


## THE GASTROINTESTINAL SYSTEM

The gastrointestinal system is generally divided into three segments, anterior, middle, and posterior. Each segment will be discussed separately. The anterior gut (Table 7) extends from the buccopharyngeal membrane (the stomodeum) to approximately the first half of the duodenum, and its development is complex. It includes the pharyngeal derivatives, the foregut, and that portion of the duodenum from which the liver, gall bladder and pancreas develop.

The pharyngeal gut is most easily distinguished by the branchial apparatus consisting of branchial arches from which develop the visceral skeleton including the jaws, palate and the ear ossicles, and branchial pouches and clefts from which develop the external ear, middle ear, Eustachian tube (*vide supra*), palatine tonsil, thymus, parathyroid glands, ultimobranchial body, and the thyroid gland. The major portion of this differentiation is accomplished during the third to eighth week of life. Palatal fusion is not complete until about the 12th week in man but has occurred by 12 days in the hamster. Further discussion of the pharyngeal gut will be limited to its endocrine derivatives (*vide infra*).

The foregut changes its dimensions through differential growth. The esophagus lengthens as the cervical flexure is reduced, the neck forms, and the vertebral column straightens during the seventh week. The stomach appears as a dilatation of the foregut during the fifth week and rotates 90 degrees around its longitudinal axis during the sixth week, causing its left side to face anteriorly. Similar activity begins during the fourth week in macaques and at about day 11 in rats and mice.

TABLE 7. *Development of the gastrointestinal system/time in days*

| | Intestinal Pocket | | Membranes Perforate | | Liver | | Gall Bladder | Stomach Appears | Umbilical Hernia | |
|---|---|---|---|---|---|---|---|---|---|---|
| | Foregut | Hindgut | Oral | Anal | Anlage | Epithelial Cords | | | Begins | Reduced |
| Man | 20.5 | 21.5 | 28 | 49 | 24 | 26 | 26 | 31-32 | 45 | 65 |
| Macaque | 20.5 | | 27-28 | | 24-26 | | 28-29 | 28-29 | 33-34 | 47-48 |
| Guinea Pig | 14.5 | 15.5 | | | 16 | 16.5 | 19 | 16.5 | 23 | |
| Rabbit | 8.5 | 9 | 10 | 10 | 9.5 | 10.5 | 11.5 | 10.5 | 12.5 | 20 |
| Rat | 9.5 | 11 | 10 | 15 | 11 | 11.5 | | 11.5 | 12.5 | 18 |
| Mouse | 7.8 | 8.5 | 8 | 14 | 8.8 | 9.5 | 9.7 | 11.5 | 11.0 | 16.3 |
| Hamster | 7.8 | 8 | 8.5 | 13 | 8.5 | 9 | 8.7 | 8.5 | 9.3 | 13 |
| Chick | 1.1 | 3 | 2.5 | 3 | 2.5 | 3 | 2.8 | 3 | 6 | 18 |
| Standard Stages | 13 | 15 | 15 | 31 | 16 | 16 | 17 | 18 | 27 | 34 |
| Streeter's Horizons | IX | XI | XI | XVIII | XI | XII | XII | XI-XII | XVII | XXIII |

Abbreviations: A - anal or cloacal membrane; DP - dorsal pancreas; FG - foregut or anterior intestinal portal; GB - gall bladder; H - heart; HG - hindgut or posterior intestinal portal; L - liver; O - oral or buccopharyngeal membrane; S - stomach; VP - ventral pancreas.

During this movement, a greater curvature develops through more rapid growth of the original posterior part of the stomach. The stomach completes its rotation by the seventh week around what has now become its anterioposterior axis, causing the greater curvature to face caudally and assume a position immediately anterior (ventral) to the developing transverse colon. These movements help to form the omental bursa and force the pylorus, with the attached duodenum, to the right into a position immediately anterior (ventral) to the developing metanephric kidney.

The liver appears during the fourth week in man and macaques as a single diverticulum from the duodenum, growing within the ventral mesentery to reach the septum transversum in which it proliferates forming anastomosing hepatic cords. The gall bladder and ventral pancreas bud off the now narrowed liver diverticulum (bile duct) during the fourth and fifth weeks, and the dorsal pancreas emerges from the duodenum growing into the dorsal mesentery during the fourth week. Identifiable hepatic lobes are present by the sixth week, and bile is secreted by the 12th week. The dorsal and ventral pancreatic buds, aided by both differential growth in the wall of the duodenum and by rotation of the gut, meet and fuse in the dorsal mesentery during the seventh week. This fusion occurs rapidly during days 11 to 13 in rats, days 9 to 11 in mice, and days 16 to perhaps 21 in guinea pigs. This period of development in rodents stands in vivid contrast to that in man and macaques which require about 2 weeks to complete the processes. The spleen develops from mesenchymal cells located in the dorsal mesogastrium. It assumes its definitive location anterior to the superior pole of the left metanephric kidney as the greater curvature of the stomach rotates to face caudally, forcing the dorsal mesogastrium and the spleen against the left lateral posterior wall of the abdomen.

The midgut extends from the distal half of the duodenum through the proximal two-thirds of the transverse colon. It is characterized by extraordinary elongation and rotation, the latter occurring in conjunction with an umbilical herniation. The midgut begins its elongation during the fourth to fifth week and herniates during the sixth week. It then withdraws from the cord, rotating as it does so, and assumes its normal position during the 10th week. A rotation of approximately 270 degrees occurs in a counterclockwise direction around the superior mesenteric artery. This traps the distal portion of the duodenum between the aorta and the caudal surface of the superior mesenteric artery, thus limiting further rotation. Umbilical herniation and its reduction requires about 4 weeks in primates (man and macaques) but only about 1 week in rodents. When the umbilical hernia is reduced, the sigmoid, descending, and transverse segments of the colon have attained approximately their definitive locations, while the ileocecal junction may be found superior to the superior mesenteric artery and just inferior to the liver. The cecum, appendix, and ascending colon develop by differential growth during the ensuing months, all being recognizable and definitively located by about 6 months.

The hindgut, extending from the distal third of the transverse colon to the upper part of the anal canal, is intimately associated with those changes that occur in the cloaca. The latter is at its height of development during the fourth week. Between the fifth and sixth weeks, a transverse ridge of tissue, the urorectal septum, grows caudally in a coronal plane towards the cloacal membrane. When the septum reaches the cloacal membrane (its point of contact is later described as the perineal body), the cloaca itself is divided into an anorectal canal and urogenital sinus, covered, respectively, by the anal membrane and the urogenital membrane. Elevations of mesenchymal proliferations appear surrounding the anal membrane, forming an anal pit. The anal membrane ruptures at the end of the seventh week, thus establishing the anal canal whose upper two-thirds were derived from the hindgut and whose lower one-third was derived from the anal pit. Subsequent development of the urogenital sinus is most closely associated with the appearance of the external genitalia and will be discussed under the urogenital system.


## THE UROGENITAL SYSTEM


The urogenital system, although actually two separate systems, is united both through inductive interactions during development and, in the male, through the utilization of a common discharge duct, the penile urethra. An understanding of the development of this delicately interwoven system rests on several key concepts. These are: (a) the location within the embryo of the tissue from which the urogenital system including the gonads and the adrenals will develop; (b) the utilization of the duct of the developing renal system, variously referred to as the archinephric duct, pronephric duct, mesonephric duct, or Wolffian duct, as the egress for sperm; (c) the induction of the female genital tract (paramesonephric duct) by the renal system and of the vagina by Müller's tubercle; (d) the migration of the germ cells from the yolk sac to establish the gonad; and (e) the differentiation of the external genitalia from the cloaca (17,30,44,47).

The urinary system (Table 8) develops within the intermediate mesodermal ridge which occupies a position lateral to the aorta and anterolateral to the developing vertebral column and musculature. These two ridges bulge into the coelomic cavity dorsal to the developing gut. They stretch the length of the cavity to join with one another in the region of the urogenital sinus. Three different, overlapping kidney systems develop in rapid succession. They appear in a craniocaudal progression in the intermediate mesodermal ridge between the third and fourth weeks of gestation in man, but over a 2-day period in rats (days 10–12) and mice (days 9–11). The pronephros is transitory and of little importance except in larval anamniotes such as the tadpole that have no need to conserve water (17,60).

The appearance of the mesonephros (at the level of somite 10) is characterized by a single Bowman's capsule for each segmentally arranged excretory tubule and a longitudinal collecting duct, the mesonephric duct. Initially, the mesonephric duct ends blindly just short of the cloaca but then fuses with and empties into the cloaca between 26 and 28 days. Vascular connections are made, circulation is established, and the mesonephros becomes capable of producing urine, although there is no proof that it does so in humans (40,47). The 30 or so mesonephric tubules begin to degenerate in a craniocaudal progression even as the most caudal nephrons are establishing their functional capacity. However, the mesonephros remains as a functional kidney until about the end of the third month. At 28 days, the ureteric bud, an outgrowth of the mesonephric duct close to its entrance into the cloaca, penetrates the intermediate mesodermal ridge and induces the metanephros or definitive kidney. The ureteric bud gives rise to the collecting system (the ureter, calyces, and collecting ducts) at the time that the metanephric mesoderm forms the filtering system (the nephrons). These events occur between the fifth and eighth weeks, culminating in functional capacity early in the third month of pregnancy. However, the kidney continues to modify its functional units until term or perhaps even after birth in man. As with the gastrointestinal system, the development of the renal system in rodents is concentrated during the second week, days 10 to 13 in rats and 8 to 12 in mice. The establishment of the internal "bisexual state" takes only 1 or 2 additional days.

TABLE 8. Development of the urogenital system/time in days

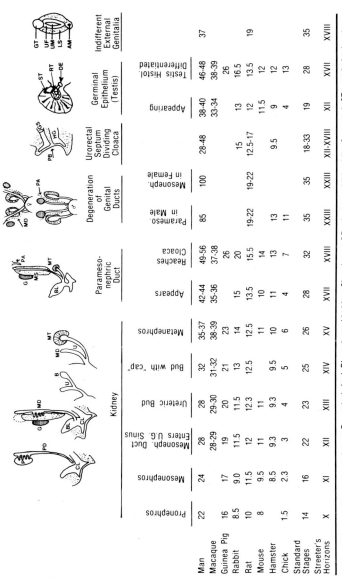

| | Pronephros | Mesonephros | Kidney — Mesoneph. Duct Enters U.G. Sinus | Kidney — Ureteric Bud | Kidney — Bud with "cap" | Kidney — Metanephros | Paramesonephric Duct — Appears | Paramesonephric Duct — Reaches Cloaca | Degeneration of Genital Ducts — Paramesoneph. in Male | Degeneration of Genital Ducts — Mesoneph. in Female | Urorectal Septum Dividing Cloaca | Germinal Epithelium (Testis) — Appearing | Germinal Epithelium (Testis) — Testis Histol. Differentiated | Indifferent External Genitalia |
|---|---|---|---|---|---|---|---|---|---|---|---|---|---|---|
| Man | 22 | 24 | 28 | 28 | 32 | 35-37 | 42-44 | 49-56 | 85 | 100 | 28-48 | 38-40 | 46-48 | 37 |
| Macaque | | | 28-29 | 29-30 | 31-32 | 38-39 | 35-36 | 37-38 | | | | 33-34 | 38-39 | |
| Guinea Pig | 16 | 17 | 19 | 20 | 21 | 23 | | 26 | | | 15 | 13 | 26 | |
| Rabbit | 8.5 | 9.0 | 11.5 | 11.5 | 13 | 14 | 15 | 20 | 19-22 | 19-22 | | 12 | 16.5 | |
| Rat | 10 | 11.5 | 12 | 12.3 | 12.5 | 12.5 | 13.5 | 15.5 | | | 12.5-17 | 11.5 | 13.5 | 19 |
| Mouse | 8 | 9.5 | 11 | 11 | | 11 | 10 | 14 | 13 | | | 9 | 12 | |
| Hamster | | 8.5 | 9.3 | 9.3 | 9.5 | 10 | 11 | 13 | 11 | | 9.5 | | 12 | |
| Chick | 1.5 | 2.3 | 3 | 4 | 5 | 6 | 4 | 7 | | | | 4 | 13 | |
| Standard Stages | 14 | 16 | 22 | 23 | 25 | 26 | 28 | 32 | 35 | 35 | 18-33 | 19 | 28 | 35 |
| Streeter's Horizons | X | XI | XII | XIII | XIV | XV | XVII | XVIII | XXIII | XXIII | XII-XVIII | XII | XVII | XVIII |

Abbreviations: AM - anal membrane; B - ureteric bud; BL - urinary bladder; CL - cloaca; DE - ductus epididymidis; G - gonad; GT - genital tubercle; HG - hindgut; LS - labioscrotal swelling; MD - mesonephric duct; MS - mesonephros; MT - metanephros; P - pronephros; PA - paramesonephric duct; PB - perineal body; PD - pronephic duct; RT - rete testis; ST - seminiferous tubule; U - ureter; UF - urogenital fold; UGS - urogenital sinus; UM - urogenital membrane.

As stated above, the urorectal septum separates the primitive urogenital sinus from the anorectal canal, this separation being completed by the seventh week. The primitive urogenital sinus may now be divided into three parts: a cranial vesicourethral canal which is continuous with the allantois; a middle (pelvic) segment; and a caudal (phallic) portion, which awaits the expression of the sex of the embryo. The wall of the urogenital sinus, into which the mesonephric ducts emptied, undergoes selective development and modeling, incorporating these ducts until their ureteric buds enter the wall of the vesicourethral canal as individual ureters. Simultaneously, the mesonephric ducts move closer together and inferiorly to enter the pelvic portion of the urogenital sinus. The vesicourethral canal dilates, forming the urinary bladder, as the allantois shrinks, loses its lumen, and becomes the urachus which extends from the apex of the bladder to the umbilicus. The mesonephric ducts and the remaining portions of the urogenital sinus undergo further modification as determined by the sex of the developing embryo.

The genital system (Table 8) in the human forms in the sixth week. It is then that the primordial germ cells complete their migration from the yolk sac into the genital ridge, establishing the gonad. It is also at this time that two pairs of genital ducts are established and the embryo is in an indifferent, bisexual state. The mesonephric duct (Wolffian duct) is now in close association with the gonad (see Endocrine System) and empties into the urogenital sinus. This structure becomes the main genital duct of the male—the ductus deferens. The paramesonephric ducts (Müllerian), from which the oviducts and uterus develop, are also in close approximation to the developing gonad and are induced within the intermediate mesodermal ridges by the mesonephric ducts. They appear between the fifth and sixth weeks as funnel-shaped invaginations of the coelomic epithelium on the anterolateral surface of the urogenital ridges parallel to the mesonephric duct. Cranially, each duct opens into the coelomic cavity (future ostium of the oviduct). Each progresses caudally, lateral to the mesonephric duct, crosses it ventrally, and grows caudomedially to meet and fuse with the paramesonephric duct from the opposite side within the pelvic mesenchyme at about 8 weeks. The two fused paramesonephric ducts continue to grow caudally until they meet the posterior wall of the urogenital sinus, a point of juncture known as Müller's tubercle.

Depending on the sex of the embryo, one of these two duct systems completes its development, and the other disappears almost completely. In the male, under the influence of the developing testis, the paramesonephric duct (Müllerian duct) disappears, and the mesonephric duct (Wolffian duct) and the urogenital sinus differentiate into their several components. The mesonephric duct becomes the epididymis, ductus deferens, and ejaculatory duct. The seminal vesicles appear as diverticula just proximal to the ejaculatory duct. The prostate gland develops from the pelvic portion of the urogenital sinus, and bulbourethral (Cowper's) glands appear as bilateral diverticula from the junction of the pelvic and phallic portions of the urogenital sinus.

In the female, the mesonephric duct disappears almost completely. At about 9 weeks, the individual paramesonephric ducts differentiate into the oviducts with their ostium, the fused ducts becoming the corpus and cervix of the uterus. At about the ninth week of gestation, the vagina begins its development from that portion of the urogenital sinus in the region of Müller's tubercle. By the fifth month, the vaginal outgrowth is canalized but remains separated from the urogenital sinus by the hymen.

The external genitalia develop as follows: the cloacal orifice, closed by a membrane, is originally surrounded by elevated cloacal folds that are continuous posteriorly and terminate in a genital tubercle anteriorly. Genital swellings appear lateral to the urethral folds, and by the end of the sixth week, the external genitalia of the male and the female are essentially identical. The cloacal folds are divided during the seventh week by the urorectal septum into anal and urethral folds. In the female, the genital tubercle enlarges to become the clitoris. The urethral folds do not fuse, becoming the labia minora, and the genital swellings enlarge to become the labia majora. The definitive urogenital sinus is modified slightly to form the urethra and the vestibule. In the male, the genital tubercle elongates into a phallus, drawing the urethral folds into a long urethral groove which fuses to form the penile portion of the urethra by the end of the third month. The pelvic part of the urogenital sinus becomes the prostatic and membranous urethra. The genital swellings enlarge, moving caudally to fuse and form the scrotum. These scrotal swellings are prepared for the descending testes during the third month. However, the testes do not complete their descent into the scrotum until between the seventh month of development and birth.

## THE ENDOCRINE SYSTEM

The endocrine system originates from the foregut directly (thyroid, thymus, parathyroid, and pancreas), from the stomodeal ectoderm in association with the central nervous system (pituitary) and from the urogenital ridge directly (gonads) or in association with the central nervous system (adrenals) (Table 9).

The thyroid gland appears between days 24 and 27 in man as an epithelial outgrowth of the endoderm from the floor of the pharyngeal gut near the origin of the tongue (future foramen cecum). It penetrates the underlying mesoderm to reach the anterior surface of the trachea at about 29 days and descends along it as a bilobed diverticulum, still connected to its pharyngeal origin by the thyroglossal duct. The thyroid reaches its definitive location at approximately 7 weeks, having spread transversely into two lobes, each lateral to the trachea, and having lost its connection to the pharyngeal gut. It begins to function at 3 to 4 months (3,21,40,46).

The thymus and parathyroid glands appear during the sixth week as endodermal outgrowths of the third and fourth pharyngeal pouches. The thymus is derived primarily from the ventral wing of each third pouch and descends to its final location in the superior mediastinum during the eighth week. During its descent, the thymus contacts the inferior parathyroid glands at their origin in the dorsal wing of each

TABLE 9. *Development of the endocrine system/time in days*

| | Pharyngeal Pouches Appear | Thyroid | Para-thyroids | Thymus | Pancreas | | | Pituitary | | Adrenal |
|---|---|---|---|---|---|---|---|---|---|---|
| | | | | | Ventral | Dorsal | Fused | Rathke's Pouch | Neuro-hypophysis | |
| Man | 28 | 24-27 | 35-38 | 30-40 | 31-32 | 28 | 40-44 | 30-34 | | 34 |
| Macaque | 24-29 | 28 | | | 29-30 | 28-29 | 35-36 | 28-29 | 30-31 | |
| Guinea Pig | 16-19 | 16.5 | | | | 17.5 | | 15.5 | 18.5 | 23 |
| Rabbit | 9-11.5 | 9.5 | | 12.5 | 11.5 | 10 | 14 | 9.5 | 12 | 18 |
| Rat | 11-13 | 11-12 | 12.5 | 12.5 | 11.5 | 11 | 13 | 10.5 | 11.5 | 12.5 |
| Mouse | 8.3-9.8 | 8.5 | 11 | 12 | 9.7 | 9.5 | 11.5 | 8.5 | 11.5 | 11 |
| Hamster | 8 | 8.5 | 9 | 9 | 9.5 | 9.5 | 11.5 | 8.5 | 10 | 10 |
| Chick | 2.1-3.5 | 1.8 | 6-8 | 6-8 | 4 | 3 | 6 | 2.2 | 3 | 3.5-7.0 |
| Standard Stages | 16-19 | 15-16 | 25-26 | 19-27 | 17 | 17 | 27 | 23 | | 23 |
| Streeter's Horizons | XI-XII | X-XI | XIV-XV | XII-XVI | XIII | XII | XVI | XII-XIII | | XIII |

Abbreviations: AC - adult cortex; B - bone; DP - dorsal pancreas; EC - embryonic cortex; FC - foramen caecum; GB - gall bladder; M - medulla; PD - pars distalis; PI - pars intermedia; PN - pars nervosa; VP - ventral pancreas.

third pouch and transfers them to the inferior pole of each lateral lobe of the developing thyroid gland where they remain. The superior parathyroid glands, derived from the ventral wing of each fourth pharyngeal pouch, attach themselves to each superior pole of the descending bilobed thyroid gland. They remain on the dorsal surface of the thyroid throughout life.

As was mentioned above, the pancreas is of double origin, arising from the endoderm in two locations on the distal portion of the foregut. The ventral pancreas buds off the liver diverticulum (bile duct) in the ventral mesentery during the fifth week. The larger dorsal pancreatic bud had already emerged from the foregut and grown rapidly into its dorsal mesentery. As the ventral origin of the bile duct begins its movement to the dorsal surface of the developing duodenum (approximately 5 weeks), it carries the ventral pancreas towards its ultimate fusion with the dorsal pancreatic bud, an event that occurs during the seventh week. As the pancreatic buds fuse, their duct systems anastomose in such a way that the main pancreatic duct (duct of Wirsung) is derived from the ducts of the ventral bud and opens into the ampulla of Vater. The accessory pancreatic duct (duct of Santorini) is formed from the ducts of the dorsal pancreas. Insulin secretion is thought to begin at approximately the fifth month (46).

The pituitary gland is derived from both the ectoderm of the stomodeum and the neuroectoderm of the diencephalon. It begins development at about 21 days with the appearance of Rathke's pouch as a dorsal outgrowth of the stomodeal portion of the pharyngeal gut just anterior to the origins of the buccopharyngeal (stomodeal) membrane. The glandular portion of the pituitary, the adenohypophysis, develops from Rathke's pouch. After losing its connection with the stomodeal vault at about 45 days, it proliferates into the pars distalis, pars tuberalis, and pars intermedia. At approximately 40 days, the infundibulum develops from the floor of the third ventricle. Reaching the adenohypophysis at about 45 days, this diverticulum, the neurohypophysis, proliferates into the pars nervosa, the median eminence, and the stalk, which remains attached to the diencephalon. It is suggested that neurosecretion begins during the fourth month as indicated by the stimulation of the thyroid through the presence of thyrotropic hormone (TSH) in the blood (61).

Components of the endocrine system derived primarily from the urogenital ridge include only the gonads (testes and ovaries). The gonads appear anteriorly and medially to the cranial pole of each mesonephros at about the level of the 7th to the 11th somite and/or nephron. The latter are modified to form a urogenital union that in the male becomes the ductuli efferentes and is represented in the female as degenerated remnants, the epoophoron (16). As indicated earlier, the gonads achieve their indifferent sexual state by about 6 weeks and become recognizable as either testes at about 7 weeks or ovaries by 10 weeks. The interstitial cells of Leydig reach their maximum development between 16 and 18 weeks in the male. The primordial follicles, oogonium surrounded by a single layer of follicular cells, appear at about 16 weeks in the female. This activity appears to be concentrated during the fourth and fifth months in man and macaques and in the second week in rodents.

The adrenals develop from both the urogenital ridge and the ectoderm of the central nervous system, specifically, migrating sympathetic cells that are of neural crest origin. The bilateral cellular aggregation of the mesoderm primordium of the fetal adrenal cortex begins at approximately 30 to 35 days between the root of the dorsal mesentery and the developing gonad. The medullary primordium appears at about 40 days as an assemblage of immature sympathetic (paraganglia) cells that begin to intermingle with and penetrate the mesodermal primordium at about 45 days, differentiating into the chromaffin cells of the adrenal medulla. Development of the definitive adrenal cortex and its physiological activity appear to be regulated by the pituitary and its secretion of ACTH (61). Differentiation of the definitive cortical zones actually begins during the late fetal period and is completed with the appearance of a recognizable zona reticularis at about 3 years postpartum (40).

## ACKNOWLEDGMENTS

Gratitude is expressed by Dr. A. G. Hendrickx and to Dr. Mary C. Williams for advice and the provision of data. Some information on rat development was provided by studies (Ian W. Monie) supported by USPHS Grant HD00419.

## REFERENCES

1. Altmann, P. L., and Dittmer, D. S. (1962): *Growth*. Federation of American Societies of Experimental Biology, Washington.

2. Anson, B. J., and Donaldson, J. A. (1973): *Surgical Anatomy of the Temporal Bone and Ear.* W. B. Saunders, Philadelphia.
3. Arey, L. B. (1974): *Developmental Anatomy, Seventh Edition.* W. B. Saunders, Philadelphia.
4. Armstrong, R. C., and Monie, I. W. (1966): Congenital defects in rats following maternal folic acid deficiency during pregnancy. *J. Embryol. Exp. Morphol.*, 16:531–542.
5. Asling, C. W., and Elia, K. J. (1964): Prenatal development of the vestibular system of the inner ear of rats. *Anat. Rec.*, 148:256.
6. Avery, M. E. (1975): Pharmacological approaches to the acceleration of fetal lung maturation. *Br. Med. Bull.*, 31:13–17.
7. Barclay, A. E., Franklin, K. J., and Prichard, M. M. L. (1945): *The Foetal Circulation.* Charles C. Thomas, Springfield, Illinois.
8. Boddy, K., and Dawes, G. S. (1975): Fetal breathing. *Br. Med. Bull.*, 31:3–7.
9. Boyden, E. A. (1976): Development of the lung in the pig-tail monkey (*Macaca nemestrina*). *Anat. Rec.*, 186:15–37.
10. Boyer, C. C. (1953): Chronology of development for the golden hamster. *J. Morphol.*, 92:1–37.
11. Boyer, C. (1968): Embryology. In: *The Golden Hamster*, edited by R. A. Hoffman, P. F. Robinson, and H. Magalhaes, pp. 73–89. Iowa State University Press, Ames, Iowa.
12. Braekevelt, C. R., and Hollenberg, M. J. (1970): The development of the retina of the albino rat. *Am. J. Anat.*, 127:281–302.
13. Conen, P. E., and Balis, J. U. (1969): Electron microscopy in study of lung development. In: *The Anatomy of the Developing Lung*, edited by J. Emery, pp. 18–48. Heinemann, London.
14. Dunnill, M. S. (1962): Postnatal growth of the lung. *Thorax*, 17:329–333.
15. Edwards, J. A. (1968): The external development of the rabbit and rat embryo. In: *Advances in Teratology*, edited by D. H. Woollam, pp. 239–263. Academic Press, New York.
16. Farris, E. J., and Griffith, J. R. (1962): *The Rat in Laboratory Investigation, Second Edition.* Haffner, New York.
17. Felix, W. (1912): The development of the urogenital system. In: *Manual of Human Embryology, Vol. 2*, edited by F. Keibel and F. P. Mall, pp. 752–979. Lippincott, Philadelphia.
18. Ferencz, F. (1969): Pulmonary arterial design in mammals. *Johns Hopkins Med. J.*, 125:207–224.
19. Haiman, M. T., and Prickett, M. (1931/32): The development of the external form of the guinea-pig (*Cavia cobaya*) between the ages of eleven days and twenty days of gestation. *Am. J. Anat.*, 49:351–373.
20. Hamburger, V., and Hamilton, H. L. (1951): A series of normal stages in the development of the chick embryo. *J. Morphol.*, 88:49–92.
21. Hamilton, W. J., and Mossman, H. W. (1972): *Human Embryology, Fourth Edition.* Heffer, Cambridge.
22. Harris, P., and Heath, D. (1977): *The Human Pulmonary Circulation, Second Edition.* Churchill-Livingston, Edinburgh.
23. Hendrickx, A. G., and Sawyer, R. H. (1975): Embryology of the rhesus monkey. In: *The Rhesus Monkey, Vol. 2*, edited by G. H. Bourne, pp. 141–169. Academic Press, New York.
24. Heuser, C. H., and Streeter, G. L. (1941): Development of the macaque embryo. *Contrib. Embryol.*, 29:15–55.
25. Heymann, M., and Rudolph, A. M. (1975): Control of the ductus arteriosus. *Physiol. Rev.*, 55:62–78.
26. Jacobsen, M. (1970): *Developmental Neurobiology.* Holt, Rhinehart, and Winston, New York.
27. Jilek, L., and Trojan, S. (1968): *Ontogenesis of the Brain.* University of Caroline, Prague.
28. Kalter, H. (1968): How should times during pregnancy be called in teratology? *Teratology*, 1:231–234.
29. Keeney, A. H. (1966): Development of vision. In: *Human Development*, edited by F. Falkner, pp. 459–464. W. B. Saunders, Philadelphia.
30. Langman, J. (1974): *Medical Embryology, Third Edition.* William & Wilkins, Baltimore.
31. McEwen, R. S. (1957): *Vertebrate Embryology, Fourth Edition.* Holt, New York.
32. McRoberts, D. D. (1934): A study of the development of the cochlea and cochlearis in the fetal albino rat. *J. Morphol.*, 56:243–265.
33. Meyrick, B., and Reid, L. M. (1977): Ultrastructure of alveolar lining and its development. In: *Development of the Lung*, edited by W. A. Hodson, pp. 135–214. Marcel Dekker, New York.
34. Minot, C. S., and Taylor, E. (1905): Normal plates of the development of the rabbit. In: *Normentafeln Zur Entwicklungsgeschichte der Wirbelthiere*, Vol. 5, edited by F. Keibel, G. Gischer, Jena.

35. Monie, I. W. (1965): Comparative development of rat, chick and human embryos. In: *Teratologic Workshop Manual (Supplement)*, pp. 146–162. Pharmaceutical Manufacturers Association, Berkeley.
36. Monie, I. W. (1970): The genesis of single umbilical artery. *Am. J. Obstet. Gynecol.*, 108:400–405.
37. Monie, I. W. (1976): Comparative development of the nervous, respiratory, and cardiovascular systems. *Environ. Health Perspect.*, 18:55–60.
38. Monie, I. W., and Khemmani, M. (1973): Absent and abnormal umbilica arteries. *Teratology*, 7:135–142.
39. Monie, I. W., Nelson, M. M., and Evans, H. M. (1957): Persistent right umbilical vein as a result of vitamin deficiency during gestation. *Circ. Res.*, 5:187–190.
40. Moore, K. L. (1973): *The Developing Human*. W. B. Saunders, Philadelphia.
41. Naeye, R. L. (1966): Development of pulmonary arteries from brith through early childhood. *Biol. Neonate*, 10:8–16.
42. Nelsen, O. E. (1953): *Comparative Embryology of the Vertebrates*. McGraw-Hill, New York.
43. O'Rahilly, R. (1973): *Development Stages in Human Embryos. Part A: Embryos of First Three Weeks (Stages 1–9) Publication 631*. Carnegie Institute, Washington.
44. O'Rahilly, R., and Meucke, E. C. (1972): The timing and sequence of events in the development of the human urinary system during the embryonic period proper. *Z. Anat. Entwickl. Gesch.*, 139:99.
45. Otis, E. M., and Brent, R. (1954): Equivalent ages in mouse and human embryos. *Anat. Rec.*, 120:33–63.
46. Patten, B. M. (1951): *Early Embryology of the Chick, Fourth Edition*. McGraw-Hill, New York.
47. Patten, B. M. (1969): *Human Embryology, Third Edition*. McGraw-Hill, New York.
48. Pei, Y. F., and Rhodin, J. A. G. (1970): The prenatal development of the mouse eye. *Anat. Rec.*, 168:105–126.
49. Rodier, P. M. (1976): Critical periods for behavioral anomalies in mice. *Environ. Health Perspect.*, 18:79–86.
50. Ruben, R. J. (1967): Development of the inner ear of the mouse: A radioautographic study of terminal mitosis. *Acta Otolaryngol. [Suppl.] (Stockh.)*, 220:1–44.
51. Rugh, R. (1968): *The Mouse: Its Reproduction and Development*. Burgess, Minneapolis.
52. Scott, J. P. (1937): The embryology of the guinea pig. 1. Table of normal development. *Am. J. Anat.*, 60:397–432.
53. Shepard, T. H. (1976): *Catalog of Teratogenic Agents, Second Edition*. Johns Hopkins University Press, Baltimore.
54. Sissman, N. J. (1970): Developmental lanumarks in cardiac morphogenesis: Comparative chronology. *Am. J. Cardiol.*, 25:141–148.
55. Snell, G. D., and Stevens, L. C. (1966): The Early Embryology of the Mouse. In: *Biology of the Laboratory Mouse*, edited by E. L. Green, pp. 205–245. Blakiston, Philadelphia.
56. Streeter, G. L. (1942): Developmental horizons in human embryos (XI–XII). *Contrib. Embryol.*, 30:211–245.
57. Streeter, G. L. (1945): Developmental horizons in human embryos (XIII–XIV). *Contrib. Embryol.*, 31:27–63.
58. Streeter, G. L. (1948): Developmental horizons in human embryos (XV–XVIII). *Contrib. Embryol.*, 32:133–203.
59. Timiras, P., Vernadakis, A., and Sherwood, N. M. (1968): Development and plasticity of the nervous system. In: *Biology of Gestation, Vol. 2*, edited by N. S. Assali, pp. 261–316. Academic Press, New York.
60. Torrey, T. W. (1954): The early development of the human nephros. *Contrib. Embryol.*, 35:175–197.
61. Tuchmann-Duplessis, H., Auroux, M., and Hoegel, P. (1974): Nervous system and endocrine glands. In: *Illustrated Human Embryology, Vol. 3*, pp. 126–136. Springer-Verlag, New York.
62. Wada, T. (1923): *Anatomical and Physiological Studies on the Growth of the Inner Ear of the Albino Rat*. Wistar Institute, Philadelphia.
63. Waterman, A. J. (1943): Studies of the normal development of the New Zealand White strain of rabbit. *Am. J. Anat.*, 72:473–515.
64. Wilson, D. B., Sawyer, R. H., and Hendrickx, A. G. (1975): Proliferation gradients in the inner ear of the monkey (*Macacca mulatta*) embryo. *J. Comp. Neurol.*, 164:23–30.
65. Witschi, E. (1956): *Development of Vertebrates*. W. B. Saunders, Philadelphia.
66. Zeman, W., and Innes, J. R. M. (1963): *Craigie's Neuroanatomy of the Rat*. Academic Press, New York.

*Developmental Toxicology*, edited by
C. A. Kimmel and J. Buelke-Sam. Raven Press,
New York © 1981.

# Comparative Placental Morphology and Function

F. Beck

*Department of Anatomy, The Medical School, University of Leicester, Leicester LE1
7RH, England*

The fact that the mammalian placenta is responsible for a multiplicity of functions is general knowledge. It provides nutrition for the conceptus, is a vehicle for the exchange of blood gases, allows fetal excretory material to be disposed of, and maintains pregnancy by a variety of hormonal mechanisms that vary from species to species. Additionally, the extraembryonic (placental) membranes protect the fetus, provide it with a stable, equable physical environment, and carry out a large number of "minor" functions, many of which are as yet little understood. In many species, it transfers immunoglobulin from the mother to her offspring and very probably transmits trophic factors that control and modulate fetal growth and differentiation. While doing all this, the placenta prevents its own rejection as a homograft and probably contributes not unsubstantially to its own demise with the accurately timed onset of parturition. Little wonder, therefore, that, in theory at least, derangement of such a complex structure can lead to dire consequences for the fetus. Clearly, when the placenta is a target organ for drugs or disease, a variety of fetal effects might be predicted. The surprising fact is perhaps that relatively few fetal effects directly attributable to placental dysfunction have been thoroughly and completely defined and investigated.

## DEFINITION AND EVOLUTION

Mossman's (26) definition of a placental relationship as an intimate apposition or fusion of fetal organs to maternal tissues for physiological interchange still serves as the most convenient one for practical purposes. In mammals, the fetal organs that contribute to the formation of placental systems are the extraembryonic membranes, and the nature of these can best be appreciated by reference to their analogs and homologs in lower forms.

The most primitive of the fetal membranes in animals is the yolk sac, the forerunner of which is represented in the anamniotes. Thus, in fish, early cleavage results in a blastoderm perched on a mass of yolk which later gradually becomes enclosed as the ectoderm, mesoderm, and an underlying periblast extend from the blastoderm to surround the yolk mass in a vascularized trilaminar yolk sac (Fig.

1). The periblast transfers nutrients to mesodermal blood vessels for utilization by the developing embryo.

Terrestrial life probably began when largely aquatic reptiles laid their eggs on dry land in order to protect them from water-bound predators. To achieve this, it was necessary to modify and strengthen the shell membranes of the eggs in order to prevent desiccation, but this in its turn inhibited gaseous interchange and excretion. To overcome this, an endodermally lined diverticulum of the hindgut, the allantois, was formed. Surrounded by vascularized mesoderm, this large sac lay in the extraembryonic coelom which developed as a split in the extraembryonic mesoderm separating an outer, somatopleuric chorion (trophoblast plus avascular mesoderm) from an endodermal, splanchnopleuric, yolk sac covered by vascularized mesoderm (Fig. 2). The allantoic mesoderm then fused with the chorionic mesoderm and served to vascularize it, thus allowing the allantoic circulation to take a large part in gaseous interchange. Another function of the allantois was to act as a repository for nitrogenous waste which could no longer diffuse into the environment as it had done in anamniotes. To this purpose, embryonic metabolism was altered, with urea being converted to insoluble uric acid for deposition in the allantoic cavity. In addition, the amniotic cavity itself developed to provide the developing conceptus with a liquid external environment contained in an ectodermally lined fluid filled sac—its amniotic cavity (Fig. 2).

These, then, are the building blocks from which the fetal parts of the placenta are constructed. Why they have become modified to sustain viviparity is of course impossible to say. Clearly the viviparous state protects the embryo in an inhospitable environment (33), but the development of the homeothermic state allows such conditions to be overcome by the incubating mechanisms used by birds. The alternative of viviparity is thus another rather than the only method of reproduction

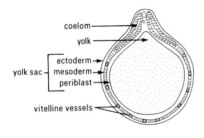

FIG. 1. Diagrammatic section through an idealized large-yolked anamniote conceptus

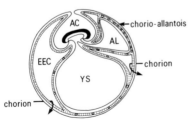

FIG. 2. Diagrammatic section showing the extraembryonic membranes of an amniote: AC, amniotic cavity; YS, yolk sac; EEC, extraembryonic coelom; AL, allantois. The disposition of the membranes is essentially that found in the typical mammalian chorionic vesicle.

in poor climatic conditions. It is not necessary to postulate that viviparity arose only in a single reptilian stock. Indeed, there is compelling evidence that this was not the case, and the diversity of extant viviparous reptiles that use homologous extraembryonic membranes to produce a similar series of placental forms suggests a good deal of parallel evolution (11,12,17,18,24,30,33). It has been suggested (31) that in mammals "monotreme-like" eggs were originally retained in the oviducts of cold-blooded therapsid reptiles. This reptilian subclass ancestral to the mammalia probably became warm-blooded somewhat later and then began to suckle their young (22). There is not even good evidence of direct evolutionary continuity from monotremes through marsupials to eutherian mammals, and it may be that the placentae of the Metatheria and Eutheria are examples of parallel evolution in different groups (see ref. 31 for discussion).

## Classification

Gross classification of the placenta by topographical characteristics is of value only insofar as it reflects histophysiological characteristics. Four main placental types fall into this form of "classification by shape."

In the diffuse placenta, the whole of the outer surface of the chorionic vesicle is made up of chorionic villi, and materno–fetal interchange is thus not concentrated in specific regions of its surface. The pig is the only species used in teratology that falls into this category. In the majority of ruminants, including sheep, the placenta is cotyledonary, the chorionic villi being restricted to circumscribed areas of the chorionic vesicle corresponding to specialized areas of the uterine wall (caruncles). The greater part of materno–fetal exchange occurs in these areas, although the intermediate smooth chorioallantois is not without function, especially over the mouths of the uterine glands in absorptive areas known as areolae. In sheep, for example, each conceptus has about 75 cotyledons. A zonary placenta is found in most carnivores and many other nonrelated groups. Here, the chorionic villi are very long and densely aggregated into a girdle around the equator of the chorionic vesicle, this being the site of much of the materno–fetal interchange. Again, however, the rest of the chorioallantois is not without function; this is especially so in the region of the hemophagous organ (13) where a great deal of extravasated maternal blood is degraded by adjacent chorion. The discoid or double discoid placenta of primates and rodents, as well as of other animals not often considered in the context of teratology, is of importance because both in man and in the rat, the fine structure allows for very close approximation of the maternal and fetal bloodstreams. This must not, however, detract the investigator from examining the function of the rest of the placental system in these species.

Diffuse and cotyledonary placentae are sometimes termed plicate (2), whereas those in which there is much thickening and reduplication of the chorion without great lateral expansion are called cumulate. The full-term cumulate placenta of man is that structure usually known as "the placenta" by obstetricians. Thus, it is important to realize that the full-term "placenta" in the topographical sense does not represent the total tissue across which materno–fetal interchange can occur (see definition of placenta above). This is particularly so in the early stages of gestation when much of organogenesis occurs. Furthermore, the cumulate placenta in many forms does not include membranes (such as the inverted yolk sac in rodents) that perform important transport functions throughout gestation.

A more logical way of classifying placental tissue is to pay attention to the form and disposition of homologous fetal membranes as described above and their relationship with the endometrium in various species.

### Yolk-Sac Placentation

This is illustrated in Fig. 1. In its simplest form, the bilaminar yolk-sac wall (omphalopleur) consists only of an outer (ectodermal) trophoblastic layer lined by endodermal cells. This nonvascular structure may come into intimate contact with the endometrium to form a simple yolk-sac placenta. Usually this system is invaded to a greater or lesser degree by mesoderm and is thus converted into a trilaminar omphalopleur which may become vascularized and form the embryonic part of a choriovitelline placenta (26).

In rodents and certain other orders, a peculiar form of yolk-sac placentation called an inverted yolk-sac placenta is formed. This will be described when the placenta of the rat is covered in detail.

### Chorionic Placentation

When the extraembryonic coelom extends into the vascular mesodermal area of the trilaminar omphalopleur, it splits the mesoderm into a vascular splanchnopleur which remains adherent to the endoderm of the yolk sac and a nonvascular somatopleur which, together with the overlying trophoblast, forms the chorion (Fig. 2). The extent to which the extraembryonic coelom penetrates the mesoderm varies greatly among Eutheria. In its complete form (as in man), the endodermal yolk sac is entirely separated from the wall of the chorionic vesicle. True chorion is never vascular. In Eutheria, it fuses at least in part with the vascular mesoderm covering the endodermal allantois to form the chorioallantois (see following section); but in some species (e.g., the rabbit and ferret), transient chorionic placentation occurs wherein extension of the allantois lags behind that of the extraembryonic coelom (Fig. 2). Indeed, chorionic placentation may occasionally (though rarely) be a permanent feature of placentation (e.g., the 13-striped ground squirrel, *Citellus tridecemtineatus*) (27).

### Chorioallantoic Placentation

In all Eutherian mammals, the allantoic mesoderm vascularizes the chorion to form the embryonic part of a ubiquitous chorioallantoic placenta. The extent to which the endodermal allantoic vesicle develops varies greatly in different species. Even in man, where it is minute, it is postulated that vascularization of the chorion is achieved by mesenchyme homologous with the allantoic mesoderm of other forms.

The fetal component of the chorioallantoic placenta invades the endometrium of many mammaliam groups to a greater or lesser extent, and, based on this property, Grosser (19,20) put forward a classification of placentae founded on microscopic anatomy that is still used today.

While in many ways constituting the most convenient grouping of placental forms available, Grosser's classification by fine structure survives only as a convenient morphological concept. Originally, it was thought that the number of layers separating the maternal and fetal bloodstreams (i.e., in the placental membrane) could be related fairly consistently to various functional parameters of the placenta, but this idea is no longer accepted. The number of layers constituting the placental membrane is not necessarily related to its thickness or its power of active or passive transmission of materials between maternal and fetal circulations.

Figure 3 illustrates the three types of placental membrane and indicates some of the variations each may exhibit in animals sometimes used in teratological studies. The epitheliochorial form (three maternal layers, three fetal layers) is found in the pig and sheep, the endotheliochorial (one maternal layer, three fetal layers) in the dog, cat, and ferret, and the hemochorial (maternal layers absent, three fetal layers) in mice, rats, hamsters, monkeys, apes, and man.

## FUNCTION IN RELATION TO STRUCTURE

### Embryonic Nutrition

A fundamental distinction exists between histiotrophic and hemotrophic embryonic nutrition. Histiotrophic nutrition results from the breakdown of maternal biopolymers by the extraembryonic membranes, whereas hemotrophic nutrition consists mainly of an interchange of solutes between the maternal and fetal circulation.

### *Histiotrophic Nutrition*

Maternal macromolecules forming the so-called histiotroph may be derived from endometrial cells, glandular secretions, and maternal blood or blood transudate. Its precise nature varies with species, but it is the only mode of nutrition available to the conceptus prior to the development of an embryonic circulation and usually persists to some extent even after circulatory establishment. Histiotrophic nutrition usually involves the breakdown of maternal macromolecules in the vacuolar system of cells of the extraembryonic membranes (6). Besides supplying the early conceptus with its metabolic needs, the same process is involved in implantation in many species. Figure 4 illustrates the process of heterosis whereby macromolecules are ingested (by phagocytosis, pinocytosis, or micropinocytosis) and digested intracellularly by means of acid hydrolases (see 14 for a comprehensive review of intracellular "digestion"). The possibility also exists that histiotroph may be broken down extracellularly (see 16 for discussion) and that the soluble breakdown products

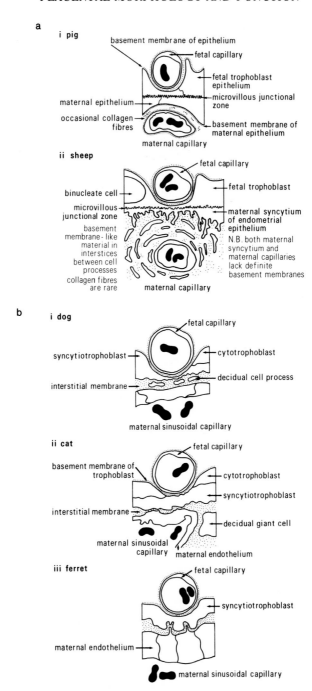

**FIG. 3. a and b.** See legend on facing page.

c

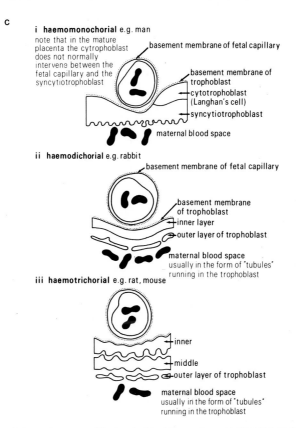

i **haemomonochorial** e.g. man

note that in the mature placenta the cytrophoblast does not normally intervene between the fetal capillary and the syncytiotrophoblast

basement membrane of fetal capillary

basement membrane of trophoblast
cytotrophoblast (Langhan's cell)
syncytiotrophoblast
maternal blood space

ii **haemodichorial** e.g. rabbit

basement membrane of fetal capillary

basement membrane of trophoblast
inner layer
outer layer of trophoblast
maternal blood space usually in the form of "tubules" running in the trophoblast

iii **haemotrichorial** e.g. rat, mouse

inner
middle
outer layer of trophoblast
maternal blood space usually in the form of "tubules" running in the trophoblast

**FIG. 3.** The placental membrane. **a**: The trophoblast has not penetrated the endometrium so that potentially three maternal cell layers are present (capillary endothelium, connective tissue stroma, and uterine epithelium). The placental membrane may be considerably thinned in regions by attenuation of the maternal stroma and fetal mesenchyme so that "intraepithelial capillaries" are present. In the sheep, this only occurs on the fetal side. **b**: The endotheliochorial placental membrane. The trophoblast has penetrated through the endometrial epithelium and connective tissue stroma and (in the form of syncytiotrophoblast) surrounds the sinusoidal maternal capillaries. In the ferret, the maternal capillary endothelium is greatly hypertrophied. **c**: The haemochorial placental membrane. The trophoblast has penetrated through all three maternal layers and is in direct contact with the maternal blood. Depending on the species, two or three layers of trophoblast may separate the maternal and fetal bloodstreams. [From Steven, ref. 31, with permission, from *Comparative Placentation*. Copyright Academic Press Inc., (London) Ltd.]

might then pass through the fetal membranes to the embryo. In special circumstances, such as the transfer of IgG from mother to young, whole macromolecules pass the placental barrier without the intervention of hydrolytic enzymes (3).

## Hemotrophic Nutrition

Hemotrophic nutrition can begin when the fetal circulation perfuses the extraembryonic membranes and, therefore, requires a certain stage of organogenesis to have

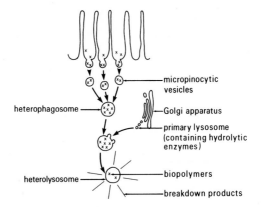

**FIG. 4.** Diagram to illustrate the process of heterosis in its simplest form. There is evidence to indicate that heterophagosomes obtain hydrolytic enzyme by fusion with secondary lysosomes (e.g., heterolysosomes) as well as with primary lysosomes as shown in the diagram. The process illustrated here is of micropinocytosis, but the uptake of macromolecules may equally well involve gross pinocytosis or even the uptake of solid particles, e.g., red blood corpuscles and endometrial cell detritus.

been reached (at least to the point of development of a beating embryonic heart). Theoretically, it can exist when the embryonic and maternal bloodstreams come into close relationship to one another either in a choriovitelline or a chorioallantoic circulation. Hemotrophic transfer of solutes may occur by simple diffusion along a chemical or electrochemical gradient. Sometimes (as in the case of glucose), the diffusion is "facilitated" by chemical or physical factors, so that while still occurring along a diffusion gradient, it is in excess of that which might be predicted by molecular size, charge, lipid solubility, etc. Other metabolites may pass across the placental membrane by active transport involving chemical alteration and a membrane carrier, and this process involves the expenditure of energy. Finally, certain materials seem to be "dragged" across the placenta by virtue of bulk flow of solvent (see 5 for a more detailed account of the factors involved in histiotrophic and hemotrophic nutrition).

## Excretion and Exchange of Blood Gases

Embryonic and fetal excretion is carried out by the extraembryonic membranes and does not require the participation of the embryonic kidneys. Human infants may be born alive with complete renal agenesis, although concomitant oligoamnios usually results in characteristic malformations (Potter's syndrome). The principal nitrogenous waste products, urea, creatinine, and creatine as well as sulfates pass across the placental membrane by simple diffusion and (when measurable) are present in similar concentrations in the fetal and maternal bloodstreams. Fetal plasma bilirubin in man is mainly unconjugated and slowly diffuses from the fetal to the maternal circulations where it is combined with plasma proteins and does not recross the placental barrier.

Blood gases also cross the placenta by simple diffusion. Most measurements of $P_{O_2}$ and $P_{CO_2}$ have been taken near term and are remarkably constant within species, although wide interspecies variations exist. There is little evidence that the fetus lives near the limits of its $O_2$ requirements. It seems that as pregnancy proceeds, blood flow per unit weight of uterus and fetus remains relatively constant, and oxygen uptake per unit mass of fetus is also unchanged. Diffusion of blood gases is rapid, so that two other factors are of importance in determining fetal blood gas levels. These are: first, the relationship of the fetal to the maternal blood flow which varies with the gestation period and species from counter-current to cross-current arrangements; second, the placental mass, particularly the amount of tissue between the maternal and fetal bloodstreams, will affect fetal blood gas concentration. It is true that the diffusion gradients are unvaried in direction, but the actively metabolic placental tissue will consume oxygen, and this may be particularly so in early gestation and in certain types of placentae (e.g., the endotheliochorial mustelid form in which the placental membrane is thick and oxygen consumption is great by the placental cells that are actively synthetic). In this context, it may be that the oxygen tension in the fetus with a placenta in which synthetic and diffusion functions are carried out in parallel (i.e., in the same cells) is lower than in forms in which these placental functions are performed in series (i.e., in specialized "exchange" and "synthetic" portions of the placenta).

### Placental Hormones

The hormonal maintenance of pregnancy varies greatly among species as do the relative contributions made by the placenta, ovary, and the other endocrine organs. Furthermore, the temporal sequence of hormone production also differs with species. The endocrinological aspects of placental function are, therefore, highly individual, and it is virtually impossible to extrapolate the results obtained from observations in one species to those of another.

In the human female, only human chorionic gonadotrophin (HCG), human chorionic somatomammotrophin (HCS), as well as estrogens and progesterone are known to be synthesized by the placenta. Heap (23) provides a well-balanced summary of the role of hormones in pregnancy in a number of species, and Thau and Lanman (32) give an excellent account of the hormonal function of the human extraembryonic membranes in normal human pregnancy.

## THE DEVELOPMENT OF THE PLACENTA IN A VARIETY OF SPECIES

### The Shrew

Placentation in the shrew (36,38) is illustrated in Fig. 5. During the early stages of placentation, the extraembryonic membranes come into topographical relationship with the endometrium in almost all possible ways. The illustration shows the simultaneous presence of an endotheliochorial, chorioallantoic placenta as well as

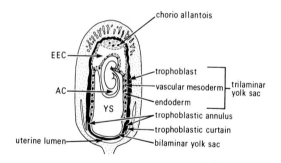

**FIG. 5.** Diagram of early placentation in the shrew showing the simultaneous presence of bilaminar and trilaminar portions of the yolk sac as well as an endotheliochorial, chorioallantoic placenta. The trilaminar yolk sac forms a transient choriovitelline placenta in this species. AC, amniotic cavity; EEC, extraembryonic coelom, YS, yolk-sac cavity. (Adapted from Wimsatt, ref. 36.)

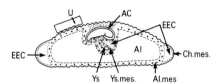

**FIG. 6.** Extraembryonic membranes in the pig: AC, amniotic cavity; Al, allantois; Al.mes., allantoic mesoderm; Ch.mes., chorionic mesoderm; EEC, extraembryonic coelom; U, uterine wall; YS, yolk-sac cavity; Ys.mes., yolk-sac mesoderm.

bilaminar and trilaminar portions of the yolk sac. The chorioallantoic placenta is concerned with hemotrophic nutrition, whereas the choriovitelline placenta as well as the placenta formed between the bilaminar yolk sac and the uterine wall probably subserve a histiotrophic function and are mainly concerned with the breakdown of endometrial "cushions." The choriovitelline placenta is able to transfer the breakdown products of ingested endometrium into the embryonic vessels of its mesoderm. In the case of the bilaminar yolk sac, however, degradation products must pass directly into its cavity. Here they presumably diffuse to a region where they are able to enter the embryonic circulation. At the extreme mesometrial pole, the bilaminar yolk sac is exposed to the uterine lumen, and here it is probably concerned with the breakdown of histiotroph in the form of uterine secretions.

The shrew is not an animal used in teratological studies, but an appreciation of its early placental relationships facilitates an understanding of the arrangements seen in the other species to be considered.

## The Pig

Figure 6 illustrates a fairly advanced stage of placentation in the pig (1,9). The chorioallantois is epitheliochorial with the areas in which the placental membrane is attenuated lying side by side with regions in which histiotrophic digestion of endometrial secretion preponderates. A histiotrophic bilaminar yolk sac is responsible for early nutrition. This is replaced by choriovitelline placentation and finally, at the early limb bud stage, by a chorioallantoic placenta which at first is still largely histiotrophic in function. Only later in gestation, and at an embryonic stage that is far more advanced than that in most other orders, does hemotrophic nutrition become important.

### The Rat

This is the species most frequently used in teratology, and its placentation therefore will be described in as much detail as space permits (31). Eccentric implantation occurs before gastrulation (5.5 days), and the embryonic mass remains relatively quiescent while trophoblast invades the decidua and the walls of the maternal capillaries. Gastrulation (between 7.5 and 8.5 days) occurs when entypy (inversion) of the germ layers has occurred because of growth of an ectoplacental cone of extraembryonic ectoderm (Fig. 7). At this stage, the embryonic disk probably derives its nutrition largely because the visceral layer of the extraembryonic endoderm (the so-called inverted yolk-sac placenta) is able to degrade macromolecules by heterosis (Fig. 4). The histiotroph comes from three sources: the maternal serum located in lacunae between trophoblastic cells, endometrial cells broken down by trophoblast, and uterine glandular secretion.

In later pregnancy, the uterine cavity near the implanted blastocyst is obliterated to reappear some days later on the antimesometrial aspect of the implantation site. At 20 somites, when embryonic head, tail, and lateral folds are well developed, the labyrinthine chorioallantoic placenta develops consequent upon fusion of the allantoic bud with the chorion, and this enables the inception of hemotrophic nutrition at about 11 to 12 days of gestation to take place, i.e., when the forelimb buds have appeared. On day 16 of pregnancy, the parietal layer of the yolk sac together with the overlying trophoblast are resorbed, leaving the visceral layer exposed to the uterine cavity where it is in an excellent position to pinocytize and degrade uterine secretions.

### The Ferret

This is a convenient laboratory carnivore that is of value in teratological work (21). It is much cheaper than a cat or a dog and can be induced to breed easily in captivity (8). The placental system is typical of the Mustelidae with central implantation occurring on day 12 of gestation. At this stage, the primitive streak is just beginning to form. The endometrial epithelium forms symplasmal masses which are penetrated by tongues of trophoblast responsible for histiotrophic nutrition. This is supplemented by absorption of uterine secretions from the mesometrial gutter. The choriovitelline placenta that soon develops (Fig. 8) and is probably largely histiotrophic in function because there is no vascularized mesoderm in the cores of the trophoblastic villi. Closure of the amniotic cavity by folding is followed by the extravasation of maternal blood into the antimesometrial portion of the implantation chamber. Here the red blood corpuscles are absorbed by trophoblastic cells in the hemophagous organ (cf, the marginal hematomata found at the placental edges in the cat and the dog) and presumably provide a source of iron for the

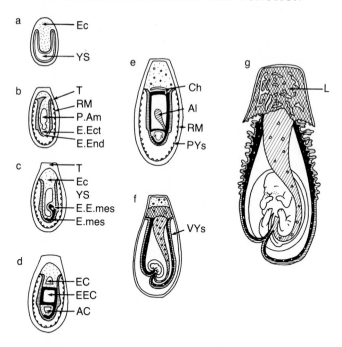

**FIG. 7.** Development of the extraembryonic membranes of the rat. **a**: At 6½ days postfertilization. The ectoplacental cone has grown so that the inner cell mass has become invaginated into the yolk-sac cavity. The latter is now horseshoe shaped. **b**: At 8 days; formation of the proamniotic cavity. A proamniotic cavity has appeared in the inner cell mass extending into the ectoplacental cone. The endoderm covering the sides of the ectoplacental cone is called the visceral layer of the yolk-sac endoderm and, in contrast to the parietal layer that is separated from the trophoblast only by an acellular layer known as Reichert's membrane, is highly pinocytic. The ectoplacental cone and the embryonic region at its apex are together known as the egg cylinder. **c**: At 9¼ days, gastrulation is well advanced. Mesoderm has migrated from the embryonic area into the region of the ectoplacental cone where ("pushing" the extraembryonic ectoderm ahead of it) it begins to subdivide the proamniotic cavity. A small extraembryonic coelom continuous with the embryonic coelom has developed. **d**: At 9½ days; division of the proamniotic cavity into three. The extraembryonic mesoderm with its contained extraembryonic coelom has grown right across the proamniotic cavity, and three cavities are apparent in the egg cylinder. They are an upper epamniotic cavity, a middle extraembryonic coelom, and a lower amniotic cavity. **e**: At 10 days; development of the allantoic bud. The embryo has begun to form head and tail folds. The allantois, an outgrowth of the endoderm in the tail fold covered by allantoic mesoderm, is growing into the extraembryonic coelom. The epamniotic cavity has collapsed; its original lower wall consists of extraembryonic ectoderm and nonvascularized mesoderm, thus forming the chorion. **f**: At 11½ days; early chorioallantoic placenta. The allantois has fused with the chorion, and a labyrinthine chorioallantoic hemochorial placenta is established. The embryo has turned so that it is now convex dorsally and has become invaginated into the extraembryonic coelom (this is sometimes incorrectly referred to as the yolk-sac cavity). **g**: At 16 days to full term; disappearance of parietal yolk sac and Reichert's membrane. The parietal layer of the yolk sac, Reichert's membrane, the adjacent trophoblast, and attenuated decidua capsularis are resorbed, and the visceral layer of the yolk sac is exposed to the cavity of the uterus. Ec, ectoplacental cone; Ys, yolk-sac cavity; T, trophoblast; P.Am, proamniotic cavity; E.Ect, embryonic ectoderm; E.End, embryonic endoderm; E.mes, embryonic mesoderm; EC, epamniotic cavity; EEC extraembryonic coelom; AC, amniotic cavity; Ch, chorion; Al, allantois; RM, Reichert's membrane; PYs, parietal yolk-sac wall; VYs, visceral yolk-sac wall; L, chorioallantoic placental labyrinth.

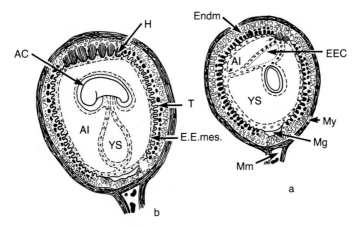

**FIG. 8.** The extraembryonic membranes of the ferret (**a**) at 19 days showing predominantly chorio-vitelline placentation. The allantois has fused with the chorion antimesometrially and begun to form an endothelial chorioallantoic placenta which is extending laterally in the direction of the *arrows*. (**b**) At 21 days, when the chorioallantoic placenta is well developed. AC, amniotic cavity; H, hemophagous organ; T, trophoblastic villus; E.E.mes., extraembryonic mesoderm; Al, allantois; YS, yolk sac; Endm, endometrium; EEC, extraembryonic coelom; Mg, mesometrial gutter; Mm, mesometrium; My, myometrium.

embryo. The allantois eventually grows into a rapidly expanding extraembryonic coelom and, fusing with the chorion, forms an endotheliochorial, chorioallantoic placenta which replaces the choriovitelline form at about 20 days (35 + somite embryo). In mustelids in particular, the placental membrane of the chorioallantois is very thick (Fig. 3), and maternal and fetal circulations are separated by some 10 μm of tissue. This must place certain constraints on the physiology of hemotrophic nutrition in these species when compared with the hemochorial arrangement in primates and rodents or even when compared with the relatively thin membrane found in regions of epitheliochorial ungulate placentae (Fig. 3). The implications of the morphological appearance of the mustelid placenta, although probably of importance, are not at all understood (Fig. 9).

## Higher Primates (Excluding Man)

Both the rhesus monkey and marmosets have been used in teratology, and their placentae have been described (1,37). The marmoset, a New World monkey, implants centrally and rapidly develops an extensive trophoblastic proliferation leading to a broad area of attachment to the endometrium. Rapid blastocyst expansion occurs, and a reticulated syncytiotrophoblast containing maternal blood lacunae penetrates the uterus lying on a basally located cytotrophoblast. The cytotrophoblast then forms villi containing a mesodermal core which penetrate the reticulated syncytiotrophoblast and, branching repeatedly, often reach to the decidual boundary. However, no cytotrophoblastic shell, characteristic of Old World monkeys, great apes, and man develops. In the second half of gestation, the superficial cells of the

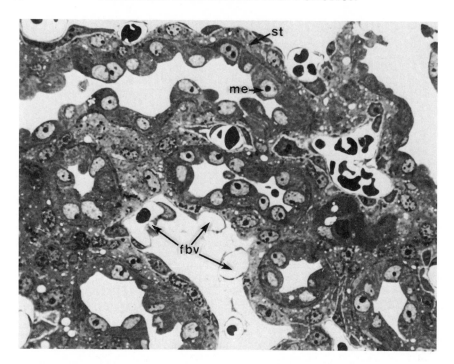

**FIG. 9.** Chorioallantoic, endotheliochorial placenta of the ferret showing trophoblastic villi with mesenchymal cores containing fetal blood vessels (fbv) and covered with syncytiotrophoblast (st). Between the trophoblastic villi there lie sinusoidal maternal blood vessels with greatly hypertrophied endothelial cells (me). The latter may greatly increase the distance between the fetal and maternal bloodstreams. Toluidine blue; ×800. (From Gulamhusein and Beck, ref. 21, with permission.)

cytotrophoblastic villi become converted into "secondary" syncytiotrophoblast co-inciding with the degeneration of the original syncytium. The placenta now looks very similar to that found in Old World monkeys with the exception of strands of syncytiotrophoblast that still often connect the villous tips. The marmoset probably depends on histiotrophic nutrition for a longer period than does the macaque, and this is reflected by the considerable proliferation of an endometrial plaque and a great deal of endometrial glandular secretion.

In the macaque, placentation is more like the human than the marmoset. Super-ficial implantation, on the ninth day of gestation, is more limited, but the trophoblast is more invasive. Chorionic villi do not penetrate a preformed reticular syncytio-trophoblast; instead, cytotrophoblastic cores bore their way into syncytiotrophoblast forming primary placental villi (Fig. 10). This is followed by penetration into the villi of vascular fetal mesoderm so that tertiary placental villi result. The macaque establishes precocious hemotrophic nutrition as soon as fetal blood begins to cir-culate in the tertiary villi, i.e., at about five somites or 22 days of gestation. This is earlier than the onset of hemotrophic nutrition in the marmoset.

Placental villi continue to differentiate, and at about 35 days, the cytotrophoblast of "anchoring" villi has penetrated the syncytiotrophoblast and, spreading laterally, has formed a cytotrophoblastic shell at the junctional zone with the decidua. Subsequently, branch villi make the histological arrangement very like that of the human placenta. The principal difference in placentation between Old World monkeys and great apes is that the former develop a well-marked epithelial plaque at the attachment site of the blastocyst. Histiotrophic nutrition is therefore more prominent in the early stages of gestation and retains its importance for a longer period.

## The Human Placenta

The human placenta is sufficiently well documented (10) for only a brief summary of its development to be given here. Implantation at about 7.5 days is interstitial, and a small plaque of trophoblast forms at the point of penetration. Histiotrophic nutrition at implantation consists of trophoblastic digestion of endometrial cells and secretions. Within 4 to 5 days of implantation, the blastocyst is already completely buried in the endometrial stratum compactum, and lacunae develop within the trophoblast. These lacunae first contain endometrial secretions; later, at about 13 days, they become interconnected and filled with sluggishly moving maternal blood (Fig. 10). Gastrulation commences 3 days later, and histiotrophic nutrition now becomes a matter of breakdown of maternal blood by syncytiotrophoblast lining the lacunae. Chorionic villi are established rather as in the macaque (see above and Fig. 10), and less than a week after gastrulation, hemotrophic nutrition commences as fetal blood vessels become established in the mesodermal cores of the villi. At this stage, the embryo is about the five-somite stage (21–22 days). As in the macaque, the cytotrophoblastic cores of "anchoring" villi grow distally toward the decidua and, breaking through the syncytiotrophoblast at the periphery of the chorionic vesicle, form a cytotrophoblastic shell at the junctional zone. This is capable of continuing histiotrophic nutrition at least until midterm mainly by absorbing the secretion of endometrial glands. In man as well as in the simian primates (see above), full development of the placental villi only occurs in a restricted area of the chorionic vesicle, the so-called chorion frondosum. This results in the discoidal form of the human placenta and the bidiscoidal placenta of the macaque. In all higher primates, the placental membrane becomes thinner with advancing gestation due to attenuation of the cytotrophoblast in the branch villi (Fig. 3).

## RELEVANCE OF COMPARATIVE PLACENTOLOGY TO TERATOLOGICAL STUDIES

Teratological investigations are usually concerned either with the mode of action of certain teratogenic agents and the light this may throw on normal development or with the testing of medicines and other environmental agents for potential teratogenicity in man. An ever-present problem in all such experiments is the applicability of the model system used to the human situation. When *in vivo* systems are evaluated, the choice of experimental animal is one of the most important factors

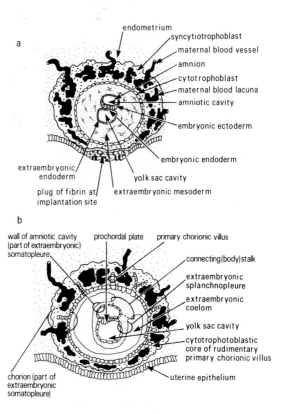

**FIG. 10.** Diagrams showing the development of the human placenta. **(a)** Following interstitial implantation, the syncytiotrophoblast has "tapped" endometrial vessels, and a sluggish circulation of maternal blood has begun through interconnecting lacunae that have developed in its substance. **(b)** Primary chorionic villi have begun to develop as cytotrophoblastic columns grown into the syncytiotrophoblast. *(contd.)*

to be considered. Teratogens will act at one or more of three potential sites: directly on the fetus, indirectly by virtue of effects produced on the mother, or on the placental system. A potential action on either the mother or the fetus requires consideration of numerous variables before an attempt to extrapolate experimental findings to man can be made. Comparative pharmacokinetics, intermediary metabolism, rate of embryonic development, and the duration of "critical periods" are but a few examples of the questions involved.

The possibility that placental function might account for interspecies variation in teratogenic response has been much neglected in the past and still is not the subject of much experimental work. Yet, from what has been said above, it is clear that enormous variations exist in placental histophysiology among species and that these variations might easily modify the teratogenic action of environmental agents.

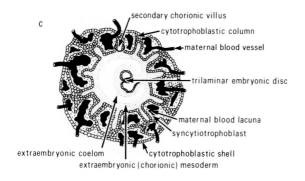

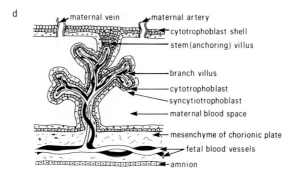

**FIG. 10 *(contd.):*** **(c)** Secondary chorionic villi develop when the primary villi acquire a mesenchymal core. The development of fetal blood vessels in the villi results in the formation of tertiary villi. **(d)** Anchoring villus and branch villi in the region of chorion frondosum. Note the presence of the cytotrophoblastic shell. (From Beck et al., ref. 7, with permission.)

In theory, the nutritive function of the extraembryonic membranes is a very likely target for the action of teratogens. Histiotrophic nutrition generally involves pinocytosis or phagocytosis of maternal macromolecules by cells of the extraembryonic membranes (6), although extracellular breakdown of maternal biopolymers by secreted enzymes or by spontaneous lysis of endometrial cells is also a possibility (see ref. 16 for discussion). Williams et al. (34) have shown that the teratogenic agent trypan blue can inhibit pinocytosis of cultured rat visceral yolk sac (the membrane the cells of which are responsible for intracellular breakdown of histiotroph) and have postulated that this may be the major factor responsible for its teratogenic action (see also ref. 4). A part of their argument depends on the fact that the teratogenic activity of the dye ceases suddenly between 10.5 and 11.5 days of gestation. This roughly coincides with the establishment of hematotrophic nutrition by the chorioallantoic placenta, an organ on which trypan blue would not be expected to have an effect. Furthermore, trypan blue does not appear to reach the embryonic tissues in any large amount if at all (35). However, some authors have suggested that small amounts do reach the embryo and that this may be significant (15). It is important to note that trypan blue exerts a teratogenic action in the ferret at 18 days of gestation (equivalent to 11.5 days in the rat), at which stage the ferret is still dependent on histiotrophic nutrition, while the rat is beginning to obtain much of its supply by the hemotrophic route. New and Brent (28) obtained very similar results to those described for trypan blue when they treated rats with anti-yolk-sac antibody.

Another way of interfering with histiotrophic nutrition is by intracellular inhibition of lysosomal enzyme. Such experiments are currently under way in our laboratory and have shown that leupeptin (a cathepsin B, H, and L inhibitor), when added in doses as low as 1 $\mu$g/ml to the medium in the rat culture system developed by New et al. (29), produces grossly malformed embryos.

Differences in the composition and thickness of the placental membrane in the chorioallantoic placentae of various species may well be related to the way in which transfer of solute between the maternal and the fetal circulation occurs (5). It is conceivable, therefore, that an environmental factor may well influence hemotrophic nutrition and placental excretion differently depending on the histophysiology of the placental membrane.

Similar factors are possibly operational with respect to respiration. Although simple diffusion will establish a gradient of oxygen and carbon dioxide between maternal and fetal circulations, it is likely that the metabolic requirements of the placental barrier itself will vary enormously, e.g., as between man and ferret (Fig. 9), because one contains so very much more tissue than the other. A secondary consequence of such a difference might clearly be in the timing of the embryonic switchover from a predominantly glycolytic and pentose shunt mechanism of energy generation to one involving maturation of the mitochondria and establishment of the Krebs cycle as an important energy source (25).

The hormonal activity of the placenta is but a facet of the general normal adaptation to pregnancy occurring in viviparous species. These adaptations vary greatly among animals, and it is likely that agents that alter hormonal synthesis and function in the placenta of one species may have no effect or an entirely different effect in another. Therefore, the teratogenic potential of such agents might well be highly specific.

## CONCLUSION

The mammalian placenta has been defined and its various forms classified with special reference to function. It is clear that a teratogenic agent acting principally on some aspect of placental function is liable to the same great species variation as are the placental membranes themselves. In this area in particular, extrapolation from one species to another must be extremely circumspect. In this context, it is perhaps most useful to think in terms not of "placental function" as an entity but on that particular aspect of function in which a perversion is suspected. The specific example of a possible effect on histiotrophic nutrition has been cited. Here an agent disrupting macromolecular pinocytosis by the extraembryonic membranes would be expected to act differently with respect to time in a species where hemotrophic nutrition is precocious in onset (as in man) when compared to one where it is relatively delayed (as in the ferret or the pig).

## ACKNOWLEDGMENT

I am grateful to the M.R.C. for a grant in aid of research.

## REFERENCES

1. Amoroso, E. C. (1952): Placentation. In: *Marshall's Physiology of Reproduction, Vol. II*, edited by A. S. Parkes, pp. 127–311. Longmans Green, London.
2. Assheton, R. (1906): The morphology of the ungulate placenta. Particularly the development of that organ in the sheep and notes upon the placenta of the elephant and hyrax. *Phil. Trans. R. Soc. Lond. (Biol.)*, 198:143–220.
3. Bangham, D. R., Hobbs, K. R., and Terry, R. J. (1958): Selective placental transfer of serum proteins in the rhesus. *Lancet*, 2:351–354.
4. Beck, F. (1979): Trypan blue induced teratogenesis. In: *Advances in the Study of Birth Defects*, edited by T. V. N. Persaud, pp. 37–51. M. T. P., Lancaster.
5. Beck, F., and Lloyd, J. B. (1977): Comparative Placental Transfer. In: *Handbook of Teratology, Vol. 3*, edited by James G. Wilson and F. Clarke Fraser, pp. 155–186. Plenum Press, New York and London.
6. Beck, F., Lloyd, J. B., and Parry, L. M. (1971): The study of endocytosis and lysosome function in embryotrophic nutrition. In: *Methods in Mammalian Embryology*, edited by J. C. Daniel, pp. 378–418. W. H. Freeman, San Francisco.
7. Beck, F. Moffat, D. B., and Lloyd, J. B. (1973): *Human Embryology and Genetics*. Blackwell, Oxford and London.
8. Beck, F., Schön, H., Mould, G., Swidzinska, P., Curry, S., and Grauwiler, J. (1976): Comparison of the teratogenic effects of mustine hydrochloride in rats and ferrets. The value of the ferret as an experimental animal in teratology. *Teratology*, 13:151–166.
9. Björkmann, N. (1970): *An Atlas of Placental Fine Structure*, Bailliere, Tindall and Cassell, London.
10. Boyd, J. D., and Hamilton, W. J. (1970): *The Human Placenta*. Heffer, Cambridge.
11. Boyd, M. M. (1942): The oviduct, foetal membranes and placentation in *Hydrodactylus maculatus* Gray. *Proc. Zool. Soc. [A]*, 112:65–104.
12. Cate-Hoedemakes, J. T. (1933): Beitrage zur Keuntuis der-plazentation bei Haien und Reptilien. *Z. Zellforsch.*, 18:229–345.
13. Creed, R. F. S., and Biggers, J. D. (1963): Development of the racoon placenta. *Am. J. Anat.*, 113:417–445.
14. de Duve, C., and Wattiaux, R. (1966): Functions of lysosomes. *Annu. Rev. Physiol.*, 28:435–492.
15. Dencker, L. (1977): Trypan blue accumulation in the embryonic gut of rats and mice during the teratogenic phase. *Teratology*, 15:179–184.
16. Finn, C. A. (1977): The implantation reaction. In: *Biology of the Uterus, second edition*, edited by R. M. Wynn, pp. 245–308. Plenum Press, New York and London.
17. Flynn, T. T. (1923): On the occurrence of a true allantoplacenta of the conjoint type in an Australian lizard. *Rec. Anat. Mus.*, 14:72–77.
18. Giacomini (1891): Sulla maniera di gestazione e sugli annessiembrionali del *Gongylus ocellatus* Forsk. *Sez. Sci. Nat.*, 3:401.
19. Grosser, O. (1909): *Eihaute und der placenta Wien and Leipzig*. Fischer, Jena.

20. Grosser, O. (1927): *Fruhentwicklung, Eihautbildung und Placentation des Menschen und der Saugetiere*. Munich. (Quoted in ref.1.)
21. Gulamhusein, A. P., and Beck, F. (1975): Development and structure of the extraembryonic membranes of the ferret. A light microscopic and ultrastructural study. *J. Anat.*, 120:349–366.
22. Halstead, L. B. (1969): *The Pattern of Vertebrate Evolution*. Oliver and Boyd, London.
23. Heap, R. B. (1972): Role of hormones in pregnancy. In: *Reproduction in Mammals, Vol. 3*, edited by C. R. Austin and R. V. Short, pp. 73–105. Cambridge University Press, Cambridge.
24. Kasturirangan (1951): Placentation in the sea snake *Enhydrina Schistora* (Daudin). *Proc. Indian Acad. Sci.* [*B*], 34:1.
25. Krowke, R., and Neubert, D. (1977): Embryonic intermediary metabolism under normal and pathological conditions. In: *Handbook of Teratology, Vol. II*, edited by J. G. Wilson and F. C. Fraser, pp. 117–151. Plenum Press, New York.
26. Mossman, H. W. (1937): Comparative morphogenesis of the fetal membranes and accessory uterine structures. *Contrib. Embryol.*, 26:129–246.
27. Mossman, H. W., and Weisenfeldt, L. A. (1939): The foetal membranes of a primitive rodent, the thirteen striped ground squirrel. *Am. J. Anat.*, 64:59.
28. New, D. A. T. (1972): Effect of yolk-sac antibody on rat embryos grown in culture. *J. Embryol. Exp. Morphol.*, 27:543–553.
29. New, D. A. T., Coppola, P. T., and Cockcroft, D. L. (1976): Improved development of head-fold rat embryos in culture resulting from low oxygen and modifications of the culture serum. *J. Reprod. Fertil.*, 48:219–222.
30. Parameswaran, K. N. (1962): The foetal membranes and placentation of *Enhydris dussumieri* (Smith), *Proc. Indian Acad. Sci.* [*B*], 56:302–327.
31. Steven, D. H. (1975): *Comparative Placentation*. Academic Press, London, New York, San Francisco.
32. Thau, R. B., and Lanman, J. T. (1975): Endocrinological aspects of placental function. In: *The Placenta*, edited by P. Gruenwald, pp. 125–144. M. T. P., Lancaster.
33. Weekes, H. C. (1935): A review of placentation among reptiles with particular regard to the function and evolution of the placenta. *Proc. Zool. Soc.*, 2:625–645.
34. Williams, K. E., Roberts, G., Kidston, M. E., Beck, F., and Lloyd, J. B. (1976): Inhibition of pinocytosis in rat yolk-sac by trypan blue. *Teratology*, 14:343–354.
35. Wilson, J. G., Shepard, T. H., and Gennaro, J. F. (1963): Studies on the site of teratogenic action of $^{14}$C-labelled trypan blue. *Anat. Rec.*, 145:300.
36. Wimsatt, W. A., and Wislocki, G. B. (1947): The placentation of the American shrews *Blarina brevicauda* and *Sorex fumeus*. *Am. J. Anat.*, 80:361–433.
37. Wislocki, G. B., and Streeter, G. L. (1938): On the placentation of the macaque (*Macaca mulatta*) from the time of implantation until the formation of the definitive placenta. *Contrib. Embryol.*, 27:1.
38. Wislocki, G. B., and Wimsatt, W. A. (1947): Chemical cytology of the placenta of two North American shrews. *Am. J. Anat.*, 81:261–307.

*Developmental Toxicology*, edited by
C. A. Kimmel and J. Buelke-Sam. Raven Press,
New York © 1981.

# The Role of Genetic Studies in Developmental Toxicology

## Fred G. Biddle

*Kinsmen Pediatric Research Centre, Alberta Children's Hospital, Calgary, Alberta T2T 5C7, and Departments of Pediatrics and Medical Biochemistry, Faculty of Medicine, University of Calgary, Calgary, Alberta, Canada T2N 1N4*

This review of genetic studies in developmental toxicity demonstrates how genetics can be a useful tool in experimental teratology. Genetic terms and methods are introduced, and examples are developed within a conceptual framework to provide visually interpretable models. The chapter is not a catalog of malformations or of strain differences; instead, it reflects an approach to the definition and interpretation of teratogenic reactions.

A teratogenic reaction in an individual presents some interesting questions. In experimental organisms belonging to a genetically homogeneous strain, what is the difference between the individual that reacts and the one that does not? When the individual is put into the context of the species, what does the reaction mean? If comparisons between species are attempted, the "standard" mouse, the "standard" rat, and so forth do not exist. How can comparisons best be made?

## CONCEPTUAL FRAMEWORK

### Norms of Reaction: Interaction and Additivity

Much energy, especially in testing and screening of potential teratogens, has been devoted to the choice of dose or dose range to be used in the test species. Consideration of results, especially for human therapeutic agents, has centered on human-equivalent dosages. A practical suggestion has been to try a broad range of doses, to look for the biological effect (any effect), and then to evaluate this effect with full knowledge of the treatment, the test species, and the use for which the compound was intended (76).

As the science of experimental teratology has evolved (and it continues to do so), there may have been a reluctance to explore the dosage range once a malformation reaction had been observed. Within a test species, for example the mouse, most reports of strain differences in teratogen-induced malformation have compared the frequencies of malformations that are produced only by a specific dose of a teratogen [e.g., the list prepared by Dagg (25)]. The use of absolute frequencies to make the comparisons is valid only if the teratogen produces the malformation by the same mechanism in all genotypes and there is an additive, linear relationship between genotypes on the frequency scale.

A practical problem arises when one strain does not respond at an arbitrarily chosen dose while other strains show intermediate frequencies of reaction or reaction in all treated embryos. If two strains happen to exhibit the malformation in all treated embryos, should they be considered equivalent? Some method is required that will relate response and dosage.

Comparisons between strains should be made with information about their *norms of reaction*. The concept of the norm of reaction and its central importance to genetics has been discussed extensively (67). Genetics is the study of the relationship between genotype, environment, and phenotype. The norm of reaction is the table of correspondence between the phenotype and genotype–environment combinations.

If norms of reaction are considered for teratogenic reactions, attention is directed toward dose–effect behaviors. Two sets of hypothetical dose–effect curves for two different genotypes, $G_1$ and $G_2$, are illustrated in Fig. 1. The curves have been drawn linearly. It must be emphasized that the phenotype is not the malformation per se in the individual, but rather, it is the frequency of the malformation in treated individuals. The dose of teratogen may be thought of as one type of environment or as one range of environments.

In Fig. 1a, the dose–effect curves are different and intersect. Therefore, depending on dosage, the two strains will have the same response or very different ones. There is *interaction* between genotype and teratogen. If only a single dose of teratogen were used to make the comparison, the genetic interpretation of the difference

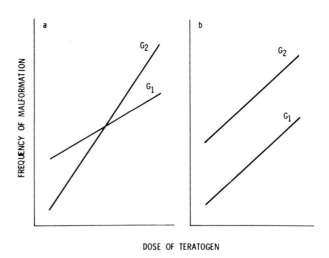

DOSE OF TERATOGEN

**FIG. 1.** Two sets of hypothetical dose–effect curves for two different genotypes ($G_1$ and $G_2$). **a:** The dose–effect curves are not parallel and demonstrate interaction between genotype and teratogen. **b:** The dose–effect curves are parallel and demonstrate an additive relationship between genotype and teratogen.

would depend on the dosage that was chosen. In Fig. 1b, the dose–effect curves of the two genotypes are parallel. The difference between genotypes on the phenotypic scale (frequency of malformation) is the same for all doses. Also, the difference between dosages is the same for all frequencies of malformation. Therefore, there is an *additive* relationship between genotype and dosage of teratogen as measured by the phenotype. In both cases, the cause of the difference between the genotypes is the subject for genetic study. Is the difference due to one or a few genes with major effect or to many genes, each with small effect? The approach taken for the genetic study and interpretation depends entirely on the dose–effect behavior.

The use of the word interaction to describe the relationship between genotype and teratogen is the familiar one also used in statistics, i.e., the departure from additivity for a particular model. "The effects of two treatments applied together cannot be predicted from the average responses of the separate factors" (93). If the dose–effect curves exhibit interaction, as in Fig. 1a, the two genotypes can be said to respond differently or to arrive at the malformation by different mechanisms. They exhibit a mutation in the response.

## Dose–Effect Models: Response and Reactivity

If the concept of norm of reaction is applied to teratogenic reactions, *appropriate* dose–effect models need to be considered (8,9). The experimenter must judge the model not only from the fit of the data to the model but also from the inferences that can be made from it.

There is no *a priori* reason why dose–effect data should fit a linear log-probit model in preference to any other model for describing binary response data such as the logistic and angular distributions (34). However, if binary response data for teratogens can be fitted to linear regression by some transformation of the response and/or dose, the concern should not be with the appropriateness of the method but with the comparisons and inferences that can be made between teratogens, between different genotypes, and between different test species. The experimental data will detect any inadequacies in the model.

A dose–effect model and its transformation to linearity permit the use of the conceptual triad of "stimulus, response, and reactivity." For a teratogenic stimulus, an important distinction can be made between response and reactivity. The slope of the dose–effect curve defines the *response*. The location of the curve on the dosage scale defines the *reactivity*.

There are several reasons for advocating dose–effect models. (a) Different kinds of mutations can be defined operationally in terms of the model: mutations in response; mutations in reactivity. (b) Genetic terms, such as additive and interaction effects, maternal effects, and specific gene–teratogen effects, can be made visually interpretable. (c) The effects of different co–treatments on teratogenesis can be defined. Additive, synergistic, or independent effects may be identified. (d) A link can be made between the teratogen, molecular biology, and embryology.

## GENETIC RESOURCES

The genetic resources potentially available to experimental teratology will be outlined before the discussion of specific examples of differences in reactions to teratogens. This will provide background for the demonstration that the exploitation of genetics as a tool in teratogenesis has only just begun.

### Mouse

An inbred strain of the mouse is equivalent to a single individual. The genetic analysis of a reaction difference between inbred strains compares only the net difference between the two strains (two individuals) and cannot be extrapolated universally to the species. However, the alternate use of random-bred or what has been called "ambigugenic" stocks in teratology is recognized as fallacious (116).

#### Inbred Strains

When the advantages of inbred strains are considered, such as replicate sampling from genetically homogeneous individuals, the resources of the mouse have hardly been touched. A recent listing (94) cites 252 distinct strains, and even these strains must represent a limited sampling of the genome of the mouse (72). Most inbred strains have never been used in teratology, but they can be used in a systematic way.

The genetic relationship has been established for 27 common inbred strains for which pedigree relations are largely unknown (99). There appear to be three clusters (Fig. 2) on the basis of genetic similarity at 16 polymorphic loci. For teratology, the 16 loci can be considered as a relatively unbiased sampling of the genome, and this clustering can be put to practical use. If a teratogenic reaction has been defined, and genetic differences in this reaction are sought, they will more likely be found between, rather than within, the clusters. Large differences in reaction between two genetically similar strains would suggest that few genes determine the trait, but,

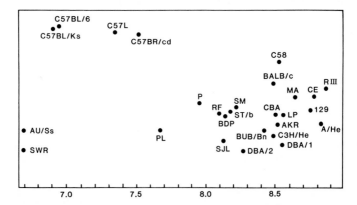

**FIG. 2.** Genetic similarity among 27 inbred strains of mice. The positions of the strains in the two dimensions were determined from an analysis of similarity matrix. (Reprinted from Taylor, ref. 99, with permission.)

if differences are found only between the clusters, the trait is more likely due to many gene differences. Figure 2 illustrates an interesting problem. The C57BL strain has been used almost as the "standard" inbred mouse, but with reference to the other strains in the figure, it appears to be genetically atypical.

## Recombinant Inbred Strains

Recombinant inbred (RI) strains are produced by crossing two highly inbred strains, raising an $F_2$ generation, and then deriving a series of separate inbred lines from $F_2$ pairs by sib matings (2). The independent inbred lines are derived without selection, and the set of RI strains from the parental pair approximates a stable segregant population. Recombinant inbred strains have become a powerful tool for the study of complex genetic traits (98) and for detecting linkage (101).

Recombinant inbred strains are useful for traits that are defined by repeated observation with many individuals. Conventional breeding tests, to study the $F_2$ and backcross generations of progeny, are not possible if each individual is tested destructively and therefore only once. Each set of RI strains represents a replicate population of recombinant genotypes of the genetic differences that are found between the two parental strains. It would be possible to study genetic differences in a teratogenic reaction that are determined by dose–effect curves. A dose–effect determination with one RI strain is equivalent to making the determination on a single mouse. Comparison between the members of a set of RI strains relative to the two parental reactions can be used to search for segregation of the genetic determinants of the difference between the parental reactions.

## Congenic Inbred Strains

Congenic strains of mice were developed as a tool for the identification and study of histocompatibility differences (92). The term congenic has come to mean mice that are produced by the introduction of a selected gene into an existing inbred strain. The congenic strain differs from the inbred strain by the particular selected allele (one or more alternate forms of a gene occupying the same genetic locus), and, depending on the number of cycles of backcrossing and available marker genes, it will also have an indeterminant amount of genetic material linked to the selected allelic difference. In contrast, coisogenic strains arise by chance mutations within an existing inbred strain.

For toxicity traits that are defined by assays of many individuals, a difference in reaction between the members of a congenic pair would suggest that a single genetic factor determined the trait. Also, the single factor would provide a marker gene for further study of the trait with other strains.

## Stocks with Defined Mutations or Physiological Variants

Modification of a teratogenic reaction might be predicted from prior knowledge of known or suspected genetic variants in physiological characteristics. Three examples appear to stand out. First, strain differences in alcohol metabolism have been associated with behavioral characteristics and, in the development of the mouse model of the fetal-alcohol syndrome, dose-dependent differences between two strains were found (18). A breeding study using three strains demonstrated that the differences in tolerance for the fetal reaction were dependent on the maternal genotype. The maternal genotype determined the maternal blood alcohol level for a defined diet intake of alcohol (19).

Second, strain differences are known in what appears to be tolerance to embryonic death induced by aromatic hydrocarbons (59). The difference may be associated with the $Ah$ locus that controls the inducibility of the cytochrome P-450 monooxygenase system that metabolizes various xenobiotic compounds. The $Ah^b$ allele determines the induction response to various hydrocarbons and is dominant to the $Ah^d$ allele (74); the $Ah$ locus has not been mapped yet. The reciprocal backcross matings of nonresponsive (AKR/N) females to responsive (AK.B6F$_1$) males and of responsive (AK.B6F$_1$) females to nonresponsive (AKR/N) males were treated with benzo($a$)pyrene (91). The activity of aryl hydrocarbon hydroxylase was assayed in surviving fetuses ($Ah^d/Ah^d$ or $Ah^b/Ah^d$) to follow segregation of the $Ah^d$ and $Ah^b$ alleles. Both maternal and embryonic genetic effects on the embryotoxicity of benzo($a$)pyrene were identified. In treated nonresponsive dams, there was a significant deficiency of responsive fetuses, and more responsive fetuses than nonresponsive fetuses were malformed. In treated responsive dams, the two embryonic genotypes were affected equally.

Third, strains have been characterized in terms of their resistance or susceptibility to cadmium-induced testicular necrosis that is determined by the $cdm$ gene. The role that this genetic difference may play in cadmium teratogenesis will be discussed further (*vide infra*).

In contrast to these directed studies, the known genetic differences in endocrine function of the mouse (89,90) have not been employed in the study of glucocorticoid teratogenesis and the obvious modifications of teratogenic reactions by stress or teratogen co-treatment.

## Other Species

The late A. W. F. Hughes (53) presented an historical perspective of experimental teratology and showed that we are stuck with catalogs of empirical observations at the point of "Stockard's second principle": similar malformations are induced in many species by many different treatments. Genetic determinants of responses and reactivities, and the comparison across species of their underlying biological causes, may point the way out of the impasse. If predictability is the objective of testing for teratogenesis, it will come only from comparative genetic teratology.

It is premature to move beyond the mouse in a discussion of genetic teratology, but there are a few reports of differences in developmental toxicity in other species such as rats (3,75) and hamsters (40,41). Possibly, as various species are used in the search for animal models of toxicity, greater familiarity with and availability of these genetic resources will be realized (1,33).

## GENETIC STUDIES

### Definitions

A genetic trait in developmental toxicity is defined as a heritable difference in a reaction between two or more individuals. After the difference has been defined as being a difference in response, reactivity, or both, the source of the difference is identified as being maternal or embryonic. The role of genetics then is to determine the cause of the difference: one gene or many. The importance of demonstrating this cannot be emphasized enough. Most molecular studies of developmental toxicity presume a single, molecular causal event; it would be helpful if the genetic evidence supported this assumption.

When strains that differ in a teratogenic reaction are crossed, differences in reaction between the reciprocal $F_1$ embryos suggest the possibility of maternal, cytoplasmic, or X-chromosome-linked effects (12). A difference in reaction between reciprocal $F_1$ male embryos but not between reciprocal $F_1$ female embryos suggests an X-chromosome-linked effect. This is supported further by a predicted difference between test-mating results of the two $F_1$ males. A difference between $F_1$ female embryos suggests a maternal effect which may be due to genetic differences between the two dams or to cytoplasmically transmitted effects. The distinction between a maternal uterine factor and a cytoplasmic factor requires a specific test-mating design (17). So far, only one clear example of a cytoplasmic effect has been described in teratology (28), but it presents a biochemical enigma. There does not appear to be a readily available molecular model to interpret it (12). Usually, a maternal genetic effect can be resolved by comparisons of the reactions of the reciprocal $F_1$ embryos with the two parental strains. In most cases, the genetic study of the cause of the maternal effect on a teratogenic reaction is complicated by embryonic genetic effects, since both are assessed by the reaction of the embryo.

### Methods

Several embryonic genetic traits of teratogenic reaction have been studied with the purpose of determining the number of genes involved. It must be emphasized that what is examined in these studies is the net genetic difference in a trait between a strain pair and not all the genetic variation in a trait that is possible for the species. For different pairs of strains, different genetic loci may be involved. This has been suggested for the cortisone–cleft palate reactivity trait of the mouse (11,108).

### Classical Breeding Studies

Classical breeding studies can be used to examine embryonic teratogenic traits because maternal effects can be kept constant by using females of one strain to test-mate males of different genotypes. The embryonic traits that have been examined in this way are 5-fluorouracil cleft palate and limb malformations (26), acetazolamide ectrodactyly (6), cortisone cleft palate (11), 6-aminonicotinamide cleft palate (7), and 6-aminonicotinamide cleft lip (55).

For a recessive autosomal trait, backcrossing (BC) to the recessive parent, and for a codominant trait, backcrossing to either parent, can be used to follow segregation. This method and the rationale for its use have been discussed elsewhere (9,11), and Fig. 3 outlines the test and the minimum number of generations that are required.

Suppose the hypothetical strain A in Fig. 3 has an embryonic reactivity that is recessive to hypothetical strain B. A number of unselected (i.e., untreated) $F_1$, $BC_1$, and $BC_2$ males are produced. The $F_1$ and $BC_1$ males are test-mated with the recessive hypothetical A strain females and several females for each male. The frequencies of the induced malformation in treated progeny from the test-mating of the $F_1$ and $BC_1$ males are compared with the treated progeny of A and B parental males that are test-mated with the A females. The frequency of the induced malformation in the test-mating progeny is expected to change from the $F_1$ males to the $BC_1$ males in the direction of the recessive parent (in this case, the hypothetical A strain). This means only that genetic factors are being recovered and fixed in the homozygous recessive state similar to the recessive inbred parent.

The number of genes involved is determined by examining the distribution of the test-mating scores of the $BC_1$ males and demonstrating *segregation* in a predicted way. The most simple hypothesis, the single gene model, should be tested first rather than assuming the complex condition of a polygenic model with many genes.

Suppose two alleles, A and B, are found at a single genetic locus that controls the observed difference between strains A and B. The A strain has the A allele, and the B strain has the B allele, and A is recessive to B. For qualitative morphological traits such as pigmentation or a protein polymorphism, segregation of the trait is expected in the progeny of the test-mated $F_1$ males because the progeny can be identified by mutually exclusive phenotypes, i.e., AA and AB types of progeny. However, for teratogenic reactivity, all that is observed is a single frequency of induced malformation, and the AA and AB individuals are indistinguishable in one litter. Nevertheless, segregation can be found by comparing the test-mating scores of individual $BC_1$ males. Those $BC_1$ males that are AA will produce only AA test progeny; $BC_1$ males that are AB will produce AA and AB test progeny. Bimodality of the test-mating scores of the $BC_1$ males is one demonstration of segregation and suggests that a single genetic factor determines the trait.

A number of biometric methods are available to analyze the distribution of test-mating scores. Simple tests of bimodality (48) can be applied to the distribution

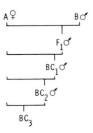

**FIG. 3.** The generalized backcross and test-mating scheme to search for embryonic genetic determinants of a difference in reaction between the hypothetical A and B strains. Suppose the A strain is recessive to the B strain for the reaction trait. $F_1$, $BC_1$, and $BC_2$ males are produced without teratogen treatment, and, in addition to the A and B strain males, they are test-mated with A-strain females. Segregation of embryonic genes for the reaction difference occurs in the test-mating progeny ($BC_1$ embryos) of the $F_1$ males, but it cannot be detected until the test-mating progeny ($BC_2$ embryos) of individual $BC_1$ males. An additional backcross generation ($BC_2$ males) is produced and test-mated ($BC_3$ embryos) in order to test independently any genetic hypothesis that is suggested by the distribution of the test-mating values of the $BC_1$ males.

of the $BC_1$ males. If a specific genetic model, such as a single gene model, is being tested, the distribution of test-mating scores from the $BC_1$ males can be compared with the distributions from the $F_1$ and the parental strain males by parametric (30,95) or nonparametric (23,24,71) methods. The test-mating values for individual $BC_1$ males will not usually fall into two mutually exclusive categories on the frequency scale. This is dependent partly on the difference in mean frequency between the two parental males or the $F_1$ and the recessive strain male and partly on the sample size of the test-mating progeny from each $BC_1$ male.

Sewall Wright's (117) charges must be remembered. "There are many cases in slow-breeding animals in which a gene has been designated on no more basis than dominance in $F_1$ of a cross between true breeding strains, a 3:1 ratio in $F_2$, and a 1:1 ratio in the backcross to the recessive strain. There is, however, no conclusive evidence for or against its existence until breeding tests have been made of the segregating generation." Thus, the test and demonstration of the single gene model can be made only with a further backcross generation (16,117). Unselected $BC_2$ males are produced. Some families of $BC_2$ males from "AA"-type $BC_1$ males should breed true when test-mated; other families of $BC_2$ males from "AB"-type $BC_1$ males should continue to exhibit segregation similar to the test-mating results from the $BC_1$ males. Therefore, there should be bimodality of the test-mating values from families of $BC_2$ males.

The backcross test-mating scheme has a number of advantages. If the A and B strains are known to differ with respect to single gene traits, such as enzyme polymorphisms or antigenic differences, these can be followed also in the breeding scheme. If association between a "marker" gene and the teratogenic trait is found, genetic linkage can be investigated further. Linkage between a known single "marker" gene and the teratogenic trait would add substance to the model. In addition, if a molecular difference is postulated to be causally associated with the teratogenic reaction, it can be tested directly in the backcross scheme.

## Other Methods

Other methods may be used to study a genetic trait in developmental toxicity once the toxic response has been defined. Usually, a molecular variable is postulated to be associated with the difference in teratogenic reaction of the parental strains. Three methods are relatively straightforward, and each will permit a test for association between the molecular variable and the teratogenic trait.

One method is to use a backcross generation directly. If the homozygous and heterozygous embryos can be phenotyped directly for the molecular trait, their reactions to the teratogen can be compared. An example of this approach is the association of embryotoxicity to benzo($a$)pyrene and the $Ah$ locus (91). If the $BC_1$ embryos cannot be typed directly, the test-mating scores for the teratogenic trait of the $BC_1$ males can be compared with the segregation of the molecular trait in the $BC_1$ males. This method was used as part of a larger breeding study with the embryonic reactivity differences to cortisone and 6-aminonicotinamide cleft palate (7,11).

A second method is a systematic strain survey using the information presented in Fig. 2. If sufficiently diverse strains are chosen, segregation of the postulated molecular variable and of the teratogenic trait should have taken place in the development of the strains. The question can be asked, are the traits associated or did they segregate independently?

The third method, the use of recombinant inbred strains, is similar in principle to a systematic strain survey in the attempt to determine association between the molecular and teratogenic traits.

## GENETIC VARIATION IN TERATOGENIC REACTIONS

Sufficient genetic data have been collected to permit a discussion of four malformation reactions of the mouse (cleft palate, exencephaly, cleft lip, ectrodactyly).

### Cleft Palate

#### Cortisone

*Genetics of the $ED_{50}$ Trait*

For a considerable time, cortisone acetate has been known to induce cleft palate in mouse embryos (4). Differences among strains in the frequency of induced cleft palate were found as more strains were tested (39). Stable differences in reaction between strains indicate genetic differences in the reaction.

The historical development of the problem of genetic differences in the cortisone cleft palate reaction was reviewed recently (9). The A/J and C57BL/6J strains differ in frequency of cortisone-induced cleft palate with A/J being more sensitive than C57BL/6J. An early genetic analysis revealed both maternal and embryonic genetic effects on the frequency of induced cleft palate, but no simple mode of inheritance appeared to explain these data (57).

A threshold model, based on normal differences in embryonic development of the palate, was proposed to interpret the apparent difference in cleft palate susceptibility between A/J and C57BL/6J to a number of teratogens (36,38). Without cortisone treatment, palate closure occurs at a later gestational age in A/J than in C57BL/6J embryos (103,111). Cortisone causes a delay in palate closure (107). Therefore, a teratogen that induced cleft palate by causing a delay in palate closure would be expected to induce a higher frequency in A/J than in C57BL/6J, because A/J normally had a later palate closure.

The strain difference in cleft palate sensitivity between A/J and C57BL/6J was reexamined systematically in a series of experiments using two teratogens, cortisone acetate and 6-aminonicotinamide (6-AN). The question asked was whether the genes that determined the difference in cleft palate sensitivity to cortisone and to 6-AN were the same. In other words, was the apparent strain difference in reaction to the two teratogens a property of the strains or a property of the teratogens.

Cortisone and 6-AN were examined separately. The dose-effect data or the norms of reaction of the strains and their reciprocal $F_1$ embryos were fitted to a normal log-tolerance distribution. The only apparent difference between A/J and C57BL/6J for cortisone and for 6-AN was in the reactivity or the $ED_{50}$ for the reaction (7,10). Therefore, there was additivity between genotype and teratogen (cf. Fig. 1b). The two strains and the $F_1$ embryos did not differ in their cleft palate response (slope of the dose–effect curves) within each teratogen. However, the slopes of the families of dose–effect curves for the two agents were significantly different (8). Figure 4 compares the cleft palate dose–effect behaviors of the A/J and SWV strains to cortisone and 6-AN. With the conceptual triad of "stimulus, response, and reactivity," these two strains, as well as C57BL/6J, differ in response (slope) to the two teratogens, and we can "assume that, at some stage, . . . [the two teratogens] . . . differed in their mode of action" (15). Nevertheless, is the genetic control of the reactivity difference between A/J and C57BL/6J embryos the same or different for the two teratogens?

For the cortisone cleft palate trait (difference in $ED_{50}$) of A/J and C57BL/6J, the maternal genetic effect was quantified. By comparing genetically equivalent reciprocal $F_1$ female embryos, twice as much cortisone is required to induce cleft palate in C57BL/6J dams as in A/J dams (10). X-chromosome-linked embryonic factors were excluded by comparing reciprocal $F_1$ male embryos and also by test-mating reciprocal $F_1$ males with the recessive A/J strain females. The $ED_{50}$ of C57BL/6J embryos was dominant or possibly overdominant to that of A/J embryos (10,11).

The breeding study used to examine the genetic control of the difference in $ED_{50}$ for cortisone was a backcross and test-mating study with the recessive A/J strain. Since additivity between genotype and teratogen had been determined, a single dose of teratogen could be used. Also, different sets of A/J females could be test-

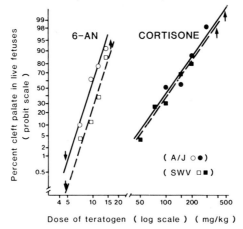

**FIG. 4.** Comparison of the dose–effect curves for cortisone (*solid symbols*) and 6-AN (*open symbols*) cleft palate in the A/J and SWV strains. The regression analysis was performed on the probit-transformed frequencies of cleft palate against log-transformed dose. By convention, the arrows indicate either 0 or 100% cleft palate response (infinite empirical probits). (Reprinted from Biddle, ref. 8, with permission.)

mated and treated with either cortisone or 6-AN. The genetic test for the question of causal difference between cortisone and 6-AN cleft palate for the A/J and C57BL/6J embryos would be independent *segregation* of the cortisone and 6-AN $ED_{50}$ traits. In practice, the genetic test of this question is made by looking for a departure from independent segregation of the two $ED_{50}$ traits. In the breeding study, $BC_1$ males (cf. Fig. 3) were test-mated with A/J females that were treated subsequently with either cortisone or 6-AN, and the results for 25 $BC_1$ males are shown in Fig. 5. There was no association between the two $ED_{50}$ traits (13) either by linear correlation or by a new test for association that does not depend on knowledge of the two underlying distributions. Therefore, the embryonic genes that determine the difference in reactivity between A/J and C57BL/6J are not the same for the two teratogens.

A minimal estimate of two or three loci with independent effects appeared to explain the difference in $ED_{50}$ to cortisone between A/J and C57BL/6J embryos (11). A single major gene difference and a polygenic model were excluded. A component of the difference between A/J and C57BL/6J embryos may be associated with or linked to the major histocompatibility *(H-2)* complex. It must be emphasized that this genetic interpretation is only relevant for the *net* difference between A/J and C57BL/6J. It cannot be extrapolated universally without testing other strains of the species. Also, the difference between A/J and C57BL/6J provides *no* information about the cause of the cleft palate response to cortisone (35,37).

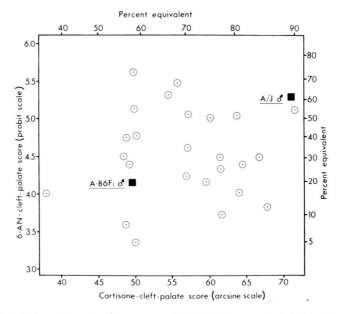

**FIG. 5.** Distribution of the test-mating scores of 25 A.AB6 $BC_1$ males (*circles*). A/J females were treated with either cortisone (*arcsine scale*) or 6-AN (*probit scale*). The mean values of the test-mating scores of the A.B6 $F_1$ and A/J males are indicated by *solid squares*. The percent equivalent to the *arcsine* and *probit scales* is indicated. (Reprinted from Biddle and Fraser, ref. 13, with permission.)

*Other Genetic Questions*

Do all strains exhibit a cleft palate reaction to cortisone with the same dose–effect characteristics? The strains that have been tested and reported to date (Table 1) appear to respond to cortisone with cleft palate in the same way; the slopes of the dose–effect curves are similar. The genetic trait is a reactivity trait, not a cleft palate response trait. If the dose–effect method is used to define the reaction operationally, no mutation or genetic difference in the cleft palate response has yet been identified.

For the genetic trait of $ED_{50}$ for cortisone cleft palate, how many different $ED_{50}$s are there? A systematic survey of a large number of genetically different mouse strains would be an approximation of the viable genotypic combinations of the mouse.

Comparisons between A/J and C57BL/6J (11) and between DBA/2J and C57BL/6J (108) suggest the reactivity trait may be determined by a few gene loci, but the linkage associations suggest there may be different loci for each strain pair. Therefore, the trait for the species may be genetically complex. If the range of $ED_{50}$s in a relatively large strain survey is described by only a few discrete values, a small number of loci, possibly with few alleles, may determine the reactivity trait. However, if the $ED_{50}$s are continuously distributed and unimodal over the dosage range (on a log scale), reactivity may be controlled by many gene loci or possibly a multiple allelic series at a few loci.

The distribution of the log $ED_{50}$ values from Table 1 appears to be unimodal when analyzed by the method of ranked normal deviates or rankits (93). This argues against relatively few loci, and the observation of "different differences" from gene-linkage associations (11,108) for individual strain pairs argues against a multiple allelic series. Nevertheless, the number of strains sampled is insignificant relative to what exists for the species, and most likely these inferences are premature.

Associations with other traits can be tested genetically once the rank order of reactivities for cortisone cleft palate has been established for a number of strains. The rationale is simple, but the test is powerful. Suppose a series of strains, such as those listed in Table 1, have been randomly picked from the existing strains of the mouse. The strains can be considered to be an independent sampling of the genome, and the genes or allelic

TABLE 1. *Strain distribution of the median effective dose for cortisone cleft palate in the mouse[a]*

| Strain | $ED_{50}$(mg/kg) | Reference |
|--------|------------------|-----------|
| SW/Fr | 50 | 106 |
| T1Wh | 75 | 108 |
| A/J | 115 | 10 |
| SWV | 122 | 10 |
| DBA/2J | 136 (140) | 108 |
| CL/Fr | 180 | 106 |
| B10.BR | 300 | 108 |
| C57BL/6J | 687 | 10 |

[a]Mice were maintained on Purina Laboratory Chow® and treated with cortisone acetate, s.c., on day 12 of gestation.

differences that control different traits are assumed to have recombined and become fixed during inbreeding of the strains. A test for association between the cortisone reactivity trait and any other genetic parameter would be similar to a test for independent segregation.

The causal relationship between the concentration of a specific cortisol-binding protein (42) and the cleft palate reactivity to glucocorticoids could be tested by a simple ranking test. If the strains are truly independent samples of the genome, a break in ranks would reject the hypothesis that the strain difference in reactivity is causally associated with the concentration of the receptor protein. In this type of test, the sample of strains must be sufficiently large so that the probability of association due strictly to chance is reduced to an acceptably low level. At least five independent strains are suggested because the probability of the association in five strains being due to chance alone is $(1/2)^5$ or 0.03.

Two problems exist with current tests for association between the concentrations of cortisol-binding protein with cleft palate reactivity (42). First, linear regression of receptor concentration on percent cleft palate is not valid if the two variables are not normally distributed. Second, the known maternal and embryonic genetic effects on the net $ED_{50}$ for glucocorticoid for each strain are assumed to be positively correlated (greater maternal effect with greater embryonic reactivity). This is not what has been observed in the A/J and C3H strains (9,10,12).

The multifactorial threshold model (38) suggests that the liability to induced cleft palate is related to a developmental threshold. The two strains in Table 1 with the lowest $ED_{50}$ have spontaneous cleft palate. Another strain, J/Glw (94), is also reported to express spontaneous cleft palate. If this strain has a low $ED_{50}$, and the spontaneous cleft palate frequencies are internally consistent with a rank ordering of $ED_{50}s$, the system affected by glucocorticoids may be the postulated threshold. However, our conceptual understanding of the maternal and embryonic control of $ED_{50}$ traits and of the genetic determination of liability for threshold traits dictates cautious interpretation.

A drawback to ranking tests should be apparent. As more variables are selected to be tested for association with the rank-ordered $ED_{50}s$, more associations will be found that are due strictly to chance, and we are back to the classic comparisons of too many variables with the historical A/J versus C57BL/6J strain pair. For example, the concentration of dexamethasone-binding proteins and the affinity of the receptors for dexamethasone from A/J and C57BL/6J embryos varied in opposite directions (85). Which of the two variables is causally associated with the embryonic difference in $ED_{50}$ for cleft palate? The extension of the study of receptor proteins to the DBA/1J and CBA/J strains (86) has not clarified their relationship to glucocorticoid cleft palate.

Rather than reject outright any association between glucocorticoid receptor concentration or kinetics and the cleft palate $ED_{50}$ trait, it would be prudent to reexamine the traits in more controlled studies. Nothing is known about the genetic control of the receptor proteins in the mouse. Since the maternal and embryonic genetic effects on the $ED_{50}$ trait are apparently separable, a backcross test-mating design with a constant maternal effect (cf. Fig. 3) may be used. The $BC_1$ males would be expected to exhibit segregation for the receptor protein trait(s) and for the embryonic $ED_{50}$ trait. The genetic test for association is made by finding a departure from independent segregation.

## Modification of the Cortisone Cleft Palate Reaction

Teratogenic reactions are known to be modified by other chemical agents, diet, stress, and so forth (37). Most studies have reported simply a change in the frequency of the teratogenic reaction with the co-treatment. Depending on the teratogen, the results of the co-treatment have been discussed in terms of additive, independent, synergistic, and interaction effects. Attention has been called to the need for biometrical procedures to evaluate the changes in teratogenic reactions and biological models to interpret such changes (9).

Diet is known to modify the cortisone cleft palate reaction (112). In the case of the A/J strain, a change from Lab Chow® to Mouse Chow® had an additive effect on the $ED_{50}$ for cortisone cleft palate (9); the diet change decreased the $ED_{50}$, but it did not alter the slope of the dose-effect curve. However, when two other strains, SW/Fr and CL/Fr, were examined (106), different results were obtained (Table 2). Again there was no alteration of the slopes of the dose-effect curves, but the change in diet decreased the $ED_{50}$ of the SW/Fr strain and increased the $ED_{50}$ of the CL/Fr strain. The reactivities changed in opposite directions with the two diets, thus indicating an interaction between diet and teratogen. These observations demonstrate that "comparisons of norms of reaction in different strains should be made only if the tested animals are on the same diet" and emphasize that "deductions about which components of the diet are important in altering a norm of reaction can be misleading if only one genotype has been tested" (106).

The rationale for the suggestion that modification of the norm of reaction should be made by dose–effect studies is provided in Fig. 6. This example is used to illustrate a conceptual problem in teratology. A pyridoxine-deficient diet during pregnancy in CFW mice was found to result in cleft palate (21%). The effects of cortisone in combination with either the deficient diet or a complete diet were then examined (70). Pyridoxine deficiency was suggested to act synergistically with cortisone at a low dose but additively at a high dose on the cleft palate phenotype. An alternative interpretation is found when the effect of cortisone is compared using only the fraction of embryos that does not express cleft palate on the pyridoxine-deficient diet. Although one must keep in mind the limitation of two-point curves, pyridoxine deficiency in CFW mice appears to act additively to lower the $ED_{50}$ for the cleft palate reaction to cortisone. There is no

TABLE 2. *Diet effects on cortisone cleft palate in the mouse*

| Strain | $ED_{50}$(mg/kg) | | Reference |
| | Lab Chow® | Mouse Chow® | |
|---|---|---|---|
| SW/Fr | 50 | 35 | 106 |
| A/J | 115 | 79 | 9 |
| CL/Fr | 180 | 220 | 106 |

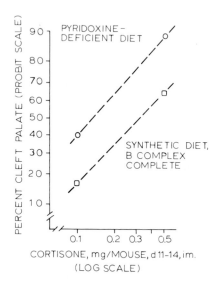

**FIG. 6.** An interpretation of the effect of pyridoxine deficiency on the cortisone cleft palate reaction of CFW mice. Percent cleft palate is plotted on a *probit scale*, and dosage is plotted on a *log scale*. The *open squares* are the cortisone cleft palate reactions with B-complex-complete diet. The *open circles* are the cleft palate reactions with pyridoxine-deficient diet but corrected for the natural cleft palate frequency (21%) that was observed with this diet alone. (Data are from Miller, ref. 70.)

obvious change in the slope of the dose–effect curve that would suggest an interaction between pyridoxine and cortisone on the cleft palate phenotype.

### 6-Aminonicotinamide

As previously discussed, 6-aminonicotinamide (6-AN) induces cleft palate (78) in the tested mouse strains, and A/J expresses a higher frequency than does C57BL/6J. Use of a nicotinamide supplement (44,79–81,110) altered the frequency of 6-AN-induced cleft palate, and the data suggested that less nicotinamide was required to protect a C57BL/6J embryo against a given dose of 6-AN than to protect an A/J embryo (37, 109). This difference in reaction to the combined effects of 6-AN and nicotinamide may or may not be genetic and should be pursued if this type of information is eventually intended for use in reducing environmental health hazards to man (73).

The difference in reactivity ($ED_{50}$) to 6-AN-induced cleft palate between A/J and C57BL/6J was examined without the nicotinamide supplement (7). There was no significant maternal effect on the reactivity of the $F_1$ embryos with a Lab Chow® diet. The difference in embryonic reactivity appeared to be determined by a three-locus, epistatic genetic model. Genetic epistasis is defined as dominance between loci. The A/J embryonic reactivity, relative to C57BL/6J, appeared to be determined by three independently segregating genetic loci that required the A/J recessive genes in the homozygous state. No association was found between the reactivity to 6-AN cleft palate and the *H-2* complex.

### Exencephaly

The interaction of teratogens with specific mutant genes has been reviewed recently (37). Most studies have compared abnormal phenotypes that are associated with a homozygous mutant gene and teratogens that induce similar malformations.

The teratogen-induced malformations, in these cases, are sometimes referred to as phenocopies of the genetic malformations. A low dose of the teratogen is tested on embryos that are heterozygous for the mutant gene and that do not normally express the "genetic" malformation. The case for interaction between the teratogen and a single "dose" of the mutant gene is made by observing a malformation that is associated only with the homozygous state of the gene. The experimental designs of most of these studies do not allow a discrimination between an additive effect and an interaction effect between gene and teratogen that is independent of a subjective evaluation of the individual term embryos. One method of discrimination was discussed in Fig. 1a.

A recent study investigated the question of gene–teratogen interaction with insulin-induced exencephaly in the mouse (21,22). Embryos that are homozygous for either of the dominant genes Crooked-tail *(Cd)* or Rib-fusion *(Rf)* normally express a low frequency of exencephaly. Insulin-induced exencephaly was examined by a dose–effect study in two inbred strains, SWV and A/J, and a difference in reactivity was found. Wild-type $(+/+)$ and heterozygous $(Cd/+$ or $Rf/+)$ males from the two mutant strains were test-mated with SWV and A/J females that were subsequently treated with insulin. From wild-type males, a single genetic class of embryos $(+/+)$ is produced; from heterozygous males, two genotypes of embryos are produced (e.g., from $Cd/+$ males, $Cd/+$ and $+/+$ embryos are produced). The slope of the dose–effect curve (norm of reaction) of the test progeny from heterozygous males was significantly different from the slope for the test progeny from the wild-type males. The mutant genes *(Cd* and *Rf)* and the teratogen interacted to produce an exencephaly response to insulin that was different from the exencephaly response of the wild-type embryos. Interaction was demonstrated simply because there was a departure from an additive relationship between the two groups of embryos in their reaction to insulin.

A possible mechanism to explain the different exencephaly responses to insulin of the heterozygous and wild-type embryos was suggested by treated embryos that were examined on days 8 to 10. During this time, the mouse embryo turns from a lordotic to a kyphotic position. Severe twisting and kinking of the hind body were found in early exencephalic embryos from the treated heterozygote crosses. No delay or abnormality in turning was found in the treated wild-type crosses. Kinking of the hind body is seen normally in mutant homozygous embryos. Stress placed on the neural folds by the kinking of the hind body in insulin-induced heterozygotes was suggested to be the different mechanism of induced exencephaly in treated heterozygotes.

## Cleft Lip

Cleft lip with or without cleft palate can occur spontaneously in the mouse and, depending on the strain, it occurs with a specific frequency (84). It should be kept in mind that the cleft palate, which occurs in mouse embryos with cleft lip, is a secondary mechanical consequence of the cleft lip (105), and the two malformations are morphogenetically distinct. Attempts to determine the genetic control of the liability to the spontaneous trait have suggested both a single recessive gene (82,83) and a polygenic model (46). Maternal genetic effects on the frequency of cleft lip have also been demonstrated (27). A threshold model based on differences in embryonic face shape has been proposed as the embryological basis for the difference between the A/J strain that expresses spontaneous cleft lip and C57BL/6J that does not (104). In contrast to the spontaneous cleft lip trait, the mouse embryo responds with cleft lip to maternal treatment with 6-aminonicotinamide (6-AN) on day 10 (79), and strain differences in the frequency of reaction are known (55,56).

The threshold model predicts that A/J embryos that are liable to spontaneous lateral cleft lip should also be sensitive to 6-AN-induced cleft lip. However, A/J embryos appear to be resistant to 6-AN with the non-cleft-lip A/J embryos being killed by the treatment (43). This apparent contradiction to the threshold model was examined in a genetic study of both the spontaneous and 6-AN-inducible cleft lip traits of the A/J and C57BL/6J strains (55,56). Dose–effect studies demonstrated strain differences in reactivity to 6-AN cleft lip and that the A/J embryo reacts, but the high frequency of 6-AN-induced resorption limits the study of cleft lip in this strain. The difference between the A/J and C57BL/6J embryos in liability to spontaneous cleft lip was *not* polygenic and appeared to be determined by either one major gene with modifiers or two loci with duplicate epistasis (the two loci must have the recessive A/J genes in the homozygous condition). More importantly, the genes that determine liability to spontaneous cleft lip segregated independently from the genes that determine the difference in reactivity to 6-AN-induced cleft lip.

The genetic study of the strain difference in the spontaneous and 6-AN-induced cleft lip traits has far-reaching implications for developmental toxicology. The so-called "mutant" and "phenocopy" are causally separable by their kinds of genetic basis. Some studies (113) have suggested that animals without treatment spontaneously express a low frequency of a given malformation but show a marked increase in incidence of the defect when teratogenic treatment is given. Similarly, the use of some strains in teratogenic screening tests has been questioned because of their predispositions to either specific spontaneous or induced defects (49). These suggestions require genetic testing.

## Ectrodactyly

### Acetazolamide

Sodium acetazolamide is a well-known teratogen in rats and mice (64) and has been reviewed (5,52). The major malformation is a postaxial reduction deformity of the forelimb with an intriguing right-sided predominance. The same postaxial forelimb deformity is induced in the golden hamster, but both forelimbs respond equally, with most fetuses being affected bilaterally; there is also some hind-limb response with left-sided predominance (61).

Dose–effect data for acetazolamide-induced ectrodactyly have been reported only for the CBA/J mouse strain (5) and the golden hamster (61), and these can be interpreted by a log-tolerance model (Fig. 7). For the golden hamster, the $ED_{50}$ was 695 mg/kg for a single i.p. injection at the time of maximum sensitivity (204 hr after mating). For CBA/J mice, two i.p. injections of acetazolamide were required to recover a sufficient number of responding fetuses; presumably this mode of treatment is required to expose the embryos to sufficient acetazolamide without being extremely toxic. The $ED_{50}$ was 801 mg/kg given at 10 a.m. and again at 4 p.m. on day 10 (the day of maximum sensitivity to the treatment for this strain). The similarity of the slopes of the dose–effect curves ($p > 0.50$) for the two species (Fig. 7) raises some interesting possibilities for comparative teratogenicity. Further discussion of this is premature, since no other data of a similar nature exist yet in experimental teratology.

When the mouse strains that have been treated with acetazolamide are compared, large genetic differences are found not only for the frequency of the ectrodactyly response but also for the day of maximum sensitivity (5,45,97). Since strains have not been compared by dose–effect, it is not known whether these differences are in reactivity, response, or both. Nevertheless, one strain, SWV, appears to be unique in that it is, so far, completely resistant to acetazolamide-induced ectrodactyly (5). Treated pregnancies that survived exhibited neither an induced resorption response nor a malformation response. Until demonstrated to be otherwise, the absolute resistance of SWV embryos can be considered to be a case of genetic interaction in the acetazolamide-induced ectrodactyly response.

The response difference between the CBA/J and SWV strain pair was studied by a conventional backcross and test-mating scheme using CBA/J mothers to control for maternal effects (6). Resistance of SWV embryos, when compared with CBA/J embryos, appeared to be a dominant trait controlled by three loci with epistasis (dominance between loci). That is, the response of CBA/J embryos appeared to

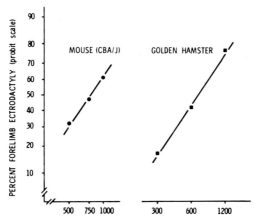

**FIG. 7.** Comparison of the dose–effect behavior of acetazolamide-induced ectrodactyly in CBA/J mice (5) and the golden hamster (61). The mice were given two i.p. injections on day 10 (10 a.m. and 4 p.m.) with the indicated doses. The hamsters were given a single i.p. injection at 204 hr after mating. The data were fitted to a linear regression of probit-transformed frequency on log dose.

depend on recessive genes for sensitivity being present in the homozygous condition at all three loci; the presence of a dominant allele at any one of the three loci conferred resistance.

It must be stressed that the three-locus model that was suggested for the CBA/J–SWV strain pair of embryos cannot be applied universally to the species. What was determined for the CBA/J and SWV strains was only the net genetic difference between the two embryonic genotypes. The cause of the apparent differences between other strains in the frequency of response and time of sensitivity is unknown.

The question of whether maternal effect differences exist between CBA/J and SWV for the acetazolamide-induced ectrodactyly trait is also unclear. The "teratogenic environment" exists in treated SWV mothers because CBA/J embryos responded with ectrodactyly when transferred to SWV mothers who were then treated with acetazolamide. The converse transfer of embryos yielded negative results. In experimental studies to determine the site of acetazolamide teratogenesis (the embryo, the placenta, or the pregnant female) (87,96), the embryo remains the resistant or responding unit.

Inhibition of carbonic anhydrase enzyme activity is the known biochemical action of acetazolamide (68,69), and controversy has centered on enzyme inhibition as the cause of teratogenesis. Thus, CBA/J and SWV have the same electrophoretic variants of the adult form of the carbonic anhydrase isoenzymes that are determined by the Car-1 and Car-2 loci (14,29). This suggests that the adult form of carbonic anhydrase is not involved in the teratogenesis of acetazolamide.

Recently, a sensitive radiotracer assay has detected carbonic anhydrase in rat embryos at the acetazolamide-sensitive stage (51). When the assay was applied to mouse embryos at day 10, CBA/J had 2.4 times the carbonic anhydrase activity of SWV, and the concentrations of acetazolamide required for 50% inhibition were $4.0 \times 10^{-9}$M and $3.3 \times 10^{-8}$M, respectively. However, in day-12 embryos that were beyond the acetazolamide-sensitive stage and in adult erythrocytes, no differences were detected between the two strains in either carbonic anhydrase activity or sensitivity to acetazolamide inhibition (50). Precipitation of cross-reacting material from day-10 CBA/J embryos and yolk sacs by antibodies against adult carbonic anhydrase I and II indicates that day-10 embryos contain a unique but transitory isoenzyme(s) (88).

These findings present the exciting possibility that an unsuspected embryonic genetic variation in the carbonic anhydrase isoenzymes is responsible for acetazolamide-induced ectrodactyly and the variations in response. The molecular difference between CBA/J and SWV in the transitory embryonic isoenzyme(s) needs to be examined further in the light of the estimated three-locus genetic model for the ectrodactyly trait. Tests with other strains that differ in the frequency and timing of sensitivity of the ectrodactyly response and the genetic test with CBA/J and SWV for possible segregation of the ectrodactyly trait and embryonic isoenzyme trait are required to demonstrate a causal association. If it stands, this may be the first demonstration of a molecular cause-and-effect relationship in teratogenesis.

An instructive application of genetics to the question of the right-sided predominance of the acetazolamide response (62) is the use of the *situs inversus (iv)* mutant of the mouse (54,63). In embryos with *situs inversus*, the laterality relationships within the embryo and the embryo within its membranes are reversed (that is, the mirror image of normal). However, the right forelimb in normal mice and the right forelimb in mice with the *situs inversus* trait were malformed. Therefore, there is no simple relationship between embryonic asymmetry and asymmetry of the acetazolamide-induced defect. It must be remembered that, in contrast to the mouse and rat, both forelimbs respond equally in the hamster (61).

### Cadmium

Cadmium is teratogenic in hamsters (31), rats (3), and mice (58) when administered parenterally in the form of an inorganic salt (32). A variety of malformations are induced by cadmium, depending on the timing of treatment, but the similarity of the postaxial forelimb ectrodactyly (3,66) to the acetazolamide malformation makes this teratogen particularly intriguing. The analogy may be superficial in that it "may be a reflection of the limited number of ways that a rodent forelimb can react to a teratogenic insult" (66).

There are also differences in the susceptibility of mouse strains to cadmium-induced testicular damage in adult mice (20,47). Some strains appear to be completely resistant to testicular necrosis, even in the lethal dosage range; only one strain, SJL/J, exhibits a variable response suggestive of a dose–effect phenomenon. Different lines of the rat and guinea pig also exhibit variable susceptibilities to testicular necrosis, but these appear to be dose-dependent differences.

In this chapter, the genetic analysis of a trait is stressed as being the prerequisite for developmental and molecular studies. The formal genetic analysis of the trait of cadmium-induced testicular damage in the mouse (102) is a particularly instructive example of how the wide range of genetic resources of this species can be used efficiently to define the genetic basis of a toxicity trait.

A survey of 45 different inbred strains with a single dose of cadmium chloride confirmed that mouse strains can be classified as either susceptible or resistant to testicular necrosis, and one strain, SJL/J, exhibited a variable response. The clear distinction between most strains with a mutually exclusive behavior suggested a single gene might control the trait. Six of the seven standard $F_1$ hybrids from the commercial production department of the Jackson Laboratory provided the progeny from four types of matings: sensitive × sensitive; reciprocal sensitive × resistant; resistant × resistant. Susceptibility was dominant to resistance, and both X- and Y-chromosome-linked inheritance were excluded. The ratios of susceptible to resistant mice in $F_2$ and backcross progeny suggested a single recessive gene, *cdm*, controls the resistance trait.

Further, the recombinant inbred strains derived from a resistant versus susceptible strain pair supported the single-gene hypothesis that was inferred from the standard strain crosses. Tests for linkage between *cdm* and the marker genes in 14 congenic strains of the resistant C57BL/10Sn strain were negative; however, standard linkage tests have now mapped the *cdm* gene in chromosome 3 (60,100).

In a study of ectrodactyly that is induced by cadmium on day 9 in the mouse (66), strains were chosen with prior knowledge of their response to testicular damage that is determined by the *cdm* locus. Three resistant strains (*cdm/cdm*) and three susceptible strains ( +/+ ) were tested, but the results were paradoxical. The strains that were resistant to testicular damage were more susceptible to cadmium-induced ectrodactyly than were the strains that were susceptible to testicular damage. The differences in sensitivity of the two groups to cadmium-induced ectrodactyly may be inversely related to the *cdm* gene ($p = 0.05$, one-tailed, Mann–Whitney U test). Also, it was noted that the *cdm/cdm* strains that are resistant to testicular damage are more susceptible to acute toxicity of cadmium (102). This may have a bearing on the embryonic differences in sensitivity to cadmium-induced ectrodactyly; however, cadmium-induced resorption, corrected for the natural resorption rate, does not appear to be related clearly to the *cdm* difference (66). Other factors than the *cdm* difference may be involved in the cadmium ectrodactyly trait. Thus, SWV is apparently completely resistant to acetazolamide ectrodactyly, and it is also resistant to cadmium-induced limb malformations at the highest tolerated dose (65). In addition, SWV is susceptible to cadmium-induced testicular damage.

It would be informative to compare mouse strains that differ in sensitivity to cadmium-induced ectrodactyly in terms of the timing of sensitivity and dose response. The ectrodactyly response of the SJL/J strain is unknown; it has a suggested dose–effect behavior to cadmium-induced testicular damage and therefore cannot be classified as either *cdm/cdm* or +/+ .

In a comparison of day-9 cadmium ectrodactyly responses among strains that differed with respect to the *cdm* gene (66), it was found that embryonic reactions may have an additional maternal genetic component. A breeding and test-mating study of the embryonic malformation and resorption responses to cadmium on day 7 suggests a major maternal genetic effect on the two variables. In addition, embryonic genetic differences modify these responses (77). Thus, C57BL/10ChPr (B10) embryos exhibit a response of exencephaly, microphthalmia–anophthalmia, orofacial clefting, and reduced mandible following cadmium exposure on day 7; NAW/Pr (NAW) embryos are relatively resistant. The induced malformation rate was greater in B10 and reciprocal $F_1$ dams than in NAW dams; the induced resorption rate was greater in the B10 mothers than in NAW mothers but was intermediate in $F_1$ mothers. Malformation scores from individual backcross females suggested the segregation of a major maternal genetic difference; the resorption scores were too variable to interpret.

A parallel study with the B10 and NAW strains suggested a molecular model for the maternal genetic effect on the resorption response to day-10 cadmium treatment (114). In embryos, cadmium was associated with a binding protein of MW 10,000 (metallothionein), and B10 embryos had more cadmium in the binding protein fraction than NAW embryos. In the placentas, cadmium was associated with a binding fraction of MW 19,000 (possibly a dimer of metallothionein and referred to as Cd-bp-D). The Cd-bp-D is produced rapidly and in large amounts in day-10 NAW dams whose embryos are relatively resistant to cadmium toxicity. However, Cd-bp-D is detectable only after 24 hr and in small amounts in day-10 B10 dams whose embryos are sensitive to cadmium toxicity. It is not detected in virgin females after cadmium exposure and is not found in day-13 or day-17 placentas from either strain.

Radioimmunoassay of serum progesterone revealed no difference between nonpregnant NAW and B10 females. On day 10, however, progesterone levels were elevated and were about 10 times higher in NAW than in B10 mice (115). NAW males are sensitive to cadmium-induced testicular necrosis, and all methods that raised the concentration of serum progesterone in NAW males caused both the production of Cd-bp-D and the absence of induced testicular necrosis. The ability to produce the Cd-bp-D protein and the interaction with the naturally elevated serum progesterone may be responsible for the NAW maternally mediated resistance to cadmium toxicity.

The test for a causal relationship between the quantitative difference (and possibly a qualitative difference) in the Cd-bp-D protein and cadmium toxicity/teratogenicity could be made genetically. Do the two traits segregate independently or are they associated? Strains that are essentially congenic for the maternal effect, or a set of recombinant inbred strains in which the maternal trait had segregated, could be tested for association between the molecular trait and the toxicity traits.

Genetic differences in the cadmium embryotoxicity traits in the mouse, by analogy with the acetazolamide response trait, provide a model in which to test causal relationships. For both teratogens, unsuspected transitory molecular systems that occur during pregnancy at the time of the index reactions appear to be involved.

## CONCLUSIONS AND SUMMARY

In developmental toxicology, identification and study of genetic differences in toxic reactions have only just begun. In the last few years, concerted genetic study of such differences in reaction to several teratogens has elucidated a few conceptual models. The interaction of dietary factors with cortisone-induced cleft palate is the first clear example of a teratogen-environment interaction. A model and interpretation of a gene–teratogen interaction have been presented using the example of insulin-induced exencephaly in the mouse. The genetic distinction and separation of the causes of spontaneous cleft lip and 6-aminonicotinamide-induced cleft lip emphasize that, if "mutant" and "phenocopy" are causally separable, it is not by "gene" versus "environment" but by their different genetic control. Examples have also been presented to show how molecular events that may be causally associated with teratogenic reactions can be evaluated directly using genetic methods.

Genetic resources available in the mouse alone have barely been touched. When taken together with the growing information in the areas of teratogenic reactions and postulated teratogenic mechanisms, these resources offer a key to clarifying the enigma of developmental toxicity. Strain surveys of differences in reactions must become an active part of teratology if comparative teratogenesis is to be a meaningful predictor of toxicity.

## ACKNOWLEDGMENTS

I should like to acknowledge the many people in genetics and teratology with whom I have had contact during the development of my explorations in experimental teratology and who have shared with me their questions, data, and interpretations. My comprehension of the problems and of their solutions reflects my historical perspective. I thank the Alberta Children's Research Foundation for support, Dr. B. A. Taylor for permission to reproduce Fig. 2, Cathy Biddle for reading various drafts of the manuscript, Marie Bruce and Eleanor Broscoe for secretarial assistance, and the Medical Audio–Visual Department of Memorial University of Newfoundland for the preparation of the figures.

## REFERENCES

1. Altman, P. L., and Katz, D. D. (1979): *Inbred and Genetically Defined Strains of Laboratory Animals, Part 1, Mouse and Rat, Part 2, Hamster, Guinea Pig, Rabbit and Chicken.* Federation of American Societies for Experimental Biology, Bethesda.
2. Bailey, D. W. (1971): Recombinant-inbred strains. An aid to finding identity, linkage, and function of histocompatibility and other genes. *Transplantation*, 11:325–327.
3. Barr, M. (1973): The teratogenicity of cadmium chloride in two stocks of Wistar rats. *Teratology*, 7:237–242.
4. Baxter, H., and Fraser, F. C. (1950): The production of congenital defects in the offspring of female mice treated with cortisone. A preliminary report. *McGill Med. J.*, 19:245–249.
5. Biddle, F. G. (1975): Teratogenesis of acetazolamide in the CBA/J and SWV strains of mice. I. Teratology. *Teratology*, 11:31–36.
6. Biddle, F. G. (1975): Teratogenesis of acetazolamide in the CBA/J and SWV strains of mice. II. Genetic control of the teratogenic response. *Teratology*, 11:37–46.
7. Biddle, F. G. (1977): 6-Aminonicotinamide-induced cleft palate in the mouse: The nature of the difference between the A/J and C57BL/6J strains in frequency of response and its genetic basis. *Teratology*, 16:301–312.
8. Biddle, F. G. (1978): Use of dose–response relationships to discriminate between the mechanisms of cleft-palate induction by different teratogens: An argument for discussion. *Teratology*, 18:247–252.
9. Biddle, F. G. (1979): Genetic studies of teratogen-induced cleft palate in the mouse. In: *Advances in the Study of Birth Defects, Vol. 1, Teratogenic Mechanisms*, edited by T. V. N. Persaud, pp. 85–111. MTP Press, Lancaster.
10. Biddle, F. G., and Fraser, F. C. (1976): Genetics of cortisone-induced cleft palate in the mouse—embryonic and maternal effects. *Genetics*, 84:743–754.
11. Biddle, F. G., and Fraser, F. C. (1977): Cortisone-induced cleft palate in the mouse. A search for the genetic control of the embryonic response trait. *Genetics*, 85:289–302.
12. Biddle, F. G., and Fraser, F. C. (1977): Maternal and cytoplasmic effects in experimental teratology: In: *Handbook of Teratology, Vol. 3, Comparative, Maternal, and Epidemiologic Aspects*, edited by J. G. Wilson and F. C. Fraser, pp. 3–33. Plenum Press, New York.
13. Biddle, F. G., and Fraser, F. C. (1979): Genetic independence of the embryonic reactivity difference to cortisone and 6-aminonicotinamide-induced cleft palate in the mouse. *Teratology*, 19:207–212.
14. Biddle, F. G., and Petras, M. L. (1967): The inheritance of a non-hemoglobin erythrocytic protein in *Mus musculus. Genetics*, 57:943–949.
15. Bliss, C. I. (1957): Some principles of bioassay. *Am. Sci.*, 45:449–466.
16. Bloom, J. L., and Falconer, D. S. (1964): A gene with major effect on susceptibility to induced lung tumors in mice. *J. Natl. Cancer Inst.*, 33:607–618.
17. Bornstein, S., Trasler, D. G., and Fraser, F. C. (1970): Effect of the uterine environment on the frequency of spontaneous cleft lip in CL/Fr mice. *Teratology*, 3:295–298.
18. Chernoff, G. F. (1977): The fetal alcohol syndrome in mice: An animal model. *Teratology*, 15:223–230.
19. Chernoff, G. F. (1977): The fetal alcohol syndrome in mice: An animal model. In: *Fifth International Conference of Birth Defects*, edited by J. W. Littlefield, pp. 61–62. Excerpta Medica, Amsterdam.

20. Chiquoine, A. D., and Suntzeff, V. (1965): Sensitivity of mammals to cadmium necrosis of the testis. *J. Reprod. Fertil.*, 10:455–457.
21. Cole, W. A. (1978): *Gene–Teratogen Interaction in Insulin-Induced Mouse Exencephaly*, M. Sc. Thesis. McGill University Library, Montreal.
22. Cole, W., and Trasler, D. G. (1980): Gene-teratogen interaction in insulin-induced mouse exencephaly. *Teratology*, 22:125–139.
23. Collins, R. L. (1967): A general nonparametric theory of genetic analysis. I. Application to the classical cross. *Genetics*, 56:551.
24. Collins, R. L. (1968): A general nonparametric theory of genetic analysis. II. Digenic models with linkage for the classical cross. *Genetics*, 60:169–170.
25. Dagg, C. P. (1966): Teratogenesis. In: *Biology of the Laboratory Mouse*, edited by E. L. Green, pp. 309–328. McGraw-Hill, New York.
26. Dagg, C. P., Schlager, G., and Doerr, A. (1966): Polygenic control of the teratogenicity of 5-fluorouracil in mice. *Genetics*, 53:1101–1117.
27. Davidson, J. D., Fraser, F. C., and Schlager, G. (1969): A maternal effect on the frequency of spontaneous cleft lip in the A/J mouse. *Teratology*, 2:371–376.
28. Diwan, B. A., and Meier, H. (1974): The inheritance of susceptibility and resistance to the teratogenic effect of 1-ethyl-1-nitrosourea in inbred strains of mice. *Tetratology*, 9:45–50.
29. Eicher, E. M., Stern, R. H., Womack, J. E., Davisson, M. T., Roderick, T. H., and Reynolds, S. C. (1976): Evolution of mammalian carbonic anhydrase loci by tandem duplication: Close linkage of *Car-1* and *Car-2* to the centromere region of chromosone 3 of the mouse. *Biochem. Genet.*, 14:651–660.
30. Elston, R. C., and Stewart, J. (1973): The analysis of quantitative traits for simple genetic models from parental, $F_1$ and backcross data. *Genetics*, 73:695–711.
31. Ferm, V. H., and Carpenter, S. J. (1968): The relationship of cadmium and zinc in experimental mammalian teratogenesis. *Lab. Invest.*, 18:429–432.
32. Ferm, V. H., and Layton, W. M. (1978): Teratogenic and mutagenic effects of cadmium. In: *Biogeochemistry of Cadmium*, edited by J. O. Nriagu. Ann Arbor Science Publishers, Ann Arbor [cited in (66)].
33. Festing, M., and Staats, J. (1973): Standard nomenclature for inbred strains of rats. *Transplantation*, 16:221–245.
34. Finney, D. J. (1971): *Statistical Method in Biological Assay*. Charles Griffen and Company, London.
35. Fraser, F. C. (1969): Gene-environment interactions in the production of cleft palate. In: *Methods for Teratological Studies in Experimental Animals and Man*, edited by H. Nishimura and J. R. Miller, pp. 34–49. Igaku Shoin, Tokyo.
36. Fraser, F. C. (1976): The multifactorial/threshold concept—uses and misuses. *Teratology*, 14:267–280.
37. Fraser, F. C. (1977): Interactions and multiple causes. In: *Handbook of Teratology, Vol. 1, General Principles and Etiology*, edited by J. G. Wilson and F. C. Fraser, pp. 445–463. Plenum Press, New York.
38. Fraser, F. C. (1977): Relation of animal studies to the problem in man. In: *Handbook of Teratology, Vol. 1, General Principles and Etiology*, edited by J. G. Wilson and F. C. Fraser, pp. 75–96. Plenum Press, New York.
39. Fraser, F. C., and Fainstat, T. D.(1951): Production of congenital defects in the offspring of pregnant mice treated with cortisone. *Pediatrics*, 8:527–533.
40. Gale, T. F. (1978): A variable embryotoxic response to lead in different strains of hamsters. *Environ. Res.*, 17:325–333.
41. Gale, T. F., and Layton, W. M. (1979): Cadmium-induced embryotoxic effects in inbred hamster strains. *Teratology*, 19:27A.
42. Goldman, A. S., Katsumata, M., Yaffe, S. J., and Gasser, D. L. (1977): Palatal cytosol cortisol-binding protein associated with cleft palate susceptibility and *H-2* genotype. *Nature*, 265:643–645.
43. Goldstein, M., Fraser, F. C., and Roth, K. (1965): Resistance of A/JAX mouse embryos with spontaneous congenital cleft lip to the lethal effect of 6-aminonicotinamide. *J. Med. Genet.*, 2:128–130.
44. Goldstein, M., Pinsky, M. F., and Fraser, F. C. (1963): Genetically determined organ specific response to the teratogenic action of 6-aminonicotinamide in the mouse. *Genet. Res.*, 4:258–265.
45. Green, M. C., Azar, C. A., and Maren, T. H. (1973): Strain differences in susceptibility to the teratogenic effect of acetazolamide in mice. *Teratology*, 8:143–146.
46. Gruneberg, H. (1952): *The Genetics of the Mouse*, pp. 363–370. Martinus Nijhoff, The Hague.

47. Gunn, S. A., Gould T. C., and Anderson, W. A. D. (1965): Strain differences in susceptibility of mice and rats to cadmium-induced testicular damage. *J. Reprod. Fertil.*, 10:273–275.
48. Haldane, J. B. S.(1952): Simple tests for bimodality and bitangentiality. *Ann. Eugenics*, 16:359–364.
49. Health and Welfare Canada (1973): *The Testing of Chemicals for Carcinogenicity, Mutagenicity and Teratogenicity.* Ottawa.
50. Hirsch, K. S., and Scott, W. J. (1979): Acetazolamide teratology: A biochemical basis for strain differences in the mouse. *Teratology*, 19:30A.
51. Hirsch, K. S., Scott, W. J., and Hurley, L. S. (1978): Acetazolamide teratology: The presence of carbonic anhydrase during the sensitive stage of rat development. *Teratology*, 17:38A.
52. Holmes, L. B., and Trelstad, R. L. (1979): The early limb deformity caused by acetazolamide. *Teratology*, 20:289–296.
53. Hughes, A. W. F. (1976): Developmental biology and the study of malformations. *Biol. Rev.*, 51:143–179.
54. Hummel, K. P., and Chapman, D. B. (1959): Visceral inversion and associated anomalies in the mouse. *J. Hered.*, 50:9–13.
55. Juriloff, D. M. (1977): *Genetics of Spontaneous and 6-Aminonicotinamide-Induced Cleft Lip in Mice*, Ph.D. Thesis. McGill University Library, Montreal.
56. Juriloff, D. M. (1980): The genetics of clefting in the mouse. In: *Etiology of Cleft Lip and Cleft Palate*, edited by M. Melnick, D. Bixler, and E. D. Shields, pp. 39–71. Alan R. Liss, New York.
57. Kalter, H. (1954): The inheritance of susceptibility to the teratogenic action of cortisone in mice. *Genetics*, 39:185–196.
58. Keino, H., and Yamamura, H. (1974): Effects of cadmium salt administered to pregnant mice on postnatal development of the offspring. *Teratology*, 10:87.
59. Lambert, G. H., and Nebert, D. W. (1977): Genetically mediated induction of drug-metabolizing enzymes associated with congenital defects in the mouse. *Teratology*, 16:147–154.
60. Lane, P. W., and Eicher, E. M. (1979): Gene order in linkage group XVI of the house mouse. *J. Hered.*, 70:239–244.
61. Layton, W. M. (1971): Teratogenic action of acetazolamide in golden hamsters. *Teratology*, 4:95–102.
62. Layton, W. M. (1974): The teratogenic effect of acetazolamide on mice with situs inversus. *Teratology*, 9:26A.
63. Layton, W. M. (1976): Random determination of a developmental process; reversal of normal visceral asymmetry in the mouse. *J. Hered.*, 67:336–338.
64. Layton, W. M., and Hallesy, D. W. (1965): Deformity of forelimb in rats; association with high doses of acetazolamide. *Science*, 149:306–308.
65. Layton, W. M., and Layton, M. W. (1977): Genetic studies of cadmium-induced limb defects in mice. *Teratology*, 15:22A–23A.
66. Layton, W. M., and Layton, M. W. (1979): Cadmium-induced limb defects in mice: Strain associated differences in sensitivity. *Teratology*, 19:229–236.
67. Lewontin, R. C. (1974): The analysis of variance and the analysis of causes. *Am. J. Hum. Genet.*, 26:400–411.
68. Maren, T. H. (1967): Carbonic anhydrase: Chemistry, physiology, and inhibition. *Physiol. Rev.* 47:595–781.
69. Maren, T. H. (1977): Use of inhibitors in physiological studies of carbonic anhydrase. *Am. J. Physiol.*, 232:F291–F297.
70. Miller, T. J. (1972): Cleft palate formation: A role for pyridoxine in the closure of the secondary palate in mice. *Teratology*, 6:351–356.
71. Mode, C. J., and Gasser, D. L. (1972): A distribution-free test for major gene differences in quantitative inheritance. *Math. Biosci.*, 14:143–150.
72. Morse, H. C. (1978): *Origins of Inbred Mice.* Academic Press, New York.
73. Nashed, N. (1976): Evaluation of a possible role for antimutagens, antiteratogens, and anticarcinogens in reducing environmental health hazards. *Environ. Health Perspect.*, 14:193–200.
74. Nebert, D. W., and Felton, J. S. (1976): Importance of genetic factors influencing the metabolism of foreign compounds. *Fed. Proc.*, 35:1133–1141.
75. Nolen, G. A. (1969): Variations in teratogenic response to hypervitaminosis A in three strains of the albino rat. *Food Cosmet. Toxicol.*, 7:209–214.
76. Palmer, A. K. (1972):Some thoughts on reproductive studies for safety evaluation. *Proc. Eur. Soc. Study Drug Toxicol.*, 14:79–90.

77. Pierro, L. J., and Haines, J. S. (1978): Cadmium-induced teratogenicity and embryotoxicity in the mouse. In: *Developmental Toxicology of Energy-Related Pollutants*, edited by D. D. Mahlum, M. R. Sikov, P. L. Hackett, and F. D. Andrew, pp. 614–626. United States Department of Energy, Oak Ridge, Tennessee.

78. Pinsky, L., and Fraser, F. C. (1959): Production of skeletal malformations in the offspring of pregnant mice treated with 6-aminonicotinamide. *Biol. Neonate*, 1:106–112.

79. Pinsky, L., and Fraser, F. C. (1960): Congenital malformations after a two-hour inactivation of nicotinamide in pregnant mice. *Br. Med. J.*, 2:195–197.

80. Pollard, D. R., and Fraser, F. C. (1968): Further studies on a cytoplasmically transmitted difference in response to the teratogen 6-aminonicotinamide. *Teratology*, 1:335–338.

81. Pollard, D. R., and Fraser, F. C. (1973): Induction of a cytoplasmic factor increasing resistance to the teratogenic effect of 6-aminonicotinamide in mice. *Teratology,* 7:267–270.

82. Reed, S. C. (1936): Harelip in the mouse. I. Effects of the external and internal environments. *Genetics*, 21:339–360.

83. Reed, S. C. (1936): Harelip in the mouse. II. Mendelian units concerned with harelip and application of the data to the human harelip problem. *Genetics*, 21:361–374.

84. Reed, S. C., and Snell, G. D. (1931): Harelip, a new mutation in the mouse. *Anat. Rec.*, 51:43–50.

85. Salomon, D. S., and Pratt, R. M. (1976): Glucocorticoid receptors in murine embryonic facial mesenchyme cells. *Nature*, 264:174–177.

86. Salomon, D. S., and Pratt, R. M. (1978): Inhibition of growth *in vitro* by glucocorticoids in mouse embryonic facial mesenchyme cells. *J. Cell. Physiol.*, 97:315–328.

87. Scott, W. J. (1970): Effects of intrauterine administration of acetazolamide in rats. *Teratology*, 3:261–268.

88. Scott, W. J., Schreiner, C. M., and Hirsch, K. S. (1979): Acetazolamide teratology: Ontogeny of carbonic anhydrase (CA) isozymes in mouse embryos. *Teratology*, 19:46A.

89. Shire, J. G. M. (1974): Endocrine genetics of the adrenal gland. *J. Endocrinol.*, 62:173–207.

90. Shire, J. G. M. (1976): The forms, uses and significance of genetic variation in endocrine systems. *Biol. Rev.*, 51:105–141.

91. Shum, S., Jensen, N. M., and Nebert, D. W. (1979): The murine *Ah* locus: In utero toxicity and teratogenesis associated with genetic differences in benzo(*a*)pyrene metabolism. *Teratology*, 20:365–376.

92. Snell, G. D. (1978): Congenic resistant strains of mice. In: *Origins of Inbred Mice*, edited by H. C. Morse, pp. 119–155. Academic Press, New York.

93. Sokal, R. R., and Rohlf, F. J. (1969): *Biometry. The Principles and Practice of Statistics in Biological Research*. W. H. Freeman, San Francisco.

94. Staats, J. (1976): Standardized nomenclature for inbred strains of mice: Sixth listing. *Cancer Res.*, 36:4333–4377.

95. Stewart, J. and Elston, R. C. (1973): Biometric genetics with one or two loci: The inheritance of physiological characters in mice. *Genetics*, 73:675–693.

96. Storch, T. G., and Layton, W. M. (1973): Teratogenic effects of intrauterine injection of acetazolamide and amiloride in hamsters. *Teratology*, 7:209–214.

97. Suzuki, M., and Takano, K. (1969): Teratogenic effect of acetazolamide in ICR mice. *Cong. Anom.*, 9:36.

98. Swank, R. T., and Bailey, D. W. (1973): Recombinant inbred lines: Value in the genetic analysis of biochemical variants. *Science*, 181:1249–1252.

99. Taylor, B. A. (1972): Genetic relationships between inbred strains of mice. *J. Hered.*, 63:83–86.

100. Taylor, B. A. (1976): Linkage of the cadmium resistance locus to loci on mouse chromosome 12. *J. Hered.*, 67:389–390.

101. Taylor, B. A. (1978): Recombinant inbred strains: Use in gene mapping. In: *Origins of Inbred Mice*, edited by H. C. Morse, pp. 423–438. Academic Press, New York.

102. Taylor, B. A., Heiniger, H. J., and Meier, H. (1973): Genetic analysis of resistance to cadmium-induced testicular damage in mice. *Proc. Soc. Exp. Biol. Med.*, 143:629–633.

103. Trasler, D. G. (1965): Strain differences in susceptibility to teratogenesis: Survey of spontaneously occurring malformations in mice. In: *Teratology: Principles and Techniques*, edited by J. G. Wilson and J. Warkany, pp. 38–55. University of Chicago Press, Chicago.

104. Trasler, D. G. (1968): Pathogenesis of cleft lip and its relation to embryonic face shape in A/J and C57BL mice. *Teratology*, 1:33–50.

105. Trasler, D. G., and Fraser, F. C. (1963): Role of the tongue in producing cleft palate in mice with spontaneous cleft lip. *Dev. Biol.*, 6:45–60.
106. Vekemans, M., and Fraser, F. C. (1978): Effects of two diets on the frequency of cortisone-induced cleft palate in mice. *Teratology*, 17:24A.
107. Vekemans, M., and Fraser, F. C. (1979): Stage of palate closure as one indication of "liability" to cleft palate. *Am. J. Med. Genet.*, 4:95–102.
108. Vekemans, M., Taylor, B. A., and Fraser, F. C. (1979): Evidence against a simple genetic model in cortisone-induced cleft palate in the mouse. *Teratology*, 19:51A–52A.
109. Verrusio, A. C. (1966): *Biochemical Basis for a Genetically Determined Difference in Response to the Teratogenic Effects of 6-Aminonicotinamide*, Ph.D. Thesis. McGill University Library, Montreal.
110. Verrusio, A. C., Pollard, D. R., and Fraser, F. C. (1968): A cytoplasmically transmitted diet-dependent difference in response to the teratogenic effects of 6-aminonicotinamide. *Science*, 160:206–207.
111. Walker, B. E., and Fraser, F. C. (1956): Closure of the secondary palate in three strains of mice. *J. Embryol. Exp. Morphol.*, 4:176–189.
112. Warburton, D., Trasler, D. G., Naylor, A., Miller, J. R., and Fraser, F. C. (1962): Pitfalls in tests for teratogenicity. *Lancet*, 2:1116–1117.
113. Wilson, J. G. (1973): *Environment and Birth Defects*. Academic Press, New York.
114. Wolkowski, R. M. (1974): Differential cadmium-induced embryotoxicity in two inbred mouse strains. 1. Analysis of inheritance of the response to cadmium and of the presence of cadmium in fetal and placental tissues. *Teratology*, 10:243–262.
115. Wolkowski-Tyl, R., and Preston, S. F. (1979): The interaction of cadmium-binding proteins (Cd-bp) and progesterone in cadmium-induced tissue and embryo toxicity. *Teratology*, 20:341–352.
116. Womack, J. E. (1979): Genetic constitution and response to toxic chemicals—an overview. *J. Toxicol. Environ. Health*, 5:49–51.
117. Wright, S. (1934): The result of crosses between inbred strains of guinea pigs differing in number of digits. *Genetics*, 19:537–551.

*Developmental Toxicology*, edited by
C. A. Kimmel and J. Buelke-Sam. Raven Press,
New York © 1981.

# Peri- and Postnatal Development of Phase I Reactions

W. Klinger, D. Müller, U. Kleeberg, and A. Barth

*Institute of Pharmacology and Toxicology, Friedrich Schiller University of Jena, DDR-69 Jena, German Democratic Republic*

Since the first reports by Jondorf et al. (46) and Fouts and Adamson (30), more than a thousand papers have been published concerning the time of appearance and the rates of development of various enzymes associated with the biotransformation of lipid-soluble xenobiotics. These foreign compounds, which are not metabolized by the highly specific enzymes of carbohydrate, lipid, or protein metabolism, would stay in the organism for weeks and months by continuous reabsorption in the gut and kidneys if they were not metabolized to more hydrophilic metabolites that are more suitable for excretion and generally less toxic. Xenobiotics are characterized by an extremely high structural variability; therefore, the enzymes responsible for their biotransformation are of low substrate specificity. Generally three major processes occur during the biotransformation of a compound:

1. Uptake into the cell, with the participation of cytoplasmic organic anion-binding acceptor or transport proteins. Excretion out of the cell of the original compound as well as of its various metabolites might result from similar mechanisms.
2. Within the cell, some reactions form reactive groups for subsequent conjugation. These reactions produce more polar metabolites ready for conjugation and are called phase I reactions.
3. Phase II reactions are conjugation reactions. The reactions of both types frequently run in parallel or stepwise. Only uptake into and excretion out of the cell and phase I reactions will be dealt with in this chapter.

The liver is considered the main organ of xenobiotic metabolism, and most phase I enzymes are located in the endoplasmic reticulum of its cells, with higher specific activity in the smooth rather than in the rough form. In the parenchymal cells of the normal adult liver, about 10 to 15% of the total protein is in the endoplasmic reticulum, and within this fraction, the final oxidase of the microsomal electron transport chain, cytochrome P-450 amounts to about 20%.

The substructure of the rat liver parenchymal cell shows an adult pattern by the fifth to seventh day of life (32). Human fetal liver parenchymal cells have attained essentially complete differentiation by the 3rd month of gestation (128). Immediately after birth, the blood supply of the liver changes (78), and this could contribute to restriction of its functional state.

In the rat, during the postnatal period, we find changing patterns in the microsomal phospholipids (112), and the phospholipid–protein quotient increases (21). The concentrations of NADP and NAD do not limit the microsomal electron transport chain in the perinatal period, and the same is true for glucose-6-phosphate dehydrogenase, which is important for the reduction of NAD and NADP (50,104).

Cytochrome P-450 and other constituents of the microsomal electron transport chain as well as P-450-dependent reactions can also be detected in kidney and lung tissue (35,85) and in other organs, but the biotransformation capacities of these organs are normally low in comparison to that of the liver. In newborn animals, these organs generally contribute little to the low total transformation capacity (67). Especially in the human fetus, very low P-450-dependent biotransformation activities have been detected in the kidney and gut (102,104), but P-450 concentration in human fetal adrenals is higher than that in the fetal liver (102,103). Correspondingly, the biotransformation capacity of fetal adrenals is high. Nevertheless, pharmacokinetic data in human newborns indicate a low total biotransformation capacity. Extrahepatic biotransformation plays a considerable role in the case of hydrolytic enzymes and of N-hydroxylation, which is not P-450 dependent and can be demonstrated to have high activity in the lung (8). Because of the preponderance of hepatic biotransformation, only the age dependence of drug metabolism in the liver will be dealt with here.

## HEPATIC TRANSPORT FUNCTION

Transfer of xenobiotics from blood into bile requires specific transport systems for hepatic uptake and biliary excretion as well as cytoplasmic proteins for binding and storage. Each of the steps was found to have its own developmental pattern, and it was demonstrated that the importance of transfer steps for the overall transport via hepatocytes changes with aging (15,53). Bile secretion begins at about the same stage of development as does glucuronidation. In rats, bile pigment is detectable in the small intestine 1 day before birth, whereas the bile canaliculi develop earlier (107). In newborn animals, especially rats, overall hepatic excretory function is low, and the excretion of organic acids (including bile acids and neutral xenobiotics) develops postnatally to reach maximum capacity at an age of 30 days (5,15, 29,52–55,121). Thereafter, the excretion capacity declines (5,6,121). Individual steps of the overall hepatic excretion will be dealt with separately.

### Hepatic Uptake and Storage

Hepatic uptake rate is dose dependent and saturable (29). Kinetics and competitive inhibition phenomena between endogenous compounds such as bilirubin and bile acids, and various drugs, such as rifampicin, bromsulfophthalein (BSP), indocyanine green (ICG), and glycosides, support the concept of carrier-mediated transport (2,15,

70,100). However, simple diffusion with subsequent binding to cytoplasmic acceptor proteins cannot be ruled out. Competition studies suggest at least four independent hepatic uptake systems responsible for handling of organic anions, bile acids, organic cations, and neutral substances (2,56,101).

In adult animals, the initial hepatic ICG uptake capacity is about 10 times larger than the excretory capacity (41,100). Therefore, hepatic uptake cannot be rate limiting for overall drug transport (69). In 20-day-old rats, hepatic eosine uptake capacity is only half of that seen in adults (29). Also, for the acids ICG and BSP and the neutral substances ouabain, digoxin, and digitoxin, hepatic uptake capacity is considerably lower in young and newborn animals than in adults (5,15,39–41,53,55,56,100,123).

In newborn rats, immature hepatic uptake leads to accumulation of drugs in plasma and might contribute to an increased lethality (53,55). Nonhemolytic hyperbilirubinemia in newborns is at least in part caused by a low rate of hepatic uptake of bilirubin (40).

Inducers such as phenobarbital (PB), spironolactone, and pregnenolone-16α-carbonitrile enhance the hepatic clearance of ouabain in neonates, whereas 3-methylcholanthrene (3-MC) is ineffective. The polychlorinated biphenyls (PCBs) also stimulate ouabain uptake. This has been shown only in 15-day-old rats, whereas no stimulation effect could be demonstrated in adults (14).

Cytoplasmic acceptor or transport protein Y (ligandin) binds organic anions (72,73) and may determine the net flux of organic anions from plasma into the liver (74,75). The concentration of this protein develops postnatally in rats, guinea pigs, and primates (54,86). The small amount of ligandin in newborns can contribute to the immaturity of hepatic transport function but does not seem to be rate limiting in young animals. After pretreatment with PB, the BSP-binding capacity of liver cytosol was enhanced in 20-day-old rats and was accompanied by increased BSP clearance (86), but this effect was not found in adults.

According to Meijer et al. (82), PB increases dibromsulfophthalein plasma clearance without influencing hepatic uptake of the dye, but the induction of ligandin diminished the reflux back into the blood. Thus, the significance of ligandin is questioned (54,55). 3-Methylcholanthrene and PB markedly enhanced the ligandin content of the liver without an increase of the ICG clearance (80,95). Ouabain uptake is age-dependent as well, but ouabain is not bound to ligandin (54,55).

## Excretion

Bauer (12) divided compounds that are excreted into bile into three classes according to their bile/plasma concentration ratios. Substances with a ratio of about 1 are considered to be excreted passively. Ratios smaller than 1 are found if diffusion is hindered by molecular weight or size. Substances with ratios higher than 1 are considered to be transported actively into bile (55). As for hepatic uptake, different transport systems of hepatic excretion are postulated for acids, bases, neutral compounds, bile acids, and metals (55). Considering the maximal hepatic transport capacity (*Tm*) for organic anions such as eosine, ICG, and BSP, decreased excretion into bile is detectable in newborn animals (5,29,41,52,53,58). Using ICG, we found the following *Tm* values for 10-, 30-, and 260-day-old male rats: 20.6, 145, and 79.6 μg/kg body weight per min, respectively (5). According to Fischer et al. (29) and Varga and Fischer (121), in rats younger than 30 and older than 120 days, hepatic transport capacity for eosine was markedly lower than that of 30- and 60-day-old rats.

After PB pretreatment, the enhancement of biliary excretion of some organic anions and of bile flow showed no parallelism (28,55). In our experiments, PB was able to increase the biliary excretion of ICG only in 20- and 30-day-old rats (5). There are probably several mechanisms responsible for the increase in biliary excretion after PB treatment of developing animals (55). The most important factor may be the stimulation of so-called transport units available for carrying drugs from blood plasma via hepatocytes into bile.

Hepatic transport function in infantile as well as in very old animals is lower than in adults (51). However, in adult and young, liver storage capacity was found to be higher than excretory capacity, which indicates that at all postnatal ages, overall hepatic transport into bile is limited by the small rate of transport from liver into bile (5,56).

However, the investigations of Cagen et al. (14) and Cagen and Gibson (15) demonstrate the importance of hepatic uptake in the maturation of the drug elimination process in developing animals.

## PHASE I REACTIONS

In man and in laboratory animals with long gestation periods (e.g., guinea pigs and rabbits), an early differentiation and morphologic development of the liver is accompanied by a prenatal development of phase I reactions and inducibility by inducers of the phenobarbital type in the late gestation period (for review, see 8,64,65,102,103).

In animals with short gestation periods (e.g., rats), development and differentiation of the liver continue after birth, and phase I reactions primarily develop postnatally. Phenobarbital induction with hypertrophy of the smooth endoplasmic reticulum is not demonstrable or is demonstrable only in some litters. Inducers of the 3-MC type, which produce little if any hypertrophy of the smooth endoplasmic reticulum, are potent inducers even in the early fetal rat liver. Therefore, the ontogeny of phase I reactions as well as age-dependent inducibility by PB and 3-MC will be considered.

### Cytochrome P-450-Dependent Monooxygenases

Among the phase I reactions, the P-450-dependent mixed function oxidases (MFO), now named monooxygenases, play a dominant role. Several hundred papers have been published concerning the time of appearance and the rates of these MFO in various mammalian species and different organs and tissues. Moreover, much research has been undertaken to determine whether liver microsomal enzymes of fetuses or newborns were induced by treatment of the pregnant female at various stages of gestation in order to attain either an earlier appearance or a more rapid enhancement of enzyme activity in fetal life. These investigations have shown that, in most laboratory animals, the monooxygenases are apparently absent or barely detectable in fetal organs, especially in the fetal liver, until just before birth (for review, see 64,65,103). This is true of all reaction types of monooxygenation as the following examples show.

### Hydroxylation of Aromatics

The age course of the hydroxylation of aniline, acetanilide, strychnine, phenazone, amphetamine, coumarin, biphenyl, chlorpromazine, zoxazolamine, and other substrates by liver microsomes of various species has been determined (8,64,65,-102,103). Generally, low or barely detectable metabolism is found prenatally, and, depending on duration of gestation, the activities start to develop a few days before birth (longer gestation periods) or immediately after birth.

### Hydroxylation of Aliphatics

This same pattern is seen for aliphatics, the most common substrates being hexobarbital and pentobarbital. The duration of action of these two substrates—sleeping time—has often been used as a measure of biotransformation. This is possible since both substrates are completely metabolized, and no age-dependent sensitivity of the central nervous system could be demonstrated with regard to these drugs' hypnotic action (61).

Like aromatics, aliphatic compounds are rarely hydroxylated in the fetus; only in the human fetus have remarkable activities been demonstrated (102). Hydroxylation reaches maximum levels before sexual maturation and declines thereafter.

### N-*Dealkylation*

This is a special case of *N*-hydroxylation of secondary and tertiary amines. The hydroxylation products are unstable, and free primary and secondary amines, respectively, and aldehydes are formed. Here again, we find the typical developmental pattern with certain differences regarding species and substrate.

The most common substrates evaluated have been aminopyrine, benzphetamine, *N*-monomethylnitraniline, dimethylaniline, methylphenobarbital, and ethylmorphine (62,64,94,102,103).

### O-*Dealkylation*

This reaction has been investigated most extensively with codeine and nitroanisole as substrates (64,94,102,103). If the age course and the age-dependent induction of the P-450-dependent monooxygenation of different substrates are compared, marked quantitative differences can be observed (Fig. 1).

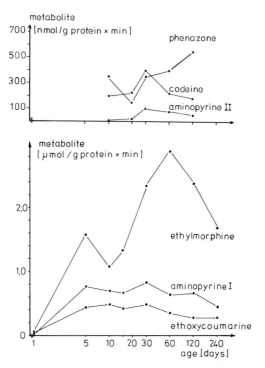

**FIG. 1.** Developmental changes in activities of phenazone hydroxylase, codeine-O-demeth-ylase, aminopyrine-N-demethylase first step (to form formaldehyde and monomethylamino-phenazone) and second step (to form formaldehyde and 4-aminophenazone) in 9,000 g liver supernatant and of ethylmorphine-N-demethylase and ethoxycoumarin-O-demethylase in liver homogenate of male rats of different ages. (Data were partially derived from refs. 62,64.)

On investigating these differences in more detail, and especially the two steps of aminopyrine N-demethylation in relation to age and inducibility, we have found indications of the existence of different cytochrome species in different age groups, i.e., more than one $K_m$ value for a single substrate and age-dependent changes of $K_m$ and $K_i$ values (62,63). Recently the existence of various P-450 subspecies with different developmental patterns has been shown directly in the rabbit (3).

In order to find the reasons for the age dependence of drug monooxygenation, the components and reactions of the microsomal electron transport chain have been investigated. The reaction sequence of this chain may briefly be described as follows (26; Fig. 2).

An organic substrate (S) reacts with the low-spin form of the ferric cytochrome P-450 to form a high-spin ferric P-450–substrate complex. This complex undergoes a one-electron reduction to a ferrous P-450–substrate complex. The ferrous–substrate complex can react with either carbon monoxide to form the familiar ferrous–carbon monoxide complex typified by the characteristic absorbance band at 450 nm or with oxygen to form a ternary complex of heme iron, oxygen, and substrate. The ferrous P-450–substrate–oxygen complex then undergoes a second stage of reduction, and

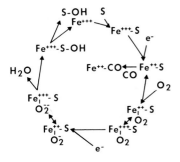

**FIG. 2.** Cyclic reduction and oxidation of P-450 during interaction with a substrate and oxygen. (Derived from Estabrook *et al.*, ref 26.) Fe, P-450 with valence state of iron; S, substrate; S-OH, hydroxylated substrate.

the cycle is completed by insertion of one atom of the bound molecular oxygen into the organic substrate concomitant with the formation of water and splitting off the hydroxylated substrate.

The total concentration of P-450 as a function of age was determined by a number of authors. In some studies, a distinct postnatal increase in P-450 concentration was observed in various species (7,31,47,81,109–111,118), whereas others found relatively small changes after the first week of life (16,20,25,34,71,85). It is evident that total cytochrome P-450 concentration is responsible neither for the age dependence of drug oxidation nor for the age-dependent induction by phenobarbital, because the postnatal increase in biotransformation activity is higher than that of P-450, and, in young rats, PB enhances biotransformation activity to a greater extent than it increases P-450 concentration (84).

The first step of monooxygenation is the binding of xenobiotics to the protein moiety, which is associated with spectral changes of P-450 (108). The magnitude of spectral changes is generally correlated with the rate of biotransformation activity (10,16,22,27,45,96), and spectral dissociation constants ($K_s$) are similar to $K_m$ values of the corresponding biotransformation reaction (108). A few investigations in animals of different ages demonstrate great differences in the magnitude of spectral changes between young and adult animals (16,25,113). We could demonstrate that the maximal spectral changes, caused by hexobarbital, increase considerably during postnatal development in spite of nearly constant P-450 concentration. Phenobarbital pretreatment enhances these spectral changes to a greater extent than it does total P-450 concentration in young rats (84,87,88). There was a strong correlation between the magnitude of spectral changes and the age course and inducibility of ethylmorphine *N*-demethylation (84,88). We concluded that the proportion of P-450 that can bind type I substrates (active P-450) increases during development and after induction with PB (84,87,88). This conclusion is supported by the determination of the concentration of the metyrapone-binding sites of P-450: the metyrapone-reactive portion of P-450 increases considerably with age (84,88).

The second reaction step, the NADPH-dependent reduction of P-450–substrate complex, does not seem to be responsible for the age dependence of drug oxidation (84,89). The difference in the concentration of active P-450 during postnatal development could be a result of a qualitatively different P-450 being formed or of the ratio of two or more P-450 subspecies changing. This has been demonstrated directly by electrophoresis (3).

Additionally, P-450 itself need not be totally responsible for the age differences, as changes in the microenvironment could also be of importance. Phospholipids, which are necessary for P-450 reduction (4,116) as well as for properties of microsomal membranes, do change with age. Age-dependent changes in the fatty acid composition have been described (19,42,112). However, we recently found that after solubilization and partial purification of P-450, the age dependence and induction by PB of spectral changes caused by the binding of hexobarbital to P-450 is the same as with intact microsomes (Fig. 3, white columns). This means that the portion of active P-450 is not influenced by membrane structure.

Endogenous substrates of P-450 that block P-450 binding of exogenous substrates could be responsible for age differences in the active portion of P-450. We have found that after removal of endogenous substances from solubilized P-450 by charcoal, the hexobarbital-binding P-450 portion increases by a factor of two to three in young and adult control and phenobarbital-treated rats (Fig. 3). However, age dependence of hexobarbital binding still is evident. Thus, the presence of endogenous substrates do play an important role in some aspects of the drug metabolism process, but they do not cause age differences in biotransformation.

In principle, the distinct age dependence of drug metabolism can also be demonstrated with P-448-dependent biotransformation reactions. For investigating this P-450 subspecies, the activity of aryl hydrocarbon hydroxylase (AHH) [with benzo($a$)pyrene as a substrate] was measured (18,92). The inducibility by a relatively specific P-448 inducer (3-MC) then was checked (1,11,17,37), and a relatively selective inhibitor, $\alpha$-naphthoflavone (7,8-benzoflavone, ANF) was also employed for this investigation (23,125).

A marked postnatal increase in AHH activity was found in the liver of male Wistar rats which reached maximum levels at about 60 days and thereafter declined. Pregnant rats exhibited distinctly lower activities than adult male rats. In fetal rat liver, activity is first detectable at the 17th gestation day. Up to an age of 25 days (postnatal), the hepatic activities of male and female rats cannot be distinguished. In the kidney, we did not observe such distinct age-dependent AHH activities. Our data support the schematic demonstration of postnatal AHH development in rat liver that has been presented by Lucier (76) and was derived from several investigations.

3-Methylcholanthrene administration to pregnant rats has been shown to increase AHH activity about 20-fold in fetal liver and also to a minor extent in extrahepatic tissues (93). Induction by postnatally administered 3-MC is dose dependent with regard to the maximum effect as well as its duration. The higher the dose administered, the higher and the later the maximum effect can be demonstrated, as was shown after administration of 1, 10, and 100 mg/kg 3-MC in 7-day-old rats (57). Although the specific renal AHH activity is only about 1/10 of the hepatic activity, the relative inducibility by 3-MC is higher than that observed in liver (57,65).

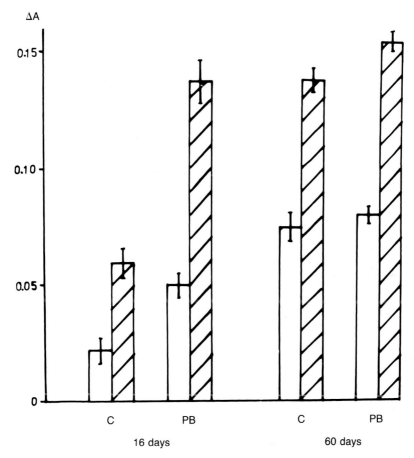

**FIG. 3.** Spectral changes after addition of hexobarbital (3 mM) to solubilized and partially purified rat liver P-450 (3.5 μM). Nontreated (C) and PB-treated (3 × 60 mg/kg) rats of different ages were used. Arithmetic means ± SEM are given. *Hatched bars*, solubilized P-450 shaken with charcoal before hexobarbital addition; *open bars*, no charcoal.

α-Naphthoflavone inhibits P-448-mediated activities when added to the incubation mixture during the *in vitro* determination of AHH activity. In our experiments, ANF has been added at a concentration of $10^{-4}$ M to samples from control or 3-MC-induced rats of different ages. The results of these studies are given in Fig. 4.

In control animals up to 30 days of age, no distinct influence of ANF on constitutive AHH is observed (in 5-day-old rats even a stimulation has been demonstrated). However, in adult animals, an inhibition of about 50% was detected. But in the 3-MC-induced rats of all age groups, the ANF-mediated inhibition was in the range of 50 to 70%. Therefore, we conclude that the newly synthetized cytochrome in induced animals belongs to the P-448 subspecies.

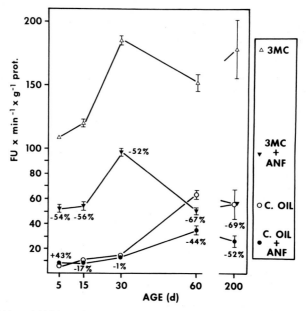

**FIG. 4.** Inhibition of AHH activity in liver 10,000 × *g* supernatant by addition of ANF (10⁻⁴ M) to the incubation mixture. Male rats of different ages received 80 mg/kg 3-MC i.p. or the solvent only (10 ml corn oil/kg). Arithmetic means ± SD are given. Relative changes of AHH by ANF are shown at the symbols. FU, fluorimetric units.

A striking stimulatory effect of ANF in neonates has also been described by Wiebel and Gelboin (124). The suggestion of the existence of a special kind of "neonatal" benzo(*a*)pyrene hydroxylating P-450 seems to be possible. Further evidence for typical pecularities of P-450 in the neonatal period is offered by Iba et al. (43) who reported that the well-known refractoriness of fetal hepatic MFO toward PB induction in rats but not toward 3-MC can be overcome by simultaneous administration of PB plus 3-MC. Moreover, 3-MC suppresses the PB-mediated induction of NADPH–cytochrome c reductase in neonates (36).

In 10-day-old male rats, the typical 3-MC-mediated induction process with enhancement of DNA-dependent RNA polymerase activity (13,33) and protein synthesis (91) can be characterized in more detail. The free and engaged forms of the nucleolar RNA polymerase are stimulated, and an interconversion process between these functional forms seems to play an important role in the extranucleolar RNA polymerase B (60). Additionally, the nucleolar and nucleoplasmic protein kinases are stimulated (117), and the 3-MC-dose-dependent AHH induction can be inhibited by actinomycin D, also in a dose-dependent manner (59).

Aryl hydrocarbon hydroxylase activity plays an important role in chemical carcinogenesis (38,83,89). With respect to the target DNA molecule, the nuclear AHH activity (49,77,106,122) may play a significant role; this AHH shows a comparable ontogenetic developmental pattern: barely detectable activities in the fetus rise considerably postpartum (97).

In the balance of toxifying–detoxifying enzymes for carcinogenic polycyclic hydrocarbons, epoxide hydrolase is very important. In fetal and neonatal rat liver, epoxide hydrolase activities are barely detectable, the main development occuring postnatally (98,115).

### Dehydrogenation (Ethanol Oxidation)

Alcohol dehydrogenase (ADH) develops mainly during the postnatal period. The full isoenzyme pattern also develops mainly during postnatal life (68,105).

### Oxidative Deamination

The monoamine oxidase (MAO) age course in different organs of different species has been investigated by several laboratories. Because various forms (isoenzymes) show different maturational patterns, perinatal and postnatal development has been found to be substrate, organ, and species dependent (9,44,79,99,114,120).

### N-Hydroxylation

The developmental patterns of these oxidations vary in different species, and there are marked differences between P-450-dependent (20) and flavin-containing amine oxidases (119,127). P-450-dependent N-hydroxylation in rats shows a first peak 2 to 3 days after birth and a second higher one after 27 days. In rabbits, a continuous increase occurs, with maximum activity attained at an age of about 40 days (20). The flavin enzyme increases in mice sharply during the first 3 days after birth; thereafter only small enhancement rates are observed (127).

## Reduction

Although information is available on ring reduction (nicotine, estrogens) and on aldehyde reduction, only nitro- and azoreduction will be discussed here.

### Nitroreduction

The process of nitroreduction can be demonstrated with microsomes as well as with P-450-free cytosol. With the cytoplasmic fraction, no definite postnatal developmental pattern has been observed (66). In whole liver homogenate or microsomes, low or nonmeasurable activities have been found in neonates, followed by a postnatal increase. With the onset of sexual maturity, a decrease in nitroreduction rates has been observed (90). Again, substrate and species differences are remarkable.

### Azoreduction

In principle, the same age course has been observed for the azoreduction of neoprontosil and p-dimethylazobenzene (30,48,109). These data are derived from older publications, as no recent publications on this topic have appeared.

## Hydrolysis

The existence of various esterases is demonstrated through the use of different substrates. Investigations on age-dependent hydrolytic activity have been carried out with α-naphthylacetate, procaine, pethidine, urethane, carisoprodol, and meprobamate, as well as with the amides isocarboxacide and cyclophosphamide. As was found for the hydroxylation of hexo- and pentobarbital, the age-dependent actions of their hydrolytic pathways and the activities correlate well with pharmacokinetic data of these substrates (24,64,126). Major developmental changes can be observed after birth with maximum activities found in young adults, before or at the beginning of sexual maturation. Thereafter the activities of the systems usually decline.

## CONCLUSIONS

All biotransformation reactions discussed in this chapter, including uptake into the liver cell, storage, P-450-dependent and other phase I reactions, and, finally, excretion out of the cell, have a low activity in the perinatal period. The main organ for biotransformation in the perinatal period is usually the liver, just as in adults. However, relatively high activities have been found in the lung for *N*-oxidation of secondary and tertiary amines and in different organs and tissues, especially in blood, for hydrolysis.

The development of these reactions begins before birth in animals with long gestation periods and immediately after birth in animals with shorter gestation periods. The low biotransformation activity in the perinatal period is not a result of insufficient cofactor availability, and it can be enhanced by induction. In all species, the 3-MC type of induction is possible even before birth, whereas the PB type of induction occurs later. The mechanism(s) that regulate this ontogenetic development are not known.

## ACKNOWLEDGMENTS

These investigations were supported by Forschungprojekt Perinatologie des Ministeriums für Gesundheitswesen der DDR. We are indebted to Mrs. E. Karge and Mrs. I. Triebel for skillful assistance and to G. Grohmann, Sylvia and K. D. Spiegler, H. Steinert, and R. Volkmann, who carried out the investigations with AHH and ethoxycoumarin in partial fulfillment of their M. D. degree. The manuscript was typed by Mrs. Gisela Säumel.

## REFERENCES

1. Alvares, A. P., Schilling, G., Levin, W., and Kuntzman, R. (1967): Studies on the induction of CO-binding pigments in liver microsomes by phenobarbital and 3-methylcholanthrene. *Biochem. Biophys. Res. Commun.*, 29:521–526.
2. Anwer, M. S., and Hegner, D. (1978): Effect of organic anions on bile acid uptake by isolated rat hepatocytes. *Hoppe Seylers Physiol. Chem.*, 359:1027.
3. Atlas, S. A., Boobis, A. R., Felton, J. S., Thorgeirsson, S. S., and Nebert, D. W. (1977): Ontogenetic expression of polycyclic aromatic compound-inducible monooxygenase activities and forms of cytochrome P-450 in rabbit. *J. Biol. Chem.*, 252:4712–4721.

4. Autor, A. P., Kuschnik, R. M., Heidema, J. K., van der Hoeven, T. A., Duppel, W., and Coon, M. J. (1973): Role of phospholipid in the reconstituted liver microsomal mixed function oxidase system containing cytochrome P-450 and NADPH-cytochrome P-450 reductase. *Drug Metab. Dispos.*, 1:156–161.
5. Barth, A., and Klinger, W. (1979): Die biliäre Ausscheidung von Indocyaningrun bei Ratten verschiedenen Alters und ihre Beeinflussung durch Phenobarbital. *Wiss. Z. Humboldt Universitat (Berl.)*, XXVIII:413–414.
6. Barth, A., Zaumseil, J., and Klinger, W. (1977): Gallenfluss und Gallensäureausscheidung bei männlichen Wistarratten (Jena) verschiedenen Alters. *Z. Versuchstierkd.*, 19:26–35.
7. Basu, T. K., Dickerson, J. W. T., and Parke, D. V. W. (1971): Effect of development on the activity of microsomal drug-metabolizing enzymes in rat liver. *Biochem. J.*, 124:19–24.
8. Bend, J. R., James, M. O., Devereux, T. R., and Fouts, J. R. (1975): Toxication–detoxication systems in hepatic and extrahepatic tissues in the perinatal period. In: *Basic and Therapeutic Aspects of Perinatal Pharmacology*, edited by P. L. Morselli, S. Garattini, and F. Sereni, pp. 229–243. Raven Press, New York.
9. Blatchford, D., Holzbauer, M., Grahame-Smith, D. G., and Youdim, M. B. H. (1976): Ontogenesis of enzyme systems deaminating different monoamines. *Br. J. Pharmacol.*, 57:279–293.
10. Bohn, W., Ullrich, V., and Staudinger, H. (1971): Species of cytochrome P-450 in rat liver microsomes with different stereoselectivity for the binding and monooxygenation. *Naunyn Schmiedebergs Arch. Pharmacol.*, 270:41–55.
11. Boobis, A. R., Nebert, D. W., and Felton, J. S. (1977): Comparison of β-naphthoflavone and 3-methylcholanthrene as inducers of hepatic cytochrome(s) P-448 and aryl hydrocarbon [benzo(a)pyrene] hydroxylase activity. *Mol. Pharmacol.*, 13:259–268.
12. Brauer, R. W. (1959): Mechanisms of bile secretion. *J.A.M.A.*, 169:1462–1466.
13. Bresnick, E. (1966): Ribonucleic acid polymerase activity in polymerase activity in liver nuclei from rats pretreated with 3-methylcholanthrene. *Mol. Pharmacol.*, 2:406–410.
14. Cagen, St.Z., Dent, J. G., McCormack, K. M., Richert, D., and Gibson, J. E. (1979): Effect of polybrominated biphenyls on the development of hepatic excretory function. *J. Pharmacol. Exp. Ther.*, 209:1–6.
15. Cagen, St.Z., and Gibson, J. E. (1979): Characteristics of hepatic excretory function during development. *J. Pharmacol. Exp. Ther.*, 210:15–21.
16. Cohen, G. M., and Mannering, G. J. (1974): Sex-dependent differences in drug-metabolism in the rat. III. Temporal changes in type I binding and NADPH-cytochrome P-450 reductase during sexual maturation. *Drug. Metab. Dispos.*, 2:285–292.
17. Conney, A. H. (1967): Pharmacological implications of microsomal enzyme induction. *Pharmacol. Rev.*, 19:317–366.
18. Conney, A. H., Miller, E. G., and Miller, J. A. (1957): Substrate-induced synthesis and other properties of benz-pyrene hydroxylase in rat liver. *J. Biol. Chem.*, 228:753–766.
19. Dallner, G., Siekevitz, P., and Palade, G. E. (1965): Phospholipids in hepatic membranes during development. *Biochem. J.*, 20:142–148.
20. Dallner, G., Siekevitz, P., and Palade, G. E. (1965): Synthesis of microsomal membranes and their enzymic constituents in developing rat liver. *Biochem. Biophys. Res. Commun.*, 20:135–141.
21. Dallner G., Siekevitz, P., and Palade, G. E. (1966): Biogenesis of endoplasmic reticulum membranes: I. Structural and chemical differentiation in developing rat hepatocyte. *J. Cell Biol.*, 30:73–96.
22. Degkwitz, E., Ullrich, V., and Staudinger, H. J. (1969): Metabolism and cytochrome P-450 binding spectra of ( + )- and ( − )-hexobarbital in rat liver microsomes. *Hoppe Seylers Z. Physiol. Chem.*, 350:547–553.
23. Diamond, L., and Gelboin, H. V. (1969): Alpha-naphthoflavon: An inhibitor of hydrocarbon cytotoxicity and microsomal hydroxylase. *Science*, 166:1023–1025.
24. Ecobichon, D. J., and Stephens, D. S. (1973): Perinatal development of human blood esterases. *Clin. Pharmacol. Ther.*, 14:41–47.
25. Eling, T. E., Harbison, R. D., Becker, B. A., and Fouts, J. R. (1970): Kinetic changes in microsomal drug metabolism with age and diphenylhydantoin treatment. *Eur. J. Pharmacol.*, 11:101–108.
26. Estabrook, R. W., Matsubara, T., Mason, J. I., Werringloer, J., and Baron, J. (1973): Studies on the molecular function of cytochrome P-450 during drug metabolism. *Drug Metab. Dispos.*, 1:98–110.

27. Feller, D. R., and Lubawy, W. C. (1973): Interactions of the hexobarbital enantiomers with rat liver microsomes. *Pharmacology*, 9:129–137.
28. Fischer, E., Varga, F., Gregus, Z., and Gogl, A. (1978): Bile flow and biliary excretion rate of some organic anions in phenobarbital-pretreated rats. *Digestion*, 17:211–220.
29. Fischer, E., Barth, A., Varga, F., and Klinger, W. (1979): Age dependence of hepatic transport in control and phenobarbital-pretreated rats. *Life Sci.*, 24:557–562.
30. Fouts, J. R., and Adamson, R. H. (1959): Drug metabolism in the newborn rabbit. *Science*, 129:897.
31. Fouts, J. R., and Devereux, T. R. (1972): Developmental aspects of hepatic and extrahepatic drug-metabolizing enzyme systems: Microsomal enzymes and components in rabbit liver and lung during the first month of life. *J. Pharmacol. Exp. Ther.*, 183:458–468.
32. Franke, H., and Klinger, W. (1967): Untersuchungen zum Mechanismus der Enzyminduktion: X. Die Wirkung von Barbital auf die Substruktur der Leberzellen von Ratten verschiedenen Alters. *Acta Biol. Med. Germ.*, 18:99–119.
33. Gelboin, H. V. (1967): Carcinogens, enzyme induction, and the gene action. *Adv. Cancer Res.*, 10:1–81.
34. Gram, T. E., Guarino, A. M., Schroeder, D. H., and Gillette, J. R. (1969): Changes in certain kinetic properties of hepatic microsomal aniline hydroxylase and ethylmorphine deethylase associated with postnatal development and maturation in male rats. *Biochem. J.*, 113:681–685.
35. Gram, T. E., Sikic, B. I., Litterst, C. L., Mimnaugh, E. G., Drew, R., and Siddik, Z. H. (1978): The role of the lung in the metabolism and disposition of xenobiotics. In: *Industrial and Environmental Xenobiotics*, edited by J. R. Fouts and I. Gut, pp. 53–58. Excerpta Medica, Amsterdam, Oxford.
36. Guenthner, T. M., and Mannering, G. (1977): Induction of hepatic mono-oxygenase systems in fetal and neonatal rats with phenobarbital, polycyclic hydrocarbons and other xenobiotics. *Biochem. Pharmacol.*, 26:567–575.
37. Haugen, D. A., Coon, M. J., and Nebert, D. W. (1976): Induction of multiple forms of mouse liver cytochrome P-450. Evidence for genetically controlled *de novo* protein synthesis in response to treatment with β-naphthoflavone or phenobarbital. *J. Biol. Chem.*, 251:1817–1827.
38. Heidelberger, C. Y. (1975): Chemical carcinogenesis. *Annu. Rev. Biochem.*, 44:79–121.
39. Heimann, G., and Roth, B. (1975): Untersuchungen zur Reifung der Transportmechanismen der Leber für anionische Farbstoffe mit Hilfe der Indocyaningrün-Kinetik. *Klin. Wochenschr.*, 53:935.
40. Heimann, G., Roth, B., and Gladtke, E. (1977): Indocyaningrün-Kinetik bei Neugeborenen mit transitorischer Hyperbilirubinämie. *Klin. Wochenschr.*, 55:451–456.
41. Hwang, S. W., and Dixon, R. L. (1973): Perinatal development of indocyanine green biliary excretion in guinea pigs. *Am. J. Physiol.*, 225:1454–1459.
42. Iba, M. N., Soyka, L. F., and Schulman, M. P. (1975): Differential inhibition of drug metabolism by hepatic microsomal lipids of neonatal and adult rats. *Biochem. Biophys. Res. Commun.*, 65:870–876.
43. Iba, M. N., Soyka, L. F., and Schulman, M. P. (1977): Characteristics of the liver microsomal drug-metabolizing system of newborn rats. *Mol. Pharmacol.*, 13:1092–1104.
44. Inagaki, C. Y., and Tanaka, C. Y. (1974): Neonatal and senescent changes in L-aromatic amine acid decarboxylase and monoamine oxidase activities in kidney, liver, brain and heart of the rat. *Jpn. J. Pharmacol.*, 24:439–446.
45. Jansson, I., Orrenius, S., Ernster, L., and Schenkman, J. B. (1972): A study of the interaction of a series of substituted barbituric acids with the hepatic microsomal monooxygenase. *Arch. Biochem. Biophys.*, 151:391–400.
46. Jondorf, W. R., Maickel, R. P., and Brodie, B. B. (1959): Inability of newborn mice and guinea pigs to metabolize drugs. *Biochem. Pharmacol.*, 1:352–354.
47. Kato, R. (1966): Possible role of P-450 in the oxidation of drugs in liver microsomes. *J. Biochem. (Tokyo)*, 59:574–583.
48. Kato, R., and Takanaka, A. (1968): Metabolism of drugs in old rats: I. Activities of NADPH-linked electron transport and drug-metabolizing enzyme system in liver microsomes of old rats. *Jpn. J. Pharmacol.*, 18:381–388.
49. Khandwala, A. S., and Kasper, C. B. (1973): Preferential induction of aryl hydrocarbon hydroxylase activity in rat liver nuclear envelope by 3-methylcholanthrene. *Biochem. Biophys. Res. Commun.*, 54:1241–1246.

50. Kimura, H., and Yamashita, M. (1972): Studies on microsomal glucose-6-phosphate dehydrogenase of rat liver. *J. Biochem.*, 71:1009–1014.
51. Kitani, K., Kanai, S., Miura, R., Morita, Y., and Kasahara, M. (1978): The effect of ageing on the biliary excretion of ouabain in the rat. *Exp. Gerontol.*, 13:9–17.
52. Klaassen, C. D. (1972): Immaturity of the newborn rats hepatic excretory function for ouabain. *J. Pharmacol. Exp. Ther.*, 183:520–526.
53. Klaassen, C. D. (1973): Hepatic excretory function in the newborn rat. *J. Pharmacol. Exp. Ther.*, 184:721–728.
54. Klaassen, C. D. (1975): Biliary excretion of drugs: Role of ligandin in newborn immaturity and in the action if microsomal enzyme inducers. *J. Pharmacol. Exp. Ther.*, 195:311–319.
55. Klaassen, C. D. (1975): Biliary excretion of xenobiotics. *CRC Crit. Rev. Toxicol.*, 4:1:29.
56. Klaassen, C. D. (1978): Independence of bile acid and ouabain hepatic uptake: Studies in the newborn rat. *Proc. Soc. Exp. Biol. Med.*, 157:66–69.
57. Kleeberg, U., Barth, A., Roth, J., and Klinger, W. (1975): On the selectivity of aryl hydrocarbon hydroxylase induction after 3-methylcholanthrene pretreatment. *Acta Biol. Med. Germ.*, 34:1701–1705.
58. Kleeberg, U., Fischer, E., Gregus, Z., Klinger, W., and Varga, F. (1979): Effect of 3-methylcholanthrene on the biliary excretion of bromsulphthalein and eosine in newborn rats. *Acta Physiol. Acad. Sci. Hung.*, 53:363–367.
59. Kleeberg, U., Grohmann, G., Volkmann, R., Steinert, H., and Klinger, W. (1980): *In vivo* and *in vitro* inhibition of 3-methylcholanthrene-induced aryl hydrocarbon hydroxylase activity in rat liver by actinomycin D and 7,8-benzoflavone. *Pol. J. Pharmacol.*, 31:675–681.
60. Kleeberg, U., Szeberenyi, J., Juhasz, P., Tigyi, A., Klinger, T. W. (1980): Hepatic nuclear free and engaged RNA polymerases in young rats pretreated with 3-methylcholanthrene. *Arch. Toxicol. (Berl.) [Suppl.]*, 4:370–372.
61. Klinger, W. (1970): Toxizität, narkotische Wirkung, Aufwachkonzentration im Blut, Elimination aus dem Blut und Biotransformation von Hexobarbital bei Ratten unterschiedlichen Alters nach Induktion mit Barbital und nach $CCl_4$-Schädigung. *Arch. Int. Pharmacodyn. Ther.*, 184:5–18.
62. Klinger, W. (1971): [Age-dependence of enzyme induction by drugs] (Rus). *Farmakol. Toksikol.*, 34:199–209.
63. Klinger, W. (1972): [Kinetics of *N*-demethylation of amidopyrine by liver supernatant of newborn and adult rats under the influence of barbital, phenobarbital and phenylbutazone] (Rus). *Farmakol. Toksikol.*, 35:63–68.
64. Klinger, W. (1973): Biotransformation in der Leber. In: *Entwicklungspharmakologie*, edited by H. Ankermann, pp. 51–126. VEB Verlag Volk und Gesundheit, Berlin.
65. Klinger, W., Muller, D., and Kleeberg, U. (1978): Induction and its dependence on development. In: *The Induction of Drug Metabolism*, edited by R. W. Estabrook and F. Lindenlaub, pp. 517–544. F. K. Schattauer Verlag, Stuttgart, New York.
66. Klinger, W., Muller, D., Reichenbach, F., Kleeberg, U., Lubbe, H., and Rein, H. (1975): Developmental aspects of the microsomal electron-transport chain in the rat. In: *Basic and Therapeutic Aspects of Perinatal Pharmacology*, edited by P. L. Morselli, S. Garattini, and F. Sereni, pp. 255–264. Raven Press, New York.
67. Klinger, W., and Traeger, A. (1973): Extrahepatische Biotransformation. In: *Entwicklungspharmakologie*, edited by H. Ankermann, pp. 99–103. VEB Verlag Volk und Gesundheit, Berlin.
68. Krasner, J., Erikson, M., and Yaffe, S. J. (1974): Developmental changes in mouse liver alcohol dehydrogenase. *Biochem. Pharmacol.*, 23:519–522.
69. Krochmann, E. (1974): *Uber die Aufnahme von ³H-Digitoxin und ³H-Ouabain in Leberschnitte von Ratte und Maus und den Einfluss von Probenecid*. Med. Diss., Universität Hamburg, Hamburg.
70. Kroker, R. (1977): Influence of rifamycin on hepatic uptake and secretion of bile acids. *Naunyn Schmiedebergs Arch. Pharmacol.*, 297:R8.
71. Kuenzig, W., Kamm, J. J., Boublik, M., Jenkins, F., and Burns, J. J. (1974): Perinatal drug metabolism and morphological changes in the hepatocytes of normal and phenobarbital treated guinea pigs. *J. Pharmacol. Exp. Ther.*, 191:32–44.
72. Levi, A. J., Gatmaitan, Z., and Arias, I. M. (1969): Deficiency of hepatic organic anion-binding protein as a possible cause of nonhemolytic unconjugated hyperbilirubinemia in the newborn. *Lancet*, 2:139–142.

73. Levi, A. J., Gatmaitan, Z., and Arias, I. M. (1969): Two hepatic cytoplasmic protein fractions, Y and Z, and their possible role in the hepatic uptake of bilirubin, sulfobromophthalein, and other anions. *J. Clin. Invest.*, 48:2156–2167.

74. Levi, A. J., Gatmaitan, Z., and Arias, I. M. (1970): Deficiency of hepatic organic anion-binding protein, impaired organic anion uptake by liver and "physiologic" jaundice in newborn monkeys. *N. Engl. J. Med.*, 283:1136–1139.

75. Levine, R. I., Reyes, H., Levi, A. J., Gatmaitan, Z., and Arias, I. M. (1971): Phylogenetic study of organic anion transfer from plasma into the liver. *Nature [New Biol.]*, 231:277.

76. Lucier, G. W., Lui, E. M. K., and Lamartiniere, C. A. (1979): Metabolic activation/deactivation reactions during perinatal development. *Environ. Health Perspect.*, 29:7–16.

77. Lutz, W. K., and Schlatter, C. Y. (1979): *In vivo* covalent binding of chemicals to DNA as a short-term test for carcinogenicity. *Arch. Toxicol. (Berl.) [Suppl.]*, 2:411–415.

78. Martius, G., Zimmer, F., and Fackler, F. (1957): Untersuchungen uber die Leistungsfähigkeit der Leber in den ersten Lebenstagen. *Arch. Gynäkol.*, 188:539–545.

79. Maura, G., Vaccari, A., Gemignani, A., and Cugurra, F. (1974): Development of monoamine oxidase activity after chronic environmental stress in the rat. *Environ. Physiol. Biochem.*, 4:64–79.

80. McDevitt, D. G., Nies, A. S., and Wilkinson, G. R. (1977): Influence of phenobarbital on factors responsible for hepatic clearance of indocyanine green in the rat: Relative contributions of induction and altered liver blood flow. *Biochem. Pharmacol.*, 26:1247–1250.

81. MacLeod, S. M., Renton, K. W., and Eade, N. R. (1972): Development of hepatic microsomal drug-oxidizing enzymes in immature male and female rats. *J. Pharmacol. Exp. Ther.*, 183:489–498.

82. Meijer, D. K. F., Vonk, R. J., Keulemans, L., and Weitering, J. G. (1977): Hepatic uptake and biliary excretion of dibromosulphthalein. Albumin dependence, influence of phenobarbital and nafenopin pretreatment and the role of Y and Z protein. *J. Pharmacol. Exp. Ther.*, 202:8–21.

83. Miller, E. C. (1978): Some current perspectives on chemical carcinogenesis in humans and experimental animals: Presidential address. *Cancer Res.*, 38:1479–1496.

84. Müller, D. (1977): *Der Einfluss des Lebensalters und des Induktors Phenobarbital auf die Cytochrom-P-450-abhängige Monooxygenierung von Arzneimitteln in der Rattenleber.* Dissertation B, Friedrich-Schiller-Universität, Jena.

85. Müller, D., Förster, D., Dietze, H., Langenberg, R., and Klinger, W. (1973): The influence of age and barbital treatment on the content of cytochrome P-450 and b₅ and on the activity of glucose-6-phosphatase in microsomes of rat liver and kidney. *Biochem. Pharmacol.*, 22:905–910.

86. Müller, D., and Klinger, W. (1974): The influence of age, phenobarbital and carbontetrachloride on the bromsulphthalein binding to cytosol of various organs and on the bromsulphthaleine elimination from blood. *Acta Biol. Med. Germ.*, 32:211–218.

87. Müller, D., and Klinger, W. (1976): The binding of hexobarbital and aniline to cytochrome P-450 of liver microsomes from control and phenobarbital-treated rats of different ages. *Acta Biol. Med. Germ.*, 35:627–633.

88. Müller, D., and Klinger, W. (1978): The influence of age and of the inducer phenobarbital on the cytochrome P-450 dependent monooxygenation of drugs in rat liver. *Pharmazie*, 33:397–400.

89. Müller, D., Lübbe, H., and Klinger, W. (1975): The NADPH-dependent cytochrome P-450 reduction in liver microsomes of rats of different ages with and without phenobarbital pretreatment. *Acta Biol. Med. Germ.*, 34:1333–1337.

90. Müller, D., Reichenbach, F., and Klinger, W. (1971): Die Aktivität der Nitroreduktase und deren Induzierbarkeit durch Barbital in der Leber von Ratten verschiedenen Alters. *Acta Biol. Med. Germ.*, 27:605–609.

91. Nebert, D. W. (1970): Microsomal cytochromes b₅ and P-450 during induction of aryl hydrocarbon hydroxylase activity in mammalian cell culture. *J. Biol. Chem.*, 245:519–527.

92. Nebert, D. W., and Gelboin, H. V. (1968): Substrate-inducible microsomal aryl hydrocarbon hydroxylase in mammalian cell culture. I. Assay and properties of induced enzyme. *J. Biol. Chem.*, 243:6242–6249.

93. Nebert, D. W., and Gelboin, H. V. (1969): The *in vivo* and *in vitro* induction of aryl hydrocarbon hydroxylase in mammalian cells of different species, tissues, strains, and developmental and hormonal states. *Arch. Biochem. Biophys.*, 134:76–89.

94. Neims, A. H., Warner, M., Loughnan, P. M., and Aranda, J. V. (1976): Developmental aspects of the hepatic cytochrome P-450 monooxygenase system. *Annu. Rev. Pharmacol. Toxicol.*, 16:427–445.

95. Nies, A. L., McDevitt, D. G., and Wilkinson, G. R. (1975): Effect of drug concentration and enzyme inducers on indocyanine green clearance in the rat. In: *Sixth International Congress of Pharmacology*, Helsinki, p. 384.
96. Nordhoek, J., van den Berg, A. P., Savenije-Chapel, E. M., and Koopman-Kool, E. (1976): Metabolism of hexobarbital enantiomers and interaction with cytochrome P-450 in male and female mice and rats. *Hoppe Seylers Z. Physiol. Chem.*, 357:1045–1046.
97. Nunnink, J. C., Chuang, A. H. L., and Bresnick, E. (1978): The ontogeny of nuclear aryl hydrocarbon hydroxylase. *Chem. Biol. Interact.*, 22:225–230.
98. Oesch, F. (1976): Differential control of rat microsomal "aryl hydrocarbon" monooxygenase and epoxide hydratase. *J. Biol. Chem.*, 251:79–87.
99. Parvez, H., Gripois, D., and Parvez, S. (1976): Corticosteroid influence on the postnatal development of monoamine oxidase activity in the young rat. *Biol. Neonate.*, 28:326–335.
100. Paumgartner, G. (1975): The handling of indocyanine green by the liver. *Schweiz. Med. Wochenschr.*, [Suppl.], 17:1–30.
101. Paumgartner, G., and Reichen, J. (1975): Different pathways for hepatic uptake of taurocholate and indocyanine green. *Experientia*, 31:306–308.
102. Pelkonen, O. (1977): Transplacental transfer of foreign compounds and their metabolism by the foetus. In: *Progress in Drug Metabolism, Vol. 2*, edited by J. W. Bridges and L. F. Chasseaud, pp. 119–161. Wiley, London.
103. Pelkonen, O. (1978): Prenatal and Neonatal Development of Drug and Carcinogen Metabolism. In: *The Induction of Drug Metabolism*, edited by R. W. Estabrook and F. Lindenlaub, pp. 507–516. F. K. Schattauer Verlag, Stuttgart, New York.
104. Pelkonen, O., Arvela, P., and Kärki, N. T. (1971): 3,4-Benzpyrene and *N*-methylaniline metabolizing enzyme in the immature human foetus and placenta. *Acta Pharmacol. Toxicol. (Kbh.)*, 30:385–395.
105. Räihä, N. C. R., and Pikkarainen, P. H. (1971): The development of alcohol dehydrogenase and its isoenzymes. In: *Metabolic Changes Induced by Alcohol*, edited by G. A. Martini and C. Bode, pp. 1–7. Springer Verlag, Berlin, Heidelberg, New York.
106. Rogan, E. G., Mailander, P., and Cavalieri, E. (1976): Metabolic activation of aromatic hydrocarbons in purified rat liver nuclei: Induction of enzyme activities and binding to DNA with and without formation of active oxygen. *Proc. Natl. Acad. Sci. U.S.A.*, 73:457–461.
107. Sandström, B. (1972): The inception time of bile secretion during development of the liver in chicken and rat. *Acta Hepatogastroenterol.*, 19:170–172.
108. Schenkman, J. B., Remmer, H., and Estabrook, R. W. (1967): Spectral studies of drug interaction with hepatic microsomal cytochrome. *Mol. Pharmacol.*, 3:113–123.
109. Short, C. R., and Davis, L. E. (1970): Perinatal development of drug-metabolizing enzyme activity in swine. *J. Pharmacol. Exp. Ther.*, 174:185–196.
110. Short, C. R., Maines, M. D., and Westfall, B. A. (1972): Postnatal development of drug-metabolizing enzyme activity in liver and extrahepatic tissue of swine. *Biol. Neonate*, 21:54–68.
111. Short, C. R., and Stith, R. D. (1973): Perinatal development of hepatic microsomal mixed function oxidase activity in swine. *Biochem. Pharmacol.*, 22:1309–1319.
112. Sinclair, A. J. (1974): Fatty acid composition of liver lipids during development of rat. *Lipids*, 9:809–818.
113. Sladek, N. E., Chaplin, M. D., and Mannering, G. J. (1974): Sex-dependent differences in drug metabolism in the rat. IV. Effect of morphine administration. *Drug Metab. Dispos.*, 2:293–300.
114. Stanton, H. C., Cornejo, R. A., Mersmann, H. J., Brown, L. J., and Mueller, R. L. (1975): Ontogenesis of monoamine oxidase and catechol-*O*-methyl-transferase in various tissues of domestic swine. *Arch. Int. Pharmacodyn. Ther.*, 213:128–144.
115. Stoming, T. A., and Bresnick, E. (1974): Hepatic epoxide hydrase in neonates and partially hepatectomized rats. *Cancer Res.*, 34:2810.
116. Strobel, H. W., Lu, A. Y. H., Heidema, J., and Coon, M. J. (1970): Phosphatidyl choline requirement in the enzymatic reduction of hemoprotein P-450 in fatty acid, hydrocarbon, and drug hydroxylation. *J. Biol. Chem.*, 245:4851–4854.
117. Szeberenyi, J., Kleeberg, U., and Gaal, J. (1980): Hepatic nuclear protein kinases in young rats pretreated with 3-methylcholanthrene. *Arch. Toxicol. (Berl.) [Suppl.]*, 4:373–375.
118. Tredger, J. M., Chhabra, R. S., and Fouts, J. R. (1976): Postnatal development of mixed function oxidation as measured in microsomes from the small intestine and liver of rabbits. *Drug Metab. Dispos.*, 4:17–24.

119. Uehleke, H. (1973): The role of cyt P-450 in the *N*-oxidation of individual amines. *Drug. Metab. Dispos.*, 1:299–313.
120. Vaccari, A., Cugurra, F., and Maura, G. (1972): Development of tissue monoamine oxidase activity in the newborn rat. *Arch. Int. Pharmacodyn. Ther.*, 196:314.
121. Varga, F., and Fischer, E. (1978): Age-dependent changes in blood supply of the liver and in the biliary excretion of eosine in rats. In: *Liver and Aging*, edited by K. Kitani, pp. 327–340. Elsevier/ North-Holland Biomedical Press, Amsterdam.
122. Vaught, J., and Bresnick, E. (1976): Binding of polycyclic hydrocarbons to nuclear components *in vitro*. *Biochem. Biophys. Res. Commun.*, 69:587–591.
123. Whelan, G., Hoch, J., Schenker, S., and Combes, B. (1970): Impaired hepatic disposition of sulfobromophthalein sodium in neonatal guinea pigs: Nature of the defect. *J. Lab. Clin. Med.*, 76:775–789.
124. Wiebel, F. J., and Gelboin, H. V. (1975): Aryl hydrocarbon [benzo(*a*)pyrene] hydroxylase in liver from rats of different age, sex, and nutritional status. *Biochem. Pharmacol.*, 24:1511–1515.
125. Wiebel, F. J., Leutz, J. C., Diamond, L., and Gelboin, H. V. (1971): Aryl hydrocarbon benzo(*a*)pyrene hydroxylase in microsomes from rat tissues: Differential inhibition and stimulation by benzoflavones and organic solvents. *Arch. Biochem. Biophys.*, 144:78–86.
126. Windorfer, A., Kuenzer, W., and Urbanek, R. (1974): The influence of age on the activity of acetylsalicylic acid-esterase and protein-salicylate binding, *Eur. J. Clin. Pharmacol.*, 7:227–231.
127. Wirth, P. J., and Thorgeirsson, S. S. (1978): Amine oxidase in mice—sex differences and developmental aspects. *Biochem. Pharmacol.*, 27:601–603.
128. Zamboni, L. (1965): Electron microscopic studies of blood embryogenesis in humans: I. The ultrastructure of the fetal liver. *J. Ultrastruct. Res.*, 12:509–524.

*Developmental Toxicology*, edited by
C. A. Kimmel and J. Buelke-Sam. Raven Press,
New York © 1981.

# Developmental Aspects of Drug Conjugation

## George W. Lucier

*National Institute of Environmental Health Sciences, Research Triangle Park,
North Carolina 27709*

The process of xenobiotic biotransformation is often divided into two parts. Phase I pathways include the cytochrome P-450-dependent monooxygenase system which catalyzes oxidative reactions such as arene oxide formation, *N*- and *C*-hydroxylation, *N*-dealkylation and desulfuration. Depending on the substrate metabolized, these reactions can result in the conversion of an inactive precursor to an electrophilic metabolite capable of binding covalently to nucleophilic nitrogen, oxygen, or sulfur atoms of cellular macromolecules such as DNA, RNA, or protein (51). It is widely accepted that macromolecules can be damaged from this interaction and thereby initiate various forms of toxicity including carcinogenesis, mutagenesis, and teratogenesis. Phase 2 reactions include the pathways of glucuronidation, sulfation, glutathione conjugation, and *N*-acetylation. Conjugation pathways of xenobiotic metabolism are generally considered a detoxication step because these reactions render the molecule less lipophilic and more excretable. However, conjugation reactions can, in some cases, produce reactive electrophilic metabolites (5,38,39) or can stimulate activation reactions by lessening the influence of product inhibition of arene oxide formation (13). A general scheme illustrating the possible roles of activation/deactivation reactions is presented in Fig. 1, and the dual role of some common drug metabolizing enzyme reactions is tabulated in Table 1.

The purpose of this perspective review on the development of conjugative enzymes is fourfold: (a) to describe the ontogeny of the important conjugative pathways in experimental animals and humans, including information on the complex regulatory mechanisms involved in the developmental onset of enzyme synthesis and the maintenance of adult levels of enzyme activity; (b) to evaluate the ways

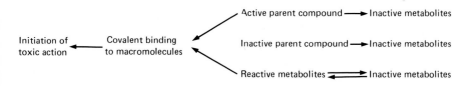

**FIG. 1.** Diagrammatic pathways for metabolic activation/deactivation of foreign chemicals.

TABLE 1. *Dual role of drug-metabolizing reactions*

| Enzyme Reaction | Activation | Deactivation |
|---|---|---|
| Epoxidation | + | + |
| Hydroxylation | + | + |
| Glucuronidation | + | + |
| Epoxide hydration | + | + |
| Sulfation | + | + |

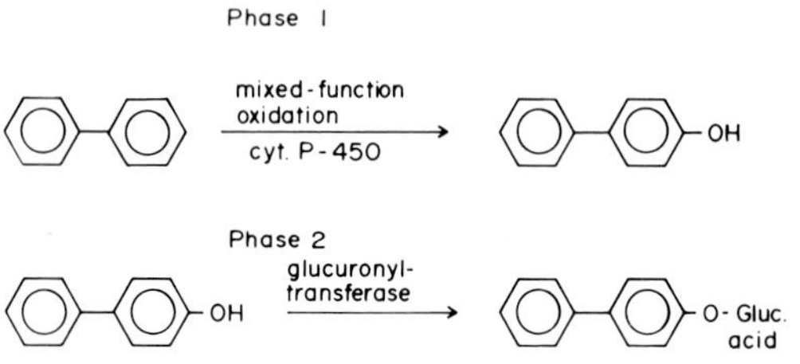

FIG. 2. Schematic representation of glucuronidation of hydroxylated biphenyl.

in which the ontogeny of conjugative processes can be altered, such as enzyme induction or hormonally mediated changes in the sex differentiation of enzyme synthesis; (c) to review the pharmacological and toxicological significance of age-dependent function of conjugative enzymes using the polychlorinated biphenyls (PCBs) and diethylstilbestrol (DES) as examples; and finally, (d) to summarize the experimental problems associated with studies dealing with the role of conjugation reactions in developmental toxicity, including the importance of age-dependent changes in the balance between activation and deactivation systems.

## ONTOGENY OF CONJUGATIVE REACTIONS

### UDP Glucuronyltransferase

One of the more important and routinely measured conjugative enzymes is UDP glucuronyltransferase (UDPGT). A schematic representation of UDPGT catalysis of drug conjugation is presented in Fig. 2; enzyme activity requires the presence of the cofactor UDP glucuronic acid (UDPGA).

A schematic composite of UDPGT ontogeny for one group of substrates in rat liver is summarized in Fig. 3A (18,23,26,32,52). For this group of substrates, the onset of UDPGT activity occurs 5 days prior to birth followed by a dramatic increase in activity such that glucuronidation rates at birth exceed adult levels. Substrates exhibiting this characteristic developmental profile of glucuronidation rates include 2-aminophenol, 2-aminobenzoate, 4-nitrophenol, 1-naphthol, 4-methylumbellifer-one, and 5-hydroxytryptamine (25,26,52,54). A second group of substrates have a qualitatively different ontogeny, and these are termed Group II substrates. Rat

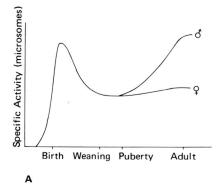

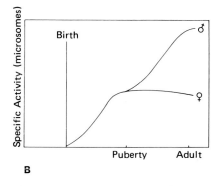

A

B

**FIG. 3.** Developmental pattern of glucu-ronidation of (**A**) Group I substrates and (**B**) Group II substrates.

liver microsomal UDPGT does not have detectable activity towards Group II sub-strates until the day prior to birth, and adult activities are not reached until the end of the first postnatal week (Fig. 3B). Group II substrates include bilirubin, testos-terone, β-estradiol, estrone, DES, phenolphthalein, morphine, and chloramphenicol (25,26,52,54).

In addition to developmental patterns, the concept of functional heterogeneity of UDPGT is supported by several other criteria. These are outlined in Table 2 and include differences in tissue distribution of UDPGT, inducibility by 2,3,7,8-te-trachlorodibenzo-*p*-dioxin, neonatal response to glucocorticoids, route of glucu-ronide excretion, and submicrosomal distribution (25,54). In general, Group I glucuronidation rates are high in extrahepatic tissues such as kidney and reproductive tract, whereas Group II substrates are, for the most part, glucuronidated slowly or not at all by extrahepatic microsomal preparations (26). Hepatic UDPGT activity towards Group I substrates in neonatal and adult rats is induced by pretreatment with TCDD and 3-methylcholanthrene but not phenobarbital, whereas Group II substrates are induced only by phenobarbital-type inducers (53). These studies suggest that induction of hepatic UDPGT activity towards Group I substrates seg-regates with the induction of cytochrome P-448-dependent monooxygenases, whereas Group II UDPGT inducibility segregates with the response of the cytochrome P-450 system. These findings suggest the possibility of a functional coupling for hepatic monooxygenase and UDPGT in the endoplasmic reticulum.

Studies assessing the functional heterogeneity of UDPGT in neonatal and adult liver have implicated molecular characteristics of the substrate as the critical factors in determining which UDPGT catalyzes glucuronidation of a given substrate. In general, Group I substrates have a lower molecular weight and are less lipophilic than Group II substrates. This relationship was further expanded by Wishart and Dutton using a series of alkylated phenols. A limiting configuration was defined for glucuronidation of Group I substrates by UDPGT in which the length of alkyl side chains determined which form of UDPGT acted on the substrate (54). Other studies have demonstrated that substrates having steroidal activity exhibit glucuronidation characteristics of Group II substrates, whereas those not having steroidal activity are glucuronidated as Group I substrates (26).

Although clear evidence has been documented for the functional heterogeneity of hepatic UDPGT, corresponding demonstration of physical heterogeneity is not conclusive. Enzyme purification studies have separated multiple forms of UDPGT, but these proteins may not correspond to the available evidence on functional differences based on substrate glucuronidation rates (3,4).

Much of the work on the mechanisms for the developmental onset of UDPGT has been conducted and reviewed by Dutton (10). These studies have established a critical role for glucocorticoids in the onset of UDPGT activity towards Group I substrates. Evidence for glucocorticoid inducibility of at least one form of fetal hepatic UDPGT includes (a) premature fetal onset of Group I UDPGT by dexamethasone administration to pregnant rats, (b) prevention of developmental onset by fetal hypophysectomy of rats, and (c) correlation of developmental onset with fetal synthesis of active glucocorticoids. Although Group I UDPGT is induced prematurely in rat fetuses by dexamethasone, this treatment will not initiate Group II UDPGT synthesis (52).

Developmental patterns for UDPGT in extrahepatic tissues vary considerably. In general, extrahepatic tissues in fetuses of experimental animals do not contain

TABLE 2. *Criteria for functional heterogeneity of UDP glucuronyltransferase*

| Criteria | Group I substrates | Group II substrates |
|---|---|---|
| Developmental peak at birth | + | − |
| Induction of glucuronidation by TCDD | + | − |
| Glucuronidation by extrahepatic tissues | + | − |
| Glucuronides excreted predominately in urine | + | − |
| Induction of hepatic glucuronidation in fetal rats by glucocorticoids | + | − |

significant UDPGT (31). For example, the developmental peak for Group I UDPGT is not seen in fetal rabbit, rat, or guinea pig kidney and lung (31). Enzyme activity in these tissues usually appears by the first week after birth, and adult levels are approached during the second postnatal week. These studies suggest that the differential ages for the onset of detectable UDPGT activities in different tissues are probably related to tissue-specific activation of UDPGT synthesis.

UDP glucoronyltransferase activity is present in nuclear as well as microsomal preparations (12), but no information is available on organelle-specific ontogeny in humans or experimental animals of either the monooxygenase or UDPGT system. In contrast to experimental animals, human fetal liver contains little or no UDPGT activity (44). No information is available concerning the existence or ontogeny of multiple forms of UDPGT in human fetuses.

### Sulfotransferase

Sulfotransferase (ST) is a family of cytosolic enzymes that catalyze the transfer of active sulfate from 3′-phosphoadenosine-5′-phosphosulfate (PAPS) to steroids and xenobiotics (43). Sulfation is generally considered a detoxication reaction, but the sulfate ester of the *N*-hydroxy metabolite of acetylaminofluorene (AAF) is a reactive electrophile (38,39). Moreover, the sulfate conjugates of several other compounds can bind covalently to cellular macromolecules including *N*-hydroxy-phenacetin and *N*-hydroxy-2-acetylaminonaphthalene (38). In addition, the glucuronide of *N*-hydroxyphenacetin binds covalently to protein but at a slower rate than the corresponding *N*-*O*-sulfate metabolite (38). It is difficult to assess the relative importance of conjugates in some forms of carcinogenesis because of the concentration of conjugates in body fluids. For example, the susceptibility of the bladder to the carcinogenic activity of aromatic amines may be related to the high concentration of conjugates in the urine. In addition to sulfation of foreign chemicals, the formation of sulfate esters of steroid hormones is integral to some steroidogenic pathways (16,17).

Although data on the ontogeny of sulfotransferase is limited, ontogeny and partial purification studies have demonstrated enzyme multiplicity (48). Sexual differentiation of sulfotransferase is substrate dependent for sulfation of a variety of glucocorticoids and steroids (48). The possible importance of sulfation and glucuronidation pathways in the initiation of mutagenic and carcinogenic reactions and the role of these enzymes in regulation of hormone action coupled with the recent findings of multiple UDPGT and ST forms make it difficult to evaluate the contribution of sulfates and glucuronides to developmental toxicity. Because of these complexities, the metabolic pathways of each chemical need to be investigated at several developmental stages with the ultimate goal of determining levels of toxic metabolites at the target site.

### Glutathione *S*-Aryl Transferase

The microsomal monooxygenase system catalyzes epoxide formation (arene or alkene oxides) of a wide range of olefinic and aromatic chemicals. As discussed at the beginning of this chapter, epoxides are often reactive intermediates, since they can bind covalently to DNA, RNA, and proteins to presumably initiate a toxic response, e.g., carcinogenesis, mutagenesis, teratogenesis, or organ-specific toxicity. Epoxides can be further metabolized by epoxide hydratase to form a diol or conjugated with glutathione by a complex of cytosolic enzymes termed collectively glutathione transferases. Both epoxide-metabolizing enzymes function as deactivation pathways (40), although epoxide diols of benzpyrene are also highly reactive and potentially toxic metabolites as illustrated in a general scheme for the metabolism of benzpyrene by both oxidative and conjugative pathways (Fig. 4).

Comparative developmental studies in mice, guinea pigs, and rabbits have demonstrated that ontogeny of epoxide hydratase and glutathione S-transferases is organ specific; liver, lung, intestine, and kidney were investigated (19). Both glutathione S-aryl transferase and glutathione S-epoxide transferase exhibited similar developmental patterns in any one organ. Of particular interest from a toxicological viewpoint was the finding that activities of pulmonary glutathione transferases were similar in both fetal and adult rabbits and guinea pigs. In contrast, epoxide hydratase activities were low in fetal tissues, and the ontogeny of this microsomal enzyme was similar to the development of aryl hydrocarbon hydroxylase and other monooxygenase components (19,41). However, the balance between epoxide formation and epoxide deactivation is age dependent and may be related to age-dependent differences in susceptibility to organ-specific toxicity.

## MODIFICATIONS OF ONTOGENY

The microsomal monooxygenase system and many of the conjugative enzymes, most notably UDPGT, can be induced or repressed by a wide variety of chemicals such as polycyclic hydrocarbons, halogenated aromatics, barbiturates, and hormones. Considerable information is also available on the perinatal effects of these chemicals on metabolic activation/deactivation reactions following transplacental and/or lactational exposures. In this chapter, two mechanisms whereby the devel-

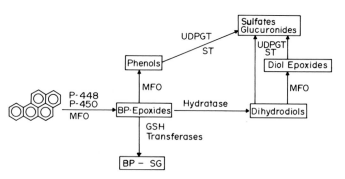

**FIG. 4.** Metabolic pathways for benzo(a)pyrene. Abbreviations are as follows: BP, benzo(a)pyrene; MFO, mixed function oxidases; GSH, glutathione; UDPGT, UDP glucuronyltransferase; ST, sulfotransferase; BP-SG, glutathione conjugate of benzo(a)pyrene.

opmental patterns of drug-metabolizing enzymes can be altered will be reviewed and discussed. One of these mechanisms involves perinatal alteration of enzyme activity as a direct result of the interaction of inducing chemicals with the cellular machinery that regulates protein synthesis in target cells. This effect does not persist long after the inducing chemical has been metabolized and/or excreted. The second mechanism is commonly termed imprinting. This mechanism deals with the ability of neonatal rat hormones to permanently and irreversibly alter subsequent hepatic metabolic competence in adulthood.

### Perinatal Induction

Polycyclic hydrocarbons and many halogenated aromatics such as the polychlorinated biphenyls (PCBs), 2,3,7,8-tetrachlorodibenzo-*p*-dioxin (TCDD), DDT, chlordecone (Kepone®), and several others are inducers of hepatic and extrahepatic monooxygenases in adult experimental animals. The capacity of these same chemicals to induce the monooxygenase system and UDPGT has also been investigated in developing animals. In general, induction characteristics in perinatal systems are similar to those observed in mature animals. For example, the potent inducing agent, TCDD, stimulates activity of aryl hydrocarbon hydroxylase (AHH), cytochrome P-448, and UDPGT and represses activity of oxidative dealkylation reactions in postnatal rats of all ages (2,28,32).

Distinct structure–activity relationships have been defined for the ability of pure PCB congeners to induce activity of either cytochrome P-450- or cytochrome P-448-dependent monooxygenase reactions (14). Induction of UDPGT correlates more closely with induction of cytochrome P-448 (42), whereas only cytochrome P-450 inducers are capable of stimulating glutathione transferase activity (1,22). Similar structure–activity relationships are expressed in early postnatal and immature rats (27). For example, 3,4-3′,4′-tetrachlorobiphenyl (4-CB) induces cytochrome P-448, AHH, biphenyl hydroxylase, and UDPGT (Group I and Group II) in rat liver, whereas 2,4,5-2′,4′,5′-hexachlorobiphenyl (6-CB) induces cytochrome P-450, aminopyrine demethylation, ethylmorphine demethylation, $16\alpha$-hydroxylation of testosterone, glutathione *S*-aryl transferase, and, to a slight extent, Group I UDPGT. Activity of the steroid-metabolizing enzyme, $5\alpha$-reductase is repressed in newborn rats by exposure to 4-CB but is unaffected by 6-CB. Structure–activity relationships are similar for the response of hepatic and extrahepatic tissues to PCB inductive actions. These findings demonstrate that precise structure–activity relationships exist for the ability of halogenated aromatics to induce or repress activities of specific hepatic enzyme systems during development as well as in adult animals.

Effects of chemicals on enzyme development of offspring following treatment of pregnant animals may result either from lactational or transplacental exposures. To assess the contribution of each route of exposure on developmental pharmacology and toxicity, cross-fostering protocols are routinely used. These types of studies have been employed to investigate the effects of halogenated aromatics on enzyme development (27,32). Aryl hydrocarbon hydroxylase is inducible in fetal livers following treatment of pregnant rats with 3μg TCDD/kg on days 5, 10, or 15 of gestation. The magnitude of induction of hepatic AHH in offspring of rats treated with TCDD during gestation is greater than that seen in fetal livers. This increased level of induction postnatally appears to be related to lactational exposure to TCDD. Subsequent tissue distribution studies revealed that relatively small quantities of TCDD pass the placenta compared to greater amounts of TCDD secreted in milk (24). Moreover, the level of TCDD-mediated induction of the drug-metabolizing enzymes appears to be directly related to the TCDD body burden independent of developmental stage. Similar studies on the perinatal pharmacology of pure PCB congeners demonstrated that PCBs, like TCDD, pass the placenta and are secreted in high concentrations in milk (30; G. W. Lucier, *unpublished observations*). Induction of placental and fetal AHH and UDPGT by chemicals is of potential importance to developmental toxicity, since fetal exposure to reactive metabolites may be regulated by the balance between activation/deactivation reactions in placental and fetal tissue.

During recent years, considerable attention has been focused on the mechanism of induction of AHH and UDPGT by polycyclic hydrocarbons and halogenated aromatics. A specific hepatic cytosolic receptor, analogous to receptors for steroid hormones, has been characterized which binds those polycyclics and organohalogens capable of inducing cytochrome P-448 and UDPGT (46). Inducers of the cytochrome P-450 system do not bind to the receptor. This binding protein possesses the criteria usually assigned to receptors: high affinity for ligand ($K_d$ of approximately $10^{-10}$ M); finite capacity; high degree of binding specificity; and translocation of ligand–receptor complex to the nucleus. Studies on the genetic regulation of UDPGT and AHH in inbred strains of mice have suggested the possibility of a common receptor in the regulation of both enzyme induction processes and have shown that the level of receptor corresponds with the magnitude of hepatic AHH and UDPGT-induction by polycyclics (42,45,46).

Ontogeny studies have detected significant amounts of receptor protein in fetal and newborn liver (7). Biochemical and functional characteristics of the receptor appear similar in both neonatal and adult liver. The quantity of receptor during development corresponds to the magnitude of induction of AHH by polycyclics (7). Although ontogeny studies of receptor have not been conducted in extrahepatic tissues, the receptor protein has been detected in those tissues that are responsive to the inductive actions of TCDD (6).

## Imprinting of Hepatic Enzymes

Activational effects, such as enzyme induction or repression, are reversible responses and reflect direct action that requires the presence of the effector. In contrast, organizational effects are developmental responses that occur during a limited critical period of fetal or early postnatal development and produce permanent effects manifested in adults. Expression of organizational effects usually occurs with the onset of sexual differentiation and can result in higher enzyme activities in one sex than the other. This process has been defined as "programming" or "imprinting." Examples of sexual differentiation of hepatic UDPGT (both Group I and Group II enzymes) are illustrated in Fig. 3. Aryl hydrocarbon hydroxylase undergoes a similar developmental pattern as characterized by the absence of sex differences in pre-pubertal rats and markedly higher enzyme activities in postpubertal males.

The mechanism for the imprinting process is not entirely clear but seems to be initiated during a critical period of development immediately following birth (11,15,36). It has been postulated (11,15,36) that adult masculine-type metabolism is dependent on neonatal androgen exposure. Conversion of androgen to estrogen can take place in neural tissues of fetal and neonatal rats, and this conversion might be required for androgen action in the neonatal brain (36). Furthermore, it has been suggested that $\alpha$-fetoprotein, which is an effective binder of some estrogens but a poor binder of testosterone, can prevent exposure of the neonatal female brain to circulating estrogens. The expression and maintenance of the organization mechanism is dependent on the pituitary–hypothalamic axis (9,20,23,29). It, therefore, appears that the hormonal environment during a critical period of development may result in latent, but permanent and irreversible, effects on hepatic metabolic activation/deactivation systems.

Various methods have been used to alter the hormonal milieu in newborn rats. The most common procedure is neonatal castration followed by hormone replacement, usually administration of testosterone proprionate during days 2 to 6 following birth. Using this protocol, data have been generated which reveal that the sensitive period for androgen-induced imprinting of the apparent $K_m$ of ethylmorphine $N$-demethylase differs from the imprinting of $V_{max}$ and androgen responsiveness of enzyme in subsequent adult rats (8).

Later studies have investigated the imprinting of the monooxygenase system by a chemically mediated reversible castration procedure. Methadone administered to neonatal rats significantly reduces circulating androgen levels during the critical period of brain differentiation (33). This procedure resulted in the feminization of the apparent $K_m$ for ethylmorphine $N$-demethylation in subsequent adult males; no changes in $K_m$ were evident in immature rats of either sex or adult females. Moreover, $V_{max}$ was not changed in immature or mature rats of either sex. Circulating androgen levels and gonadal development in adult males exposed neonatally to methadone were not different from controls, suggesting that methadone-mediated feminization of liver enzymes must involve mechanisms other than effects on androgen biosynthesis in subsequent adults.

Sex differences in rat hepatic conjugative enzymes also appear to be imprinted neonatally by androgens. Glutathione transferase and UDPGT activities are feminized in adult males that were castrated immediately after birth (21,23). In contrast, castration of adult males did not feminize enzyme activity. Hypophysectomy of adult rats results in lowered UDPGT activities and elevated glutathione transferase activities. Therefore, the pituitary is responsible for positive modulation in the former and negative modulation in the latter. Hypophysectomy of adult rats also abolished sex differences of these enzymes implicating the role of the pituitary in the expression of sex differences in hepatic conjugative enzyme activity (21,23). Furthermore, implantation of an ectopic pituitary under the kidney capsule of hypophysectomized rats was capable of reversing the feminizing effects of hypophysectomy on hepatic glutathione S-transferase (21) but not on UDPGT, suggesting that different regulatory models are operative for the sex differentiation of these two conjugative pathways. The maintenance of sex differences in glutathione transferase activity appears to be regulated by a hypothalamic inhibiting factor that is programmed for by neonatal androgens (21). Pituitary regulation of UDPGT sex differences appears also to involve a hypothalamic releasing factor (23).

The hormonal environment can also be changed neonatally by administering synthetic and natural hormones to newborn rats, and these changes can alter hepatic sex differentiation. For example, pharmacological doses of either DES or testosterone proprionate administered to newborn rats prevented the subsequent sex differentiation of hepatic monooxygenases and UDPGT (23,34). This treatment adversely affected gonadal development, but endocrine measurements demonstrated that the mechanism for altered sex differentiation must involve more than gonadal effects. A schematic representation of endocrine control of hepatic metabolism is given in Fig. 5.

The most important consequence of imprinting (both normal and altered) of hepatic metabolism involves the role of metabolic factors in the production of groups at risk to hepatotoxicity and/or liver-mediated forms of organ-specific toxicity. For example, adult male rats that had received testosterone or DES only during the neonatal period exhibited decreased sensitivity (feminization) towards the hepatotoxic effects of cadmium as measured by effects on hepatic enzymes (34) and histological evaluations (E. M. K. Lui, *personal communication*). The sex-dependent response to cadmium is under pituitary–hypothalamic control and is associated with the amount of cadmium-sensitive forms of cytochrome P-450 (29,35). These types of studies suggest that hormone action during a critical period of early development might irreversibly program sensitivity or resistance to toxic reactions including carcinogenesis. In fact, previous studies have demonstrated that neonatal exposure to estrogens increases the incidence of N-hydroxy-N-2-fluorenylacetamide

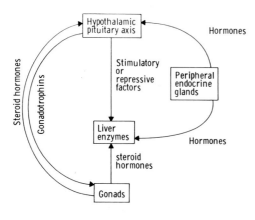

**FIG. 5.** Postulated mechanisms for the endocrine regulation of hepatic enzyme synthesis as a consequence of the imprinting of pituitary control of hepatic function by neonatal hormones.

(N-OH FAA)-induced hepatocarcinogenesis in adult animals exposed to the carcinogen in diet (50). The increase in carcinogenesis appears to be at least in part related to alterations in rate of detoxification of N-OH FAA via the glucuronide pathway (49). These studies provide further evidence for the importance of endocrine status during development in determining susceptibility to carcinogenesis.

### Role of Conjugative Enzymes in Developmental Pharmacology

Perinatal developmental patterns alone have limited value. However, experiments have been performed to determine if the perinatal developmental patterns of conjugative enzymes exert a regulatory function in perinatal pharmacokinetics. For example, studies involving administration of $^3$H-DES to pregnant mice demonstrated that fetal glucuronidation of DES plays an important role in fetal accumulation of radioactivity (25,47). Radioactivity at the later stages of gestation was primarily in the form of glucuronides, and these glucuronides must have been formed in the fetal compartment, since glucuronides are too polar to pass the placenta. During the early gestational ages, when fetal DES UDPGT activities are low or undetectable, only small amounts of $^3$H-DES glucuronide were present in fetal tissues. As hepatic DES UDPGT activities increase, levels of $^3$H-DES glucuronide in the fetal compartment increase concomitantly. This finding might have toxicological significance in that DES glucuronide should not be readily cleared from the fetal compartment and DES could be liberated from the fetal DES-glucuronide pool by β-glucuronidase. Further studies are needed to ascertain the balance between activation (37) and deactivation reactions of DES during different stages of development to gain a clearer understanding of the role of metabolic factors in transplacental toxic effects of DES and other hormonally-active chemicals.

A similar role for UDPGT has been proposed for the regulation of PCB disposition in fetal rats (25,30). Perinatal disposition studies revealed that glucuronide metabolites of hydroxylated PCBs accumulate in the fetal compartment. Glucuronides formed in the fetus will not pass back to the maternal compartment because of the polar nature of glucuronides (17).

It is concluded that the perinatal development of UDPGT plays an important role in the pharmacology (Fig. 6) and perhaps toxicity of many foreign chemicals. This enzyme system also appears to function in the metabolic regulation of steroid hormones during development and is sensitive to chemical insult in newborn as well as adult animals.

## CONCLUSIONS

The role of activation/deactivation reactions in drug disposition and developmental toxicology is not well understood and is complicated by a large number of variables not encountered in mature systems. Some of these variables are as follows:

1. Different developmental patterns of specific enzymes that cause the balance between activation/deactivation reactions for substrate metabolism to fluctuate dramatically in an age-dependent manner.

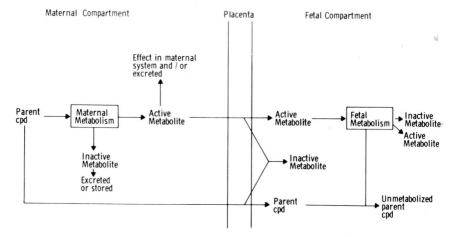

**FIG. 6.** Role of maternal, placental, and fetal tissues in the generation and retention of active and inactive metabolites of foreign compounds. In general, the fetal compartment is not capable of excreting metabolities, which means that in some cases there is fetal accumulation of both active and inactive metabolites.

2. Relative importance of maternal and fetal metabolism: does metabolic activation of specific toxins occur in the maternal or fetal compartment?

3. The role of maternal and placental metabolism in placental transfer of chemicals as influenced by changes in molecular polarity.

4. Relative importance of hepatic and extrahepatic metabolism during development as a determinant of age-dependent differences in organ-specific toxicity.

5. Chemical- and disease-mediated alterations in developmental patterns of enzyme systems as related to the generation of groups at risk to toxicity.

6. Sex differences in developmental patterns that may lead to sex-dependent as well as age-dependent differences in toxicity.

7. Extrapolation of animal data to the human condition as complicated by species differences in ontogeny of key enzyme systems.

## REFERENCES

1. Baars, A. J., Jansen, M., and Breimer, D. D. (1978): The influence of phenobarbital, 3-methylcholanthrene, and 2,3,7,8-tetrachlorodibenzo-*p*-dioxin on glutathione *S*-transferase activity of rat liver cytosol. *Biochem. Pharmacol.*, 27:2487–2494.
2. Berry, D. L., Zachariah, P. K., Namkung, M. J., and Juchau, M. R. (1976): Transplacental induction of carcinogen hydroxylating systems with 2,3,7,8-tetrachlorodibenzo-p-dioxin. *Toxicol. Appl. Pharmacol.*, 36:569–584.
3. Billings, R. E., Tephly, T. R., and Tukey, R. H. (1978): The separation and purification of estrone and *p*-nitrophenol UDP glucuronyltransferase activities. In: *Conjugation Reactions in Drug Biotransformation*, edited by A. Aitio, pp. 365–376. Elsevier/North-Holland, Amsterdam.
4. Bock, K. W., Kittel, J., and Dosting, D. (1978): Purification of rat liver UDP glucuronyl-transferase. In: *Conjugation Reactions in Drug Biotransformation*, edited by A. Aitio, pp. 357–364. Elsevier/North-Holland, Amsterdam.
5. Cardona, R. A., and King, C. M. (1976): Activation of the *O*-glucuronide of the carcinogen *N*-hydroxy-*N*-2-fluorenylacetamide by enzymatic deacetylation *in vitro*: Formation of fluorenylamine–tRNA adducts. *Biochem. Pharmacol.*, 25:1051–1056.

6. Carlstedt-Duke, J. M. B. (1979): Tissue distribution of the receptor for 2,3,7,8-tetrachlorodibenzo-*p*-dioxin in the rat. *Cancer Res.*, 39:3172–3176.
7. Carlstedt-Duke, J. M. B., Elfstrom, G., Hozberg, B., and Gustaffson, J. A. (1979): Ontogeny of the rat hepatic receptor for 2,3,7,8-tetrachlorodibenzo-*p*-dioxin and its endocrine independence. *Cancer Res.*, 39:4653–4656.
8. Chung, L. W. K. (1977): Characteristics of neonatal androgen-induced imprinting of rat hepatic microsomal monooxygenases. *Biochem. Pharmacol.*, 26:1979–1984.
9. Denef, C. (1974): Effect of hypophysectomy and pituitary implants at puberty on the sexual differentiation of testosterone metabolism in rat liver. *Endocrinology*, 94:1577–1582.
10. Dutton, G. J. (1975): Control of UDP glucuronyltransferase activity. *Biochem. Pharmacol.*, 24:1835–1841.
11. Einarsson, K., Gustaffson, J. A., and Stenberg, A. (1973): Neonatal imprinting of liver microsomal hydroxylation and reduction of steroids. *J. Biol. Chem.*, 248:4987–4997.
12. Elmamlouk, T. H., Mukhtar, H., and Bend, J. R. (1980): The nuclear envelope as a site of glucuronyltransferase in rat liver; properties of and effect of inducers on enzyme activity. *J. Pharmacol. Exp. Ther.* (*in press*).
13. Fahl, W. E., Shen A. L., and Jefcoate, C. R. (1978): UDP-Glucuronyl transferase and the conjugation of benzo(*a*)pyrene metabolites to DNA. *Biochem. Biophys. Res. Commun.*, 85:891–899.
14. Goldstein, J. A. (1977): Separation of pure polychlorinated biphenyl isomers into two types of inducers on the basis of induction of cytochrome P-450 or P-448. *Chem. Biol. Interact.*, 17:69–84.
15. Gustaffson, J. A., Gustaffson, S., Sundberg-Ingleman, M., Pousette, A., Stenberg, A., and Wrange, O. (1974): Sexual differentiation of hepatic steroid metabolism in the rat. *J. Steroid Biochem.*, 5:855–861.
16. Gustaffson, J. A., and Sundberg, M. I. (1975): Regulation of a steroid sulfate-specific hydroxylase system in female rat liver microsomes. *J. Biol. Chem.*, 250:1711–1718.
17. Hadd, M. E., and Blickenstaff, R. T. (1969): *Conjugates of Steroid Hormones.* Academic Press, New York.
18. Henderson, P. T. (1971): Metabolism of drugs in rat liver during the perinatal period. *Biochem. Pharmacol.*, 20:1225–1232.
19. James, M. O., Foureman, G. L., Law, F. C., and Bend, J. R. (1977): The perinatal development of epoxide-metabolizing enzyme activities in liver and extrahepatic organs of guinea pig and rabbit. *Drug Metab. Dispos.*, 5:19–28.
20. Kramer, R. A., Greiner, J. W., Runbaugh, R. C., Sweeney, T. D., and Colby, H. D. (1979): Requirement of the pituitary gland for gonadal hormone effects on hepatic drug metabolism in rats. *J. Pharmacol. Exp. Ther.*, 208:19–23.
21. Lamartiniere, C. A. (1980): The role of the hypothalamic–hypophyseal–gonadal axis in the regulation of hepatic glutathione *S*-transferases in the rat. *Endocrinology (in press)*.
22. Lamartiniere, C. A., Dieringer, C. S., and Lucier, G. W. (1979): Altered ontogeny of glutathione-*S*-transferase by 2,4,5-2',4',5'-hexachlorobiphenyl in rat liver. *Toxicol. Appl. Pharmacol.*, 51:233–238.
23. Lamartiniere, C. A., Dieringer, C. S., and Lucier, G. W. (1979): Altered sexual differentiation of hepatic UDP glucuronyltransferase by neonatal hormone treatment. *Biochem. J.*, 180:313–318.
24. Lucier, G. W. (1976): Perinatal development of conjugative enzyme systems. *Environ. Health Perspect.*, 18:25–34.
25. Lucier, G. W. (1978): Perinatal development of UDP glucuronyltransferase: Pharmacological and toxicological considerations. In: *Conjugation Reactions in Drug Biotransformation*, edited by A. Aitio, pp. 167–178. Elsevier/North-Holland, Amsterdam.
26. Lucier, G. W., and McDaniel, O. S. (1977): Steroid and non-steroid UDP glucuronyltransferase: Glucuronidation of synthetic estrogens as steroids. *J. Steroid Biochem.*, 8:867–872.
27. Lucier, G. W., and McDaniel, O. S. (1979): Developmental toxicology of the halogenated aromatics: Effects on enzyme development. *Ann. N. Y. Acad. Sci.*, 320:449–457.
28. Lucier, G. W., McDaniel, O. S., Hook, G. E. R., Fowler, B. A., Sonawane, B. R., and Faeder, E. (1973): Effects of TCDD on rat liver microsomal enzymes. *Environ. Health Perspec.*, 5:199–209.
29. Lucier, G. W., McDaniel, O. S., and Lui E. M. K. (1980): Pituitary regulation of the sexual dimorphic response to cadmium. Toxicology Meeting, Washington, D.C., March 1980, Abstr. 372.

30. Lucier, G. W., Schiller, C. M., McDaniel, O. S., and Matthews, H. B. (1978): Structural requirements for the accumulation of PCB metabolites in the fetal intestine. *Drug Metab. Dispos.*, 6:584–590.
31. Lucier, G. W., Sonawane, B. R., and McDaniel, O. S. (1977): Glucuronidation and deglucuronidation reactions in hepatic and extrahepatic tissues during perinatal development. *Drug. Metab. Dispos.*, 5:279–287.
32. Lucier, G. W., Sonawane, B. R., McDaniel, O. S., and Hook, G. E. R. (1975): Postnatal stimulation of hepatic microsomal enzymes following administration of TCDD to pregnant rats. *Chem. Biol. Interact.*, 11:15–26.
33. Lui E. M. K., Gregson, J., and Lucier, G. W. (1980): Altered sex differentiation of hepatic ethylmorphine *N*-demethylation by methadone induced reduction in neonatal androgen levels. *Pediatr. Pharmacol.*, 1:187–196.
34. Lui E. M. K., and Lucier, G. W. (1980): Neonatal feminization of hepatic monooxygenase in adult male rats: Altered sexual dimorphic response to cadmium. *J. Pharmacol. Exp. Ther.*, 212:211–216.
35. Lui E. M. K., Slaughter, S. R., Philpot, R. M., and Lucier, G. W. (1980): Cadmium sensitive cytochrome P-450 in rat liver. *Fed. Proc.*, 39(3):865.
36. McEwen, B. S. (1976): Interactions between hormones and nerve tissue. *Sci. Am.*, 235:48–58.
37. Metzler, M., and McLachlan, J. A. (1978): Oxidative metabolites of diethylstilbestrol in the fetal, neonatal and adult mouse. *Biochem. Pharmacol.*, 27:1087–1096.
38. Mulder, G. J., Hinson, J. A., and Gillette, J. R. (1977): Generation of reactive metabolites of *N*-hydroxy-phenacetin by glucuronidation and sulfation. *Biochem. Pharmacol.*, 26:189–196.
39. Mulder, G. J., Hinson, J. S., Nelson, W. L., and Thorgeirsson, S. S. (1977): Role of sulfotransferase from rat liver in the mutagenicity of *N*-hydroxy-2-acetylaminofluorene in *Salmonella typhimurium*. *Biochem. Pharmacol.*, 26:1356–1358.
40. Oesch, F. (1973): Mammalian epoxide hydrases: Inducible enzymes catalyzing the inactivation of carcinogenic and cytotoxic metabolites derived from aromatic and olefinic compounds. *Xenobiotica*, 3:305–340.
41. Oesch, F. (1975): Transplacental control of epoxide hydratase and its relationship to the control of microsomal monooxygenase. *FEBS Lett.*, 53:205–210.
42. Owens, J. (1977): Genetic regulation of UDP glucuronyltransferase. *J. Biol. Chem.*, 252:2827–2833.
43. Parke, D. V. (1968): *Biochemistry of Foreign Compounds*. Pergamon Press, New York.
44. Pelkonnen, O., Vorne, M., Jouppila, P., and Karki, N. T. (1971): Metabolism of chlorpromazine and *p*-nitrobenzoic acid in the liver, intestine, and kidney of the human foetus. *Acta Pharmacol. Toxicol. (Kbh.)*, 29:284–294.
45. Poland, A., and Glover, E. (1977): Chlorinated biphenyl induction of aryl hydrocarbon hydroxylase activity: A study of structure–activity relationship. *Mol. Pharmacol.*, 13:924–934.
46. Poland, A., Glover, E., and Kende, A. S. (1976): Stereospecific, high-affinity binding of 2,3,7,8-tetrachlorodibenzo-*p*-dioxin by hepatic cytosol: Evidence that the binding species is receptor for induction of aryl hydrocarbon hydroxylase. *J. Biol. Chem.*, 251:4936–4946.
47. Shah, H. S., and McLachlan, J. A. (1976): Fate of diethylstilbestrol in the pregnant mouse. *J. Pharmacol. Exp. Ther.*, 197:687–705.
48. Singer, S. S., Gieri, D., Johnson, J., and Sylvester, S. (1976): The enzymatic basis for the sex difference in cortisol sulfation by rat liver preparations. *Endocrinology*, 98:963–970.
49. Weisburger, E. K., Yamamoto, R. S. Glass, P. M., Grantham, R. H., and Weisburger, J. H. (1968): Effect of neonatal androgen and estrogen injection by *N*-hydroxy-2-fluorenylacetamide and on the metabolism of the carcinogen in rats. *Endocrinology*, 82:685–692.
50. Weisburger, J. H., Yamamoto, R. S., and Weisburger, E. K. (1966): Liver cancer: Neonatal estrogen enhances induction by a carcinogen. *Science*, 154:673–675.
51. Williams, R. T. (1977): Introduction to the concept of reactive intermediate. In: *Biological Reactive Intermediates*, edited by D. Jollow, J. Kocsis, R. Snyder, and H. Vainio, pp. 3–5. Plenum Press, New York.
52. Wishart, G. J. (1978): Functional heterogeneity of UDP glucuronyltransferase as indicated by its differential development and inducibility by glucocorticoids. *Biochem. J.*, 174:485–489.
53. Wishart, G. J. (1978): Demonstration of functional heterogeneity of hepatic UDP glucuronyltransferase activities after administration of 3-methylcholanthrene and phenobarbital to rats. *Biochem. J.*, 174:671–672.
54. Wishart, G. J., Campbell, M. T., and Dutton, G. J. (1978): Functional heterogeneity of UDP glucuronyltransferase. In: *Conjugation Reactions in Drug Biotransformation*, edited by A. Aitio, pp. 179–188. Elsevier/North-Holland, Amsterdam.

*Developmental Toxicology*, edited by
C. A. Kimmel and J. Buelke-Sam. Raven Press,
New York © 1981.

# Developmental Aspects of Chemical Interaction with Cellular Receptors

## G. L. Kimmel

*Developmental Mechanisms Branch, Division of Teratogenesis Research,
National Center for Toxicological Research, Food and Drug Administration,
Jefferson, Arkansas 72079*

Prenatal and early postnatal development in the mammal is comprised of critically timed events, and insult to this normal developmental pattern can lead to a number of alterations that manifest themselves as structural or functional deficits. The relationship between compound administration and developmental alteration has received considerable attention over the past two decades and has increased our knowledge of the teratogenic potential of a variety of agents. More recently, however, research in teratology has increasingly focused on characterizing the critical events of development, and Kretchmer has pointed out that "the search for mechanisms" has become an important, if not predominant, concern of the teratologist (41). Using techniques adapted from cell and molecular biology, investigators are now beginning to define a wide variety of developmental events and to examine their potential as determinants of normal and abnormal development. Wilson has listed as examples nine potential mechanisms of teratogenesis (85), and each of these can be further subdivided into events or sequential steps that could be susceptible to alteration.

This chapter will deal with one cellular event, namely, chemical interaction with target cells through specific receptors. While chemical agents can move into and around cells in a number of ways, the agent–cell interactions which modify cell function, in most cases, require binding to a specific subcellular component(s) (40,46). This can include interaction with cellular enzymes or binding directly to the cell genome, but in many cases, the cellular response is initiated through interaction with specific receptor molecules. The receptor concept was developed at the beginning of this century (40,46) and has been used to explain the interaction of many endogenous and exogenous agents (ligands) with the cell. In general, cells that respond to specific ligands are thought to contain receptors that bind these ligands and initiate events that culminate in a specific biological response. Most receptors appear to be macromolecules that are protein in nature and have a high affinity and limited capacity for a particular class of ligands. This preference for structurally distinct ligands (i.e., structural specificity) permits a high degree of biological control, since only a limited number of different ligands can bind and exert an effect. For the pharmacologist, the receptor concept provides a framework for examining the ability of ligands and cells to interact; for the toxicologist, it provides a framework for examining the importance of the ligand–cell interaction in altering normal cellular response.

It would seem that a concept, employed in pharmacology and toxicology for many years, would become an integral part of any systematic approach to investigating developmental toxicology. However, Fouts has recently stated that the "...interaction of drug and receptor is the most neglected area of developmental pharmacology..." (18). In part, this is due to a lack of well-defined models that can serve as points of reference in studies on development. In addition, the methods used to define such models in the adult are not always applicable in studies which concentrate on the perinatal period, due to limits of available biological material and to developmental factors that are not present or are of little consequence in the adult.

Attempts to solve these methodological problems and develop models to relate ligand–cell interaction and developmental toxicity have been limited. This chapter is intended to provide some examples of model systems and their applicability to developmental biology/toxicology and to encourage further work in the area of chemical interaction and perinatal development. The focus will be exclusively on specific cellular receptor systems; however, this is not intended to reduce the potential importance of other mechanisms for cell interaction, some of which are covered in other chapters in this text. While it is impossible to give examples of all systems, illustrations of both membrane and intracellular receptor systems, their ontogeny, and their potential as components in developmental toxicity are presented.

## MODELS OF CHEMICAL INTERACTION AND THEIR RELATION TO DEVELOPMENTAL TOXICOLOGY

### Plasma Membrane Interactions

The first point of cell contact for any circulating agent is the plasma membrane, and it is at this point that many agents initiate their effects. The current view of plasma membrane organization is based in large part on the fluid mosaic model of Singer and Nicolson (77) which extends and refines the classical model of Danielli and Davson (15). It focuses on the dynamic nature of the cell surface, suggesting that the plasma membrane plays an important role in the control of differentiation and cell function. In the fluid mosaic model, the membrane is proposed to be composed of a mobile phospholipid bilayer in which are embedded discrete protein components that can be observed at both the outer and inner surfaces and frequently appear to extend completely across the membrane. Certain of these proteins are thought to provide structural stability for the membrane, whereas others appear to serve as specific contact points for ligands involved with cell function (e.g., information transfer, enzymatic activity, and membrane transport).

As indicated above, a receptor is a functional unit that recognizes specific classes of compounds and, by associating with them, transfers information to initiate some cellular response. Plasma membrane receptors appear to be proteins that exhibit various degrees of lateral mobility in the membrane. Some membrane proteins are quite mobile; others appear more static, possibly due to their association with external restraints or internal membrane-associated components (e.g., microtubules, microfilaments) (57). Cuatrecasas (10,12) has proposed a mobile receptor model that addresses the dynamic nature of the fluid mosaic model and the relationship between binding and biological activity. In this model, a receptor in the unbound state exists separately from the membrane component (e.g., adenylate cyclase) which it influences. When a ligand binds to form a ligand–receptor complex, it causes an alteration in the receptor that promotes an interaction with the membrane component. Such membrane components are thought to be in close association with intracellular components important to cell function and to contractile proteins required for cell movement. Thus, the interaction of the receptor complex with the membrane component influences cellular events such as enzyme induction and membrane ion flux; and if this mechanism for ligand–receptor interaction is interrupted or altered during a critical phase in development, the potential for abnormal alterations of cell metabolism, migration, and cell–cell interaction is obvious.

### Lectins (Phytohemagglutinins)

Lectins have long been associated with cell agglutination, and recent investigations into their biochemical characteristics have demonstrated their usefulness in blood group typing and as probes of membrane structure and function (reviewed in 45,56). In general, lectins bind to plasma membrane receptors which appear to be integral membrane glycoproteins that project carbohydrate moieties from the cell surface into the extracellular space. The specificity of lectin binding appears to be related to the complex nature of these glycoproteins and is influenced by both the internal and terminal carbohydrate components of the receptor. Once lectin binding has occurred, alterations of cell surface properties leading to changes in membrane organization can be noted, and it has been proposed that these changes control aspects of cell function by influencing such events as membrane transport (12) and movement of contractile proteins (56).

In 1971, Moscona initiated studies on cell surface changes in the developing chick embryo, and the results of these and other studies have been reviewed (52,58). Moscona found that isolated chick neural retina cells, when exposed to the lectin, Concanavalin A (Con A), agglutinated in a fashion similar to neoplastic cells, demonstrating that these embryonic cells are lectin responsive. Subsequent work by Kleinschuster and Moscona (39), employing a variety of lectins at different developmental stages, began the characterization of the embryonic cell surface during maturation and differentiation. The ability of ricin and wheat germ agglutinin (WGA) to agglutinate cells was not dependent on the stage of embryonic development, although WGA would only agglutinate trypsinized cells, indicating that a trypsin-sensitive component was reducing the concentration or accessibility of the binding sites or inhibiting the activity of the WGA–receptor complex. Unlike the activity associated with ricin and WGA, agglutination by Con A was stage dependent, being greatest during early embryonic stages and progressively decreasing with age. Moscona (52) suggested that this loss of agglutination might be due to a reduction in the concentration and clustering of Con A receptors or to a change in their location and accessibility within the membrane. Further, it was suggested that changes in Con A receptors reflect the role of the cell surface in cell movement; i.e., increased agglutination at early embryonic stages coincides with increased cell motility and tissue organization, whereas at later stages, agglutination and motility have decreased as cellular maturation and differentiation proceed.

Other investigators have extended this approach to different biological systems at various developmental stages and have shown that definitive changes in the binding of lectins can occur as the fertilized ovum proceeds to the blastocyst stage as well as during development from the blastula to the gastrula stage (30,68,86), possibly reflecting the preparation of the embryo for normal implantation and development (68,86). The studies of Roberson and Oppenheimer (67) in the sea urchin embryo raise the possibility that membrane receptor patterns can vary among cell types. Their results demonstrated that in the 32-cell stage embryo, only one specific cell type, the micromere, was agglutinated by Con A. This raises the possibility that ligand–membrane receptor interactions identify and stimulate cell populations, important to specific developmental functions, such as migration or recognition which eventually lead to the definition of individual tissues and organ systems.

From these and other studies, it appears that the cell surface, its interaction with ligands, and its interaction with other cell surfaces are important to normal embryonic development. The specific nature of this control, however, is still largely undefined. Moscona (52) has reviewed several possibilities including embryonic enzyme induction, RNA and protein synthesis, cell recognition and adhesion, and tissue specificity. It is likely that all of these factors are important to normal development and that many are influenced by the interaction of ligands with membrane receptors.

The toxicity of lectins has been summarized by Nicolson (56), and apart from early studies demonstrating a lethal effect of lectins on the developing chick, few studies have concentrated on the developmental toxicity of lectins. Recently, Moran (51) demonstrated that Con A inhibits migration and differentiation in cultured neural crest cells, indicating a lectin-induced inhibition of morphogenetic function. This effect is dependent on the stage of development and appears to decrease as the cells cease migration and become differentiated. Hewitt and Elmer (29) also showed a stage-dependent change in lectin binding to mesenchymal cells that differed in different mouse strains, raising the possibility that genetic predisposition to lectin binding may be a factor in controlling the susceptibility of a system to developmental alteration. Finally, DeSesso (16) has reported that Con A causes limb and midline "closure" defects in rabbit embryos exposed intracoelomically. The response was stage dependent, and it was proposed that this was associated with developmental changes in exposed lectin receptors, which in effect would limit Con A binding to specific developmental periods.

Considerable work remains to define the normal developmental aspects of lectin binding and its relationship to toxic events. It is apparent that lectin receptors are in a dynamic state in the developing embryo and that alterations in their synthesis, movement, or interaction may have severe consequences on cell movement and tissue development. It is not apparent, however, what these consequences are. If lectin receptor mobility is altered, will normal cell–cell interaction take place, will cell movement cease, will differentiation cease or become uncontrolled? The onset of lectin receptor activity also needs further definition, and the potential for altering receptor availability during development must be investigated. Finally, as probes of membrane receptors, lectins should provide a better understanding of normal membrane function and should complement further investigation into the binding of other ligands to membrane receptors, thus providing a strong base to model the relationship of such binding to prenatal toxicity.

*Insulin*

The action of insulin on transmembrane sugar transport led Levine (44) to propose that the primary site of insulin action was at the cell membrane, specifically with a membrane receptor. Further characterization of the insulin–cell interaction indicated that insulin binds to a receptor that appears to be localized in the outer part of the plasma membrane (10,12,14). There is a specificity for insulin and insulin-related peptides, and most unrelated hormones (e.g., glucagon, ACTH, and prolactin) do not compete for insulin binding. However, as with many receptors, this specificity is not absolute. Competition for insulin binding to its receptor has been reported for both growth hormone (11) and for the lectins, Con A and wheat germ agglutinin (13). The specific cellular process(es) through which insulin exerts its control over cell function is unclear, although it is likely that a number of interacting cellular processes are involved (10,12,14). One area that has received considerable attention and appears closely related to several actions of insulin is the cyclic nucleotide system. In the mobile receptor model of Cuatrecasas (10,12), the cyclase could provide the membrane component that interacts with the insulin–receptor complex to initiate the production of cyclic AMP or GMP and the activation of protein kinase and phosphorylating enzymes. Other cellular events that may also be controlled by insulin include cellular ion flux, cyclic nucleotide-independent phosphorylation and dephosphorylation, sulfhydryl oxidation, and phospholipid turnover (14).

The effect of insulin on the developing embryo has been reviewed by Landauer (43), and the controversy over whether insulin is teratogenic by a direct action or by virtue of its effect on lowering blood glucose was discussed. Although hypoglycemia, regardless of its cause, may have a significant effect on prenatal development, Landauer (43) summarized evidence suggesting that insulin can be teratogenic by an action(s) not directly associated with a lowering of blood glucose.

Under both *in vivo* and *in vitro* conditions, insulin alters development of avian embryos at stages preceding an established circulatory system, and agents that differ in their effect on blood glucose show no consistent correlation between resulting glucose levels and teratogenic potency.

If the teratogenic action of insulin can be ascribed to a direct action on the embryonic cell, then one must propose a mechanism by which an insulin–cell interaction can occur. Although a significant amount of work has been directed to defining insulin receptors in the adult, few studies have concentrated on the ontogeny of the insulin receptor. Doetschman et al. (17) measured the binding of insulin to isolated chick embryo cells from various tissues at different embryonic stages to determine if a correlation existed between binding and developmental sensitivity to insulin. As early as day 4, insulin binding to limb buds could be detected but did not differ significantly from the binding of insulin to the remainder of the day-4 embryo. Thus, a tissue that is developmentally sensitive to insulin exposure (i.e., limb bud) did not demonstrate a marked increase in affinity for the hormone over the whole embryo. The authors suggested that this absence of tissue-specific binding may be associated with the reduced cell–cell contact found in isolated cell systems, and they showed that with cell aggregation there is an increase in the amount of insulin bound per cell, suggesting that the state of cell–cell interaction may be important to the availability and expression of the insulin receptor. Sandra and Przybylski (72) characterized the development of insulin binding to cultured chick embryo myoblasts, showing that binding occurred at all stages of myogenesis in culture. Furthermore, binding appeared to be saturable, specific, and of high affinity, and there was an increase in receptor concentration with myotube maturation.

Coupled with studies showing early embryonic insulin synthesis and secretion (6,9,58,64,65), these studies indicate that the endocrine system that mediates insulin action is established early in development. Thus, the potential for insulin to influence the development of certain tissues by interaction with a specific insulin receptor system and the possibility that alteration of this interaction could lead to abnormal development must be considered. Further studies on insulin receptor ontogeny and its association with insulin-responsive developmental events will indicate the applicability of current models of insulin action to the embryo/fetus. From such studies, cellular events associated with insulin action in the developing animal will be recognized, as well as the potential for such events to be altered by various environmental agents.

### Intracellular Interactions

Unlike agents that associate with plasma membrane receptors, some agents (e.g., steroid and thyroid hormones) enter the cell to associate with specific receptors. The model of the steroid–cell interaction, which has received considerable attention over the past 20 years (38,59), proposes that circulating steroids in equilibrium with various steroid-binding plasma proteins enter and are retained in target cells by cytoplasmic receptors. In general, each specific receptor is selective, binding ligands of a particular molecular class and excluding all others. This stereospecificity, however, is not absolute, and a number of synthetic agents, which appear to be structually dissimilar to a particular class of steroids, will nevertheless bind to the cytoplasmic receptor for that class. Once a steroid–receptor complex is formed, a temperature-dependent conformational change (activation) occurs in the receptor, promoting the movement of the complex into the nucleus. In the nucleus, the receptor interacts with the nuclear chromatin, where it is thought to affect cell function through alterations of specific RNA and protein production. While exceptions can be noted, this model appears to be generally applicable to all of the endogenous steroids, and it has been used to explain the effects of various synthetic steroids and nonsteroids that show steroidal activity.

Application of the steroid–receptor model initially focused on the normal physiological actions of steroid hormones. More recently, investigators have applied the model to abnormal situations in an attempt to determine the importance of ligand–cell interactions in alterations of normal cell function. Bullock and Bardin (7) reported a lack of androgen receptors in the testicular feminized rat and mouse and related this to the insensitivity of these animals to androgen stimulation. Sibley and Tomkins (76) have also shown that the resistance to glucocorticoid cytotoxicity of certain lymphoma cell lines may be associated with a glucocorticoid receptor deficiency. A wide range of studies has examined the correlation between sex steroid binding and the hormone responsiveness of mammary tumors and tumor cell lines (37,49,50). Also, Kupfer (42) has noted a possible role for the estrogen receptor in the reproductive effects of DDT. Thus, just as steroids interact with cells to influence their growth, differentiation, and function, it is also possible that the steroid–cell interaction (or lack of it) may promote toxic events through alterations in normal cell physiology.

### Glucocorticoids

Glucocorticoids are bound specifically in all glucocorticoid-responsive cells, and King and Mainwaring (38) and Munck and Leung (54) have recently reviewed the extensive work in this area. The binding process follows the general model for steroid–cell interaction, i.e., binding to a cytoplasmic receptor protein, translocation into the nucleus, and association with the nuclear chromatin. The glucocorticoid receptor has a high affinity for the natural glucocorticoids and an even higher affinity for some synthetic glucocorticoids such as dexamethasone and triamcinolone acetonide. Since these synthetic glucocorticoids do not bind significantly to plasma proteins that bind the natural glucocorticoids, they have permitted the determination of ligand binding solely to the glucocorticoid receptor. A number of studies have related this binding to specific biological activity (54). For example, Baxter and Tomkins (4) noted an inverse relationship between glucocorticoid binding and tyrosine aminotransferase activity in hepatoma cells. Munck and Brinck-Johnsen (53) have shown that cortisol, an active glucocorticoid, reduces glucose uptake into lymphocytes, whereas cortexolone, an inactive glucocorticoid receptor-blocking agent, abolishes this effect. Finally, as mentioned above, Sibley and Tomkins (76) have suggested that the resistance of certain lymphoma cell lines to glucocorticoid-induced cytotoxicity may be related to the absence of glucocorticoid receptors, since 79% of resistant clones tested showed little or no specific glucocorticoid binding, unlike steroid-sensitive cells; defective nuclear transfer of the steroid–receptor complex accounted for approximately 7% of the remaining resistant clones.

The initial studies on fetal glucocorticoid–cell interaction were developed around the knowledge that glucocorticoid exposure of the rabbit fetus near the end of gestation accelerated lung maturation and led to alveolar cell changes characteristic of increased pulmonary surfactant production (32,62). Independently, the laboratories of Ballard and Ballard (2) and Giannopoulos et al. (24) demonstrated that the fetal rabbit lung contains soluble receptors that will bind dexamethasone. The binding constants, sedimentation coefficients, and specificity of the fetal receptor were similar to those of the adult glucocorticoid receptor, and there was nuclear uptake of the dexamethasone–receptor complex at 37°C. Both laboratories speculated that glucocorticoids could be instrumental in stimulating surfactant production through a receptor-mediated system similar to that modeled for glucocorticoid activity in the adult. Ballard and Ballard (2) also suggested that *in utero* therapy with glucocorticoids may prove useful in preventing surfactant deficiencies in humans; however, no speculation was made relative to the possible toxic potential of such glucocorticoid exposure during pregnancy.

Following these initial experiments, Giannopoulos (21–23) continued the characterization of the glucocorticoid receptor throughout perinatal development in a variety of tissues. He demonstrated that dexamethasone binding to rat lung was high during the last 3 days of gestation, then decreased from birth until, in the adult, little or no binding was observed. This was contrary to the results seen in developing rat liver, where binding was high during the last days of gestation, decreased at birth, and then increased throughout postnatal development to adult levels. The binding specificity of the glucocorticoid receptor in fetal liver cytosol differed slightly from that in the adult (23). The fetal receptors bound corticosterone with a higher affinity than that shown for cortisol, whereas the reverse was true for the adult, suggesting that either the glucocorticoid receptor at these two ages is not identical or that additional binding components exist at certain stages of development that change the overall binding specificity of the system. Other laboratories interested in the effect of glucocorticoids on earlier developmental processes have extended this approach to other species and earlier times in gestation (25,27,69,71), and much of this work will be reviewed below. It is apparent that specific glucocorticoid receptors that show nuclear accumulation are present as early as gestation day 12 in the mouse, a time of major organogenesis (71).

The teratogenic activity of the glucocorticoids in laboratory animals is well known and has been extensively studied since it was first shown that cortisone can produce cleft palate in mice (3). Greene and Kochhar (26) have reviewed much of the work in this area and, where possible, have summarized the potential relationship between glucocorticoid action and critical events in palate formation such as glycosaminoglycan and collagen formation, programmed cell death, and midline fusion. Using the differing susceptibility of different mouse strains to glucocorticoid induction of cleft palate, Salomon and Pratt (69) and Goldman et al. (25) focused on the glucocorticoid receptor concentration of fetal palatal tissue from these strains of mice. Their studies showed a positive correlation between cleft palate incidence and the level of glucocorticoid binding. Salomon and Pratt (70) also have reported that the concentration of receptors parallels the inhibition of collagen synthesis and growth of palatal tissue or cells in culture. The studies of Kimmel et al. (36) in an adult model system have suggested that the receptor specificity may also be important to the teratogenic potential of an agent. In these studies, the competitive effect of the progestin, medroxyprogesterone acetate (MPA), for dexamethasone binding to the glucocorticoid receptor correlated with the teratogenic activity of MPA in the rat and rabbit (1). These studies indicated that differences in receptor specificity, as well as receptor concentration and translocation, must be considered when relating ligand–cell interaction and teratogenic potential. As development proceeds, this specificity may change, thus making the embryo/fetus more or less vulnerable to a particular agent.

Applying the model of steroid–cell interaction to the developing embryo, these studies suggest that the initial binding of a glucocorticoid to its receptor may be an essential step in initiating the subsequent response(s) of particular developing cells or tissues. Thus, alterations in receptor concentration, affinity, or specificity could significantly influence normal development. At the same time, studies on other aspects of glucocorticoid-induced cleft palate indicate the complex nature of the response. Reports on the relationship of species susceptibility and binding of the synthetic glucocorticoid, triamcinoline acetonide, are equivocal due to differences in methods of analysis, tissue sources, stages of development, and data interpretation (27,71); however, the results raise questions about the direct relationship of receptor concentration and teratogenicity. Pratt et al. (63) have recently reported that the homozygous brachymorphic mouse (bm/bm) is highly susceptible to cleft palate induction yet has a relatively low level of cytoplasmic glucocorticoid receptors. They suggested that the alteration of a specific gene locus, independent of receptor concentration, may result in changes in the timing of developmental events that predispose this and other strains to an increased teratogenic response. Bekhor et al. (5) concentrated on the role of triamcinolone in gene regulation and reported a block in gene activation. These data support the model of Zimmerman et al. (87) which proposed that an inhibition of RNA and protein synthesis would cause developmental processes to be out of phase and culminate in cleft palate. Bekhor et al. (5) did not address the issue of strain susceptibility; therefore, the relationship of gene activation to cleft palate is unclear.

The extent to which glucocorticoid-induced cleft palate has been studied provides a good base for future investigation of the developmental toxicity of steroids and is among the first systems to propose specific cellular and subcellular events in a teratogenic response. Nevertheless, additional studies relating genetic background to receptor concentration, specificity, and processing, to alterations in gene product

formation, to general cell/tissue development, and to phasing of critical developmental events will be required before glucocorticoid teratogenicity and its potential
impact on man can be assessed completely (see F. G. Biddle, *this volume* ).

## Estrogens

Since the early 1960s, modeling of the estrogen–cell interaction has benefited
from extensive investigation into the details of estrogen binding and the action of
estrogens at the molecular level. Reviews of these studies are numerous; two that
provide an overview of the major aspects of the model include those of King and
Mainwaring (38) and Segal and Koide (73). The estrogen–cell interaction follows
the general model proposed for all steroids; and although the receptor shows a
specificity for estrogens, compounds that vary markedly in their structure from that
of estradiol do bind to the estrogen receptor and have various estrogenic or anties-
trogenic activities. Included are compounds of the stilbene series, notably diethylstilbestrol, and a number of tricyclic antiestrogens (20). The studies of Nelson
(55) and others (reviewed in 42) have also shown that the pesticide $o,p'$-DDT is
capable of competing with estrogen receptor binding.

Investigation into the ontogeny of the estrogen receptor system has focused on
its relation to postnatal events such as puberty and the development of a mature
reproductive system. Thus, a great majority of the studies on ontogeny begin after
birth and do not address the topic of prenatal steroid receptors. In a comprehensive
review, Kaye (31) has recently detailed the experimental work on estrogen receptor
ontogeny and has included studies that deal with the prenatal development of the
estrogen receptor. In their original study, Clark and Gorski (8) demonstrated the
binding of estradiol-17β to an estrogen receptor in the postnatal rat uterus; the
receptor increased in concentration from day 2 to day 10 and then began to decline
to adult levels. A similar pattern has been reported for the binding of diethylstilbestrol to the early postnatal estrogen receptor (34). Somjen et al. (78) and McEwen
et al. (see 31) have shown that nuclear accumulation of the estrogen–receptor
complex parallels the changes in cytoplasmic receptor concentration, increasing
from immediately after birth to day 10 and then declining to adult levels. This is
true not only for the uterus but also for the pituitary and several estrogen-concen-
trating brain regions.

Studies on the prenatal ontogeny of the estrogen receptor have included a number
of animal species and a variety of tissues. Martinez-Vargas et al. (47) localized
estrogen uptake in several brain regions of the chick embryo as early as day 10,
and the series of studies by Teng and Teng (81–84) demonstrated estrogen–receptor
binding as early as day 8 in chick Müllerian duct. The sedimentation profile and
dissociation constant of the binding component in the chick Müllerian duct were
characteristic of a specific estrogen receptor, and nuclear translocation and interaction with chromatin were observed. The concentration of estrogen-binding sites
increased from day 8 to a maximum at day 12 when it plateaued. Plapinger et al.
(61) reported a specific, high-affinity estrogen receptor in the hypothalamic/amyg-

dala area of the fetal guinea pig brain, and Pasqualini et al. (60) reported cytoplasmic estrogen receptors in a number of tissues, including the kidney, uterus, lung, and testes, with nuclear localization in the kidney, uterus, and lung. In these latter studies, the pattern of development indicated a rise in receptor concentration from midgestation (day 35) to a high concentration just prior to birth. Following birth, there was a significant decrease in receptor concentration in the kidney, while the lung and uterus continued to show levels of binding comparable to those seen just prior to birth.

Studies on prenatal estrogen receptor ontogeny in the rat and mouse are complicated by the presence of α-fetoprotein (AFP) and other plasma proteins that are capable of binding estrogens. These components are present in large concentrations during late gestation and can all but obliterate any measurable estrogen–receptor interaction. A number of attempts have been made to methodologically circumvent the influence of these binding components. Using DNA-cellulose to separate the estrogen receptor from AFP, Fox et al. (19) have reported on estradiol binding in prenatal rat and mouse hypothalamus. In uterine cytosol from day-20 fetal rats, the studies of Somjen et al. (80) and Kimmel and Harmon (33) have demonstrated an estrogen-binding component, using labeled diethylstilbestrol, a ligand that has a high affinity for the specific estrogen receptor and a lower affinity for AFP (66,-75,79). The specificity of the binding showed a preference for estrogens, but the binding affinity appeared to be somewhat less than that reported in the immature rat uterus (33). Using a selective sedimentation technique to separate the specific receptor and AFP (28), Kimmel and Harmon (35) characterized the binding of the endogenous estrogen, estradiol-17β, and have also seen a variation from the specificity of the adult estrogen receptor. These results suggest that although the estrogen receptor may be present and functional in the developing reproductive tract, the ability of the receptor to interact with specific ligands may change with age.

The embryotoxic potential of prenatally administered estrogens has only recently received increased attention, largely in response to the association of human diethylstilbestrol (DES) exposure and transplacental carcinogenesis. Much of this attention focuses on DES metabolism and the ultimate tissue response; little attention has been paid to the interaction of DES with the fetal cell and the cellular events leading to the response. Shah and McLachlan (74) have shown an increased uptake of unmetabolized DES into the fetal reproductive tract over that in fetal plasma; however, the nature of this binding (whether to receptor or other component) was not determined. As noted above, studies on DES binding to fetal uterine components have been initiated (33,80) but have not yet addressed the association of binding and toxicity. In studies on another synthetic estrogen, clomiphene citrate, McCormack and Clark (48) have suggested that the developmental alterations of the reproductive tract following prenatal exposure to this long-acting estrogen may be due to the prolonged retention of the estrogen–receptor complex in the nucleus. This would lead to a sustained stimulation of events associated with the estrogenic response and promote hyperestrogenization of the target tissue. Finally, the effect of pesticides on reproductive function has been reviewed by Kupfer (42) who noted that the binding of DDT to the estrogen receptor could account for its hormonal action. Nevertheless, a direct correlation between DDT–receptor binding, as reported by Nelson (55) and others (reviewed in 42), and the toxic nature of DDT could not be made.

It is obvious from these examples that while a correlation of binding and developmental toxicity is suggested, considerable work remains in testing this concept. Studies characterizing the ontogeny of the estrogen–receptor interaction and its relation to cellular control in the fetus will have to continue in order to relate alterations of the process of interaction/action with events that culminate in a toxic manifestation.

## CONCLUSION

This review provides several examples of chemical interaction with target cells through specific receptor mechanisms and the impact this interaction may have on development. These examples are based on model systems that have been developed through extensive investigation in immature and adult biological systems. It should be understood that the description of each model system presented could be greatly extended, and the references to reviews and publications are intended to provide a base for more extensive coverage of a particular system. Investigators have also begun to characterize a number of other receptor systems, and the limits of this review should not be viewed as the borders of our knowledge.

For each example, the general model of ligand–receptor interaction and work in the area of receptor ontogeny in the embryo/fetus have been presented. It should be obvious that for most systems work in this latter area is minimal. Consequently, while theoretical relationships of ligand–receptor interaction and developmental toxicity can be developed, direct demonstration of such an association remains to be made. For investigators interested in the general concept of ligand–receptor interaction in fetal target cells, the field is in critical need of studies aimed at characterizing fetal receptors and their ontogeny. Are receptors available at the appropriate critical time in development to permit teratogen–cell interaction? Is the specificity such that binding can occur, and does specificity change with development? Will the ligand–receptor complex promote a cellular action? The answers to these questions, when considered together with our growing knowledge of cellular responses to compounds and the relation of these responses to cellular/tissue effects, should provide a strong base for understanding how normal developmental processes can be altered. The investigator interested in mechanisms of developmental toxicity will then be able to model cellular responses following exposure to an environmental agent. This should eventually place us in a better position to determine the teratogenic potential of an agent and the possible human risk. The requirements for such an approach, ranging from research support to the development of methods applicable to the prenatal situation, should be recognized and may be limiting. Nevertheless, this area of developmental toxicology should prove challenging, and the application of our knowledge to important environmental questions should, in the future, prove rewarding.

## ACKNOWLEDGMENTS

The author would like to express his appreciation to Ms. E. Sykes for her assistance in the preparation of this manuscript and to the editors, Mr. J. Harmon, Dr. D. Casciano, Dr. D. Sheehan, and Dr. W. Slikker, for their editorial comments.

## REFERENCES

1. Andrew, F. D., and Staples, R. E. (1977): Prenatal toxicity of medroxyprogesterone acetate in rabbits, rats and mice. *Teratology*, 15:25–32.
2. Ballard, P. L., and Ballard, R. A. (1972): Glucocorticoid receptors and the role of glucocorticoids in fetal lung development. *Proc. Natl. Acad. Sci. U.S.A.*, 69:2668–2672.
3. Baxter, H., and Fraser, F. C. (1950): Production of congenital defects in the offspring of female mice treated with cortisone. *McGill Med. J.*, 19:245–249.
4. Baxter, J. D., and Tomkins, G. M. (1971): Specific cytoplasmic glucocorticoid hormone receptors in hepatoma tissue culture cells. *Proc. Natl. Acad. Sci. U.S.A.* 68:932–937.
5. Bekhor, I., Mirell, C., and Anne, L. (1978): Induction of cleft palates by triamcinolone acetonide: Re-examination of the problem. *Cleft Palate J.*, 15:220–232.
6. Benzo, C. A., and Green, T. D. (1974): Functional differentiation of the chick endocrine pancreas: Insulin storage and secretion. *Anat. Rec.*, 180:491–496.
7. Bullock, L. P., and Bardin, C. W. (1972): Androgen receptors in testicular feminization. *J. Clin. Endocrinol. Metab.*, 35:935–937.
8. Clark, J.H. and Gorski, J. (1970): Ontogeny of the estrogen receptor during early uterine development. *Science*, 169:76–78.
9. Clark, W. R., and Rutter, W. J. (1972): Synthesis and accumulation of insulin in the fetal rat pancreas. *Dev. Biol.*, 29:468–481.
10. Cuatrecasas, P. (1974): Membrane receptors. *Annu. Rev. Biochem.*, 43:169–214.
11. Cuatrecasas, P., and Hollenberg, M. D. (1975): Binding of insulin and other hormones to non-receptor materials: Saturability, specificity and apparent "negative cooperativity." *Biochem. Biophys. Res. Commun.*, 62:31–41.
12. Cuatrecasas, P., and Hollenberg, M. D. (1976): Membrane receptors and hormone action. In: *Advances in Protein Chemistry, Vol. 30*, edited by C. B. Anfinsen, J. T. Edsall, and F. M. Richards, pp. 251–451. Academic Press, New York.
13. Cuatrecasas, P., and Tell, G. P. E. (1973): Insulin-like activity of concanavalin A and wheat germ agglutinin—direct interactions with the insulin receptors. *Proc. Natl. Acad. Sci. U.S.A.*, 70:485–489.
14. Czech, M. P. (1977): Molecular basis of insulin action. *Annu. Rev. Biochem.*, 46:359–384.
15. Danielli, J. F., and Davson, H. (1935): A contribution to the theory of the permeability of thin films. *J. Cell. Comp. Physiol.*, 5:495–508.
16. DeSesso, J. M. (1979): Lectin teratogenesis: Defects produced by concanavalin A in fetal rabbits. *Teratology*, 19:15–26.
17. Doetschman, T. C., Havaranis, A. S., and Herrmann, H. (1975): Insulin binding to cells of several tissues of the early chick embryo. *Dev. Biol.*, 47: 228–232.
18. Fouts, J. R. (1976): Developmental pharmacology: Overview. *Environ. Health Perspect.*, 18:3–4.
19. Fox, T. O., Vito C. C., and Wieland, S. J. (1978): Estrogen and androgen receptor proteins in embryonic and neonatal brain: Hypotheses for roles in sexual differentiation and behavior. *Am. Zool.*, 18:525–537.
20. Geynet, C., Millet, C., Truong, H., and Baulieu, E. E. (1972): Estrogens and antiestrogens, *Gynecol. Invest.*, 3:2–29.
21. Giannopoulos, G. (1973): Glucocorticoid receptors in lung. I. Specific binding of glucocorticoids to cytoplasmic components of rabbit fetal lung. *J. Biol. Chem.*, 248:3876–3883.
22. Giannopoulos, G. (1974): Variations in the levels of cytoplasmic glucocorticoid receptors in lungs of various species at different developmental stages. *Endocrinology*, 94:450–458.
23. Giannopoulos, G. (1975): Ontogeny of glucocorticoid receptors in rat liver. *J. Biol. Chem.*, 250:5847–5851.
24. Giannopoulos, G., Mulay, S., and Solomon, S. (1972): Cortisol receptors in rabbit fetal lung. *Biochem. Biophys. Res. Commun.*, 47:411–418.

25. Goldman, A. S., Katsumata, M., Yaffe, S. J., and Gasser, D. L. (1977): Palatal cytosol cortisol-binding protein associated with cleft palate susceptibility and H-2 genotype. *Nature*, 265:643–645.
26. Greene, R. M., and Kochhar, D. M. (1975): Some aspects of corticosteroid-induced cleft palate: A review. *Teratology*, 11:47–56.
27. Hackney, J. F. (1980): A glucocorticoid receptor in fetal mouse: Its relationship to cleft palate formation. *Teratology*, 21:39–51.
28. Harmon, J. R., and Kimmel, G. L. (1980): The use of selective sedimentation in the separation of estrogen binding components in the immature rat uterus. *Proceedings of the Annual Meeting, Society of Toxicology*, p. A20.
29. Hewitt, A. T., and Elmer, W. A. (1976): Reactivity of normal and brachypod mouse limb mesenchymal cells with Con A. *Nature*, 264:177–178.
30. Johnson, K. E., and Smith, E. P. (1976): The binding of concanavalin A to dissociated embryonic amphibian cells. *Exp. Cell. Res.*, 101:63–70.
31. Kaye, A. M. (1978): The ontogeny of estrogen receptors. In: *Biochemical Actions of Hormones*, Vol. 5, edited by G. Litwack, pp. 149–201. Academic Press, New York.
32. Kikkawa, J., Kaibara, M., Motoyama, E. K., Orzalesi, M. M., and Cook, C. D. (1971): Morphologic development of fetal rabbit lung and its acceleration with cortisol. *Am. J. Pathol.*, 64:423–433.
33. Kimmel, G. L., and Harmon, J. R. (1979): Characterization of a diethylstilbestrol (DES) binding component in fetal rat uteri. *Toxicol. Appl. Pharmacol.*, 48:A36.
34. Kimmel, G. L., and Harmon, J. R. (1980): Characteristics of estrogen binding of uterine cytosol during the perinatal period in the rat. *J. Steroid Biochem.*, 12:73–75.
35. Kimmel, G. L., and Harmon, J. R. (1980): Developmental changes in estrogen receptor specificity. *Teratology*, 21:49A–50A.
36. Kimmel, G. L., Hartwell, B. S., and Andrew, F. D. (1979): A potential mechanism in medroxyprogesterone acetate teratogenesis. *Teratology*, 19:171–176.
37. King, R. J. B. (1979): How important are steroids in regulating the growth of mammary tumors? In: *Biochemical Actions of Hormones, Vol. 6*, edited by G. Litwack, pp. 247–264. Academic Press, New York.
38. King, R. J. B., and Mainwaring, W. I. P. (1974): *Steroid–Cell Interactions*. University Park Press, Baltimore.
39. Kleinschuster, S. J., and Moscona, A. A. (1972): Interaction of embryonic and fetal neural retinal cells with carbohydrate-binding phytoagglutinins: Cell surface changes with differentiation. *Exp. Cell Res.*, 70:397–410.
40. Korolkovas, A. (1970): *Essentials of Molecular Pharmacology*. Wiley-Interscience, New York.
41. Kretchmer, N. (1978): Perspectives in teratologic research. *Teratology*, 17:203–212.
42. Kupfer, D. (1975): The effects of pesticides and related compounds on steroid metabolism and function. In: *CRC Critical Reviews in Toxicology, Vol. 4*, edited by L. Golberg, pp. 83–124. CRC Press, Cleveland.
43. Landauer, W. (1972): Is insulin a teratogen? *Teratology*, 5:129–136.
44. Levine, R. (1965): Cell membrane as a primary site of insulin action. *Fed. Proc.*, 24:1071–1073.
45. Lis, H., and Sharon, N. (1973): The biochemistry of plant lectins (phytohemagglutinins). *Annu. Rev. Biochem.*, 42:541–574.
46. Main, A. R. (1980): Toxicant–receptor interactions, fundamental principles. In: *Introduction To Biochemical Toxicology*, edited by E. Hodgson and F. E. Guthrie, pp. 180–192. Elsevier/North-Holland, New York.
47. Martinez-Vargas, M. C., Gibson, D. B., Sar, M., and Stumpf, W. E. (1975): Estrogen target sites in the brain of the chick embryo. *Science*, 190:1307–1308.
48. McCormack, S., and Clark, J. H. (1979): Clomid administration to pregnant rats causes abnormalities of the reproductive tract in offspring and mothers. *Science*, 204:629–631.
49. McGuire, W. L., Carbone, P. P., and Vollmer, E. P. (1975): *Estrogen Receptors in Human Breast Cancer*. Raven Press, New York.
50. McGuire, W. L., Raynaud, J. P., and Baulieu, E. E. (1977): *Progress in Cancer Research and Therapy, Vol. 4, Progesterone Receptors in Normal and Neoplastic Tissues*. Raven Press, New York.
51. Moran, D. (1974): The action of concanavalin A on migrating and differentiating neural crest cells. *Exp. Cell Res.*, 86:365–373.

52. Moscona, A. A. (1974): Surface specification of embryonic cells: Lectin receptor, cell recognition, and specific cell ligands, In: *The Cell Surface in Development*, edited by A. A. Moscona, pp. 67–99. John Wiley and Sons, New York.
53. Munck, A., and Brinck-Johnsen, T. (1968): Specific and nonspecific physico–chemical interactions of glucocorticoids and related steroids with rat thymus cells *in vitro. J. Biol. Chem.,* 243:5556–5565.
54. Munck, A., and Leung, K. (1977): Glucocorticoid receptors and mechanisms of action. In: *Receptors and Mechanisms of Action of Steroid Hormones*, edited by J. R. Pasqualini, pp. 311–397. Marcel Dekker, New York.
55. Nelson, J. A. (1974): Effects of dichlorodiphenyltrichloroethane (DDT) analogs and polychlorinated biphenyl (PCB) mixtures on 17β -[³H]estradiol binding to rat uterine receptor. *Biochem. Pharmacol.,* 23:447–451.
56. Nicolson, G. L. (1974): The interaction of lectins with animal cell surfaces. *Int. Rev. Cytol.,* 39:89–190.
57. Nicolson, G. L. (1975): Current views on the molecular organization of biological membranes. In: *Mammalian Cells: Probes and Problems*, edited by G. R. Richmond, D. F. Petersen, P. F. Mullaney, and E. C. Anderson, pp. 246–253. USERDA, Oak Ridge, Tennessee.
58. Oppenheimer, S. B. (1977): Interactions of lectins with embryonic cell surfaces. In: *Current Topics in Developmental Biology, Vol. 11*, edited by A. A. Moscona and A. Monroy, pp. 1–16. Academic Press, New York.
59. Pasqualini, J. R. (1977): *Receptors and Mechanism of Action of Steroid Hormones*. Marcel Dekker, New York.
60. Pasqualini, J. R., Sumida, C., Gelly, C., and Nguyen, B. L. (1976): Specific [³H]-estradiol binding in the fetal uterus and testis of guinea pig; quantitative evolution of [³H]-estradiol receptors in the different fetal tissues (kidney, lung, uterus, and testis) during fetal development. *J. Steroid Biochem.,* 7:1031–1038.
61. Plapinger, L., Landau, I. T., McEwen, B. S., and Feder, H. H. (1977): Characteristics of estradiol-binding macromolecules in fetal and adult guinea pig brain cytosols. *Biol. Reprod.,* 16:586–599.
62. Platzker, A. C. G., Kitterman, J. A., Tooley, W. H., and Clements, J. A. (1972): Surfactant appearance in secretion in fetal lamb lung in response to dexamethasone. *Pediatr. Res.,* 6:406.
63. Pratt, R. M., Salomon, D. S., Diewert, V. M., Erikson, R. P., Burns, R., and Brown, K. S. (1980): Cortisone-induced cleft palate in the brachymorphic mouse. *Teratogen. Carcinogen. Mutagen.,* 1:15–23.
64. Przybylski, R. J. (1967): Cytodifferentiation of the chick pancreas. 1. Ultrastructure of the islet cells and the initiation of granule formation. *Gen. Comp. Endocrinol.,* 8:115–128.
65. Rall, L. B., Pictet, R. L., and Rutter, W. J. (1979): Synthesis and accumulation of proinsulin and insulin during development of the embryonic rat pancreas. *Endocrinology,* 105:835–841.
66. Raynaud, J.-P., Mercier-Bodard, C., and Baulieu, E. E. (1971): Rat estradiol binding plasma protein (EBP). *Steroids,* 18:767–788.
67. Roberson, M., and Oppenheimer, S. B. (1975): Quantitative agglutination of specific populations of sea urchin embryo cells with concanavalin A. *Exp. Cell Res.,* 91:263–268.
68. Rowinski, J., Solter, D., and Koprowski, H. (1976): Change of concanavalin A induced agglutinability during preimplantation mouse development. *Exp. Cell Res.,* 100:404–408.
69. Salomon, D. S., and Pratt, R. M. (1976): Glucocorticoid receptors in murine embryonic facial mesenchyme cells. *Nature,* 264:174–177.
70. Salomon, D. S., and Pratt, R. M. (1978): Inhibition of growth in vitro by glucocorticoids in mouse embryonic facial mesenchyme cells. *J. Cell. Physiol.,* 97:315–327.
71. Salomon, D. S., Zubairi, Y., and Thompson, E. B. (1978): Ontogeny and biochemical properties of glucocorticoid receptors in mid-gestation mouse embryos. *J. Steroid Biochem.,* 9:95–107.
72. Sandra, A., and Przybylski, R. J. (1979): Ontogeny of insulin binding during chick skeletal myogenesis *in vitro. Dev. Biol.,* 68:546–556.
73. Segal, S. J., and Koide, S. S. (1979): Molecular pharmacology of estrogens. *Pharmacol. Ther.,* 4:183–220.
74. Shah, H. C., and McLachlan, J. A. (1976): The fate of diethylstilbestrol in the pregnant mouse. *J. Pharmacol. Exp. Ther.,* 197:687–696.
75. Sheehan, D. M., and Young, M. (1979): Diethylstilbesterol and estradiol binding to serum albumin and pregnancy plasma of rat and human. *Endocrinology,* 104:1442–1446.
76. Sibley, C. H., and Tomkins, G. M. (1974): Mechanisms of steroid resistance. *Cell,* 2:221–227.

77. Singer, S. J., and Nicolson, G. L. (1972): The fluid mosaic model of the structure of cell membranes. *Science*, 175:720–731.
78. Somjen, D., Somjen, G., King, R. J. B., Kaye, A. M., and Lindner, H. R. (1973): Nuclear binding of oestradiol-17β and induction of protein synthesis in the rat uterus during postnatal development. *Biochem. J.*, 136:25–33.
79. Somjen, G. J., Kaye, A. M., and Lindner, H. R. (1974): Oestradiol-17β binding proteins in the rat uterus: Changes during postnatal development. *Mol. Cell. Endocrinol.*, 1:341–353.
80. Somjen, G. J., Kaye, A. M., and Lindner, H. R. (1976): Demonstration of 8S-cytoplasmic oestrogen receptor in rat Mullerian duct. *Biochim. Biophys. Acta*, 428:787–791.
81. Teng, C. S., and Teng, C. T. (1975): Studies on sex-organ development: Isolation and characterization of an oestrogen receptor from chick Mullerian duct. *Biochem. J.*, 150:183–190.
82. Teng, C. S., and Teng, C. T. (1975): Studies on sex-organ development: Ontogeny of cytoplasmic oestrogen receptor in chick Mullerian duct. *Biochem. J.*, 150:191–194.
83. Teng, C. S., and Teng, C. T. (1976): Studies on sex-organ development: Oestrogen–receptor translocation in the developing chick Mullerian duct. *Biochem. J.*, 154: 1–9.
84. Teng, C. S., and Teng, C. T. (1978): Studies on sex-organ development: Changes in chemical composition and oestradiol-binding capacity in chromatin during differentiation of chick Mullerian ducts. *Biochem. J.*, 172:361–370.
85. Wilson, J. G. (1977): Current status of teratology. In: *Handbook of Teratology*, edited by J. G. Wilson and F. C. Fraser, pp. 47–74. Plenum Press, New York.
86. Yanagimachi, R., and Nicolson, G. L. (1976): Lectin-binding properties of hamster egg zona pellucida and plasma membrane and preimplantation development. *Exp. Cell Res.*, 100:249–257.
87. Zimmerman, E. F., Andrew, F. and Kalter, H. (1970): Glucocorticoid inhibition of RNA synthesis responsible for cleft palate in mice: A model. *Proc. Natl. Acad. Sci. U.S.A.*, 6:779–785.

Developmental Toxicology, edited by
C. A. Kimmel and J. Buelke-Sam, Raven Press,
New York © 1981.

# Evaluation of Fetal Growth and Development in the High-Risk Obstetrical Patient

*Anthony R. Scialli and **Sergio E. Fabro

*Columbia Hospital for Women, Washington, D.C. 20037; and
**Department of Obstetrics and Gynecology, The George Washington University,
Washington, D.C. 20037

Obstetrical care in the past 30 years has resulted in a decrease in maternal mortality from more than 80 deaths/100,000 live births to about 20 deaths/100,000 live births yearly (59). Perinatal deaths, however, have remained at about 20/1,000 births for much of the same period. Greater emphasis is now being placed on identifying and treating the fetus at high risk, resulting in a recent downward trend in perinatal mortality well below the 20/1,000 figure. The prediction of which pregnancies may be at risk is currently feasible (1,35), and treatment of these is no longer limited to early delivery, which may be detrimental for the fetus, but includes close monitoring in antenatal intensive care units (1,72). Here, testing is designed to determine at what point continued intrauterine life is too dangerous and when delivery will result in the best perinatal outcome.

The recognition of factors known to interfere with normal fetal development has led to an increase in evaluation of pregnancy in the second trimester. At this time, the gestation may be interrupted to prevent the carrying of a nonviable or poorly functioning fetus. These early methods of evaluation can similarly be used to reassure parents with a high risk of bearing abnormal children that a current pregnancy is free of developmental abnormality.

## INDICATIONS FOR EVALUATION

Evaluation of all high-risk pregnancies is not currently available because of limited resources. In addition, the discomfort and potential hazard of some methods require that specific indications exist for their use.

### High Risk of Detectable Morphological Error

Fetal dysmorphogenesis is the error most commonly investigated in pregnancies prior to the third trimester. Of diagnostic amniocenteses performed in the mid-

*131*

trimester, 80 to 90% were indicated by an increased risk for an error in fetal formation (50,57).

Chromosomal abnormalities account for most of the detectable morphological errors. Advanced maternal age is the commonest reason for women with chromosomally abnormal fetuses to have sought evaluation. The incidence of karyotypic anomalies in the pregnancies of women over the age of 35 is about 2% (16,23,-50,52,57,73), whereas over the age of 40, this incidence rises to 5% or greater (16,73). Although for many years maternal gametogenesis was considered to be at fault in causing development of a dyskaryotic infant, it has been found (48) that paternally contributed chromosomes are responsible for the abnormality in a significant number of cases. The association between chromosomal abnormalities and older women may reflect not only the tendency for the aging ovum to develop errors but also the preference of older women for older men with their seemingly similar tendency for abnormal gamete formation.

A history of a previous child with a chromosomal abnormality results in a 3% incidence of chromosomal error in a current pregnancy (50,57), whereas a parent with a balanced translocation may confer a 40% incidence of abnormality on his or her child (50).

Structural abnormalities of the fetus may occur without predictability by chromosomal study. Determination of an increased risk of these is based on prior occurrence of the anomaly in the family or on exposure to agents with known or suspected teratogenic potential. In a study of women in the second trimester of pregnancy, 10 of 122 who had previously delivered anomalous infants were found to have recurrent abnormalities among which were hydrocephaly, anencephaly, diaphragmatic hernia, duodenal atresia, polycystic kidneys, and omphalocele (32).

## High Risk of Detectable Enzymatic Error

A metabolic disorder that is genetically transmitted may be sought in pregnancies where a parent, sibling, or other close relation of the fetus is affected. The risk of acquiring such a disorder depends on its dominance and penetrance as well as on the family member in whom the disease is present. An increased risk of a congenital metabolic abnormality may also be conferred by ethnic or racial background. Tay-Sachs disease is known to occur largely in those of Ashkenazic Jewish background, sickle cell anemia in blacks, and the thalassemias in groups originating in the Mediterranean region.

## High Risk Imposed by Maternal Disease

Several disorders in the mother are known to interfere with proper fetal growth (62). Among these are hypertension, diabetes mellitus, renal insufficiency, heart disease, several autoimmune disorders, and severe anemia. Women coming into a pregnancy with these diseases usually have exposed their fetuses to pharmacologic agents during embryogenesis. More significantly, these pregnancies frequently demonstrate abnormal placental nutritive and respiratory function later in the gestation.

### High Risk Acquired During the Pregnancy

Women appearing to be healthy prior to conception may develop conditions that subject the fetus to serious risk. Among these conditions, the most prominent are the toxemias of pregnancy and red blood cell antigen isoimmunization (usually Rhesus factor D). Routine prenatal screening should result in the early detection of these disorders and their management in the high-risk unit.

Poor maternal nutrition is known to adversely influence fetal weight and has been implicated in more serious abnormalities of growth and development (81). Similarly, drug use by the mother is known to be potentially harmful to the developing embryo and fetus (15), although the nature of this risk varies widely depending on the drug, the extent to which it is used, and the timing of exposure. Maternal infection may be innocuous to the fetus; however, several infections are associated with fetal dysmorphogenesis or abnormalities of growth (13,69). Among the infectious agents known to be harmful are the Rubella virus, *Toxoplasma*, *Treponema pallidum*, cytomegalovirus, and the coxsackievirus.

Maternal exposure to ionizing radiation is potentially harmful to the fetus; however, these harmful effects (e.g., an increase in leukemia incidence) are generally seen well after birth and cannot be detected prenatally (77).

## METHODS OF EVALUATION

### Clinical Evaluation

Routine prenatal care includes examinations designed to detect and monitor high-risk situations. In addition to following the maternal condition, the pregnancy is evaluated by serial measurements of uterine size, auscultation of the fetal heart, and by asking the pregnant woman about fetal movements. A failure of uterine growth to keep pace with established norms would suggest a retardation of fetal growth. Fetal heart auscultation is useful in establishing evidence of fetal life, although late in the gestation, an abnormally slow or fast rate might suggest impaired placental function. Fetal movement as detected by the mother is a sensitive indicator of fetal health with a correlation seen between loss of fetal movement and impending fetal death (66).

### Amniocentesis

Analysis of amniotic fluid is useful in the detection of enzymatic abnormalities, chromosomal errors, neural tube defects, and in the evaluation of Rhesus factor isoimmunized pregnancies (80). Fluid is obtained by transabdominal needle puncture under sterile conditions utilizing either local anesthesia or no anesthesia. The accuracy of determinations made by amniocentesis exceeds 99% (23,50,57,73). The procedure is accepted as safe for mother and fetus with the pregnancy loss following the procedure being statistically similar to that in the general population (23,50,57,73).

Karyotyping of fetal cells in sedimented fluid is used to investigate possible chromosomal abnormalities and to establish fetal sex in pregnancies at risk for an X-linked disorder. In a large study of midtrimester diagnostic amniocenteses (57), 81.6% of procedures were performed because of a high risk of chromosomal abnormalities. Of these, 26.4% showed chromosomal errors. X-linked disease was the indication for study in 2.0% of the pregnancies, with male fetuses found in 52.4% of these.

Chromosomal analysis requires culturing of desquamated fetal cells, and failure of the cells to grow is the most troublesome source of failure of the procedure. Miskaryotyping occurs in less than 1% of cases and consists chiefly in errors in fetal sex determination (23,73).

α-Fetoprotein is, after albumin, the major protein in the fetal circulation. It reaches peak levels in fetal serum at 14 postmenstrual weeks. The levels in amniotic fluid parallel serum levels and will be increased in conditions where there is greater opportunity for the polypeptide to leak from fetal capillaries or cerebrospinal fluid into amniotic fluid. Such conditions include exomphalos, in which capillaries in extruding viscera leak protein into amniotic fluid, congenital nephrosis, in which glomerular filtration causes abnormal amounts of protein to enter fetal urine and thus amniotic fluid, and open neural tube defects, in which cerebrospinal fluid is in continuity with amniotic fluid (37).

Maternal serum contains α-fetoprotein as well and elevations in amniotic fluid levels are reflected in maternal levels. Routine screening of maternal serum levels has been advocated; however, the wide normal range in maternal samples raises the question of what should be considered an elevated value (6). It has been found (38) that investigating those women with serum α-fetoprotein levels more than three standard deviations above the mean for gestational age will lead to discovery by subsequent amniocentesis and ultrasonography of 82% of anencephalic fetuses and 47% of fetuses with spina bifida. On the basis of routine maternal screening, 4 to 6% of pregnancies had elevated α-fetoprotein in maternal blood. On a repeat measurement, half of these persisted in being elevated. Subsequent amniocentesis and ultrasonography disclosed that two-thirds of these were normal singleton pregnancies with the usual cause of the abnormal α-fetoprotein level being an error in determination of gestational age. One-fifth of the pregnancies contained congenitally normal multiple gestations. The remainder, about 13%, were abnormal pregnancies (37). Because of the low yield of true positive results, the feasibility of routine screening in the United States is still under study (46). Since women who have previously given birth to a child with a neural tube defect have a risk of recurrence of 5% (6), screening of this population by measuring amniotic fluid α-fetoprotein is advisable.

Hereditary disorders of metabolism are investigated by measuring enzyme activity in cultured fetal cells. Diseases detectable in this manner include disorders of lipid metabolism such as lipoprotein lipase deficiency, Tay-Sachs disease, and Niemann-Pick disease, disorders of porphyrin metabolism such as acute intermittent porphyria, and disorders of hormone metabolism such as 21-hydroxylase-deficient adrenogenital syndrome. The direct measurement of hexosaminidase levels in amniotic fluid has been shown to reliably predict Tay-Sachs disease (27) and may eliminate the need to culture amniotic fluid cells in screening for this disorder.

These methods of prenatal detection of abnormalities by amniocentesis permit the termination of pregnancies in which the fetus is affected and are therefore performed between the 14th and 20th weeks after the last menstrual period. Prior to this time, it is difficult to enter the small amniotic cavity reliably, and following this period, evaluation may not be completed in time to terminate the gestation legally.

Amniocentesis is also used to evaluate later pregnancies in which the mother has demonstrated isoimmunization to a red blood cell antigen. In these instances, amniotic fluid bilirubin is indirectly measured as an index of fetal hemolysis (80). Detection of significant hemolysis may lead to early delivery of the fetus or to transfusion into the fetus' peritoneal cavity of antigen-negative red blood cells.

## Fetoscopy

It has become possible to visualize the fetus and placenta directly in continuing human pregnancy by means of a small endoscope inserted into the uterus transabdominally (33). The scopes used have a maximum outer diameter of 2.7 mm (34). Direct observation of fetal morphology is possible, and early detection of abnormalities such as short-limbed dwarfism is practical (34).

Abnormalities detectable by examination of fetal blood have become the major indication for fetoscopy. Prior to use of the fetoscope, fetal blood was obtained by aspiration from the placenta utilizing a technique similar to amniocentesis with ultrasonographic placental localization. Although this technique was useful in detecting disorders such as Duchenne's muscular dystrophy (elevated fetal creatine phosphokinase), contamination with maternal blood and placental injury remained potential complications (49). Using the fetoscope, an umbilical cord vessel near the placental insertion or a placental vessel is visualized directly. The vessel is either directly aspirated (65) or punctured with collection of a mixture of blood and amniotic fluid (17). Disorders diagnosed by this technique include hemophilia (17), chronic granulomatous disease (56), $\alpha_1$-antitrypsin deficiency (36), thalassemia (34), sickle cell anemia (34), and Duchenne's muscular dystrophy. Some question has been raised, however, as to the accuracy of diagnosis in the last utilizing this technique (24). The procedure is associated with few complications; the amount of fetal blood taken is 50 to 500 $\mu$l (65).

## Ultrasonography

Imaging of uterine contents may be accomplished using sound waves that are transmitted into the mother's abdomen and reflected from tissues toward a collector. Interfaces between tissues with different sound-reflecting properties can be identified, and the information may be electronically processed and displayed pictorially on a television screen.

The chief use of this technique in obstetrics has been the determination of gestational age. Measurement of the biparietal diameter of the fetal skull correlates well with age and the accuracy and reproducibility of this technique is well established (62). The greatest discrimination power of ultrasound in biparietal diameter determination is during the period of most rapid head growth, between the 20th and 32nd postmenstrual weeks. Earlier, between 6 and 14 postmenstrual weeks, measurement of crown–rump length has been very accurate in estimating gestational age (10,64).

The identification of impaired fetal growth has been facilitated as well by ultrasonography. In most instances, fetal head growth will be maintained to a greater extent than body growth, and a ratio between the biparietal diameter and the trunk diameter or circumference may be useful in detecting early growth problems (10). Using serial measurements of biparietal diameter, growth retardation may be detected by an abnormally low increase in this parameter over a matter of weeks or may be detected at once by a diameter more than two standard deviations below the mean for gestational age (62).

Because of the tendency for head growth to be preserved even while significant intrauterine undernutrition exists, better estimates of somatic growth have been sought. Evaluation of total intrauterine volume has been accomplished by measuring the three diameters of the uterus ultrasonographically and treating it geometrically as an elliptical solid. Volume measurements thus calculated are correlated with gestational age, and a measurement 1.5 standard deviations below the mean for gestational age will identify growth-retarded babies with 75% accuracy (22). The disadvantage of this method is the difficulty in measuring accurately intrauterine diameters with the ultrasonographic technique. A small error in one diameter may be multiplied into a significant error in the volume calculation.

Fetal weight has been estimated by ultrasound measurements of various fetal parameters, most notably trunk circumference (11,31). Accuracy is best in the smaller babies, with 160 g being the average error in 1-kg fetuses (11). With this technique, 87% of fetuses under the fifth percentile for weight would be identified at 32 postmenstrual weeks (11).

Ultrasonography has also been useful in the evaluation of fetal morphology (32,83). Defects potentially discoverable include cranial and spinal abnormalities, renal cysts and obstructions, gastrointestinal obstructions, diaphragmatic hernias, omphalocele, and cardiac anomalies.

The recent development of real-time ultrasonography has enabled obstetricians to study fetal physiology with greater accuracy. This technique involves the rapid collection and display of ultrasonic data resulting in a moving picture display of the fetus. The detection of fetal limb or cardiac movement has been used to prove fetal life. Additionally, more detailed investigation of heart function is possible (83).

The detection of fetal respiration by ultrasound has been possible for nearly a decade (5), and current work is attempting to establish the role that this may play in evaluating high-risk pregnancies. Movement of the fetal thorax simulating respiration may be seen as early as the 13th postmenstrual week (14). These movements increase in frequency with gestational age (18) and are decreased by maternal hypoglycemia (43) and ethanol ingestion (19). A decrease in breathing movements has been noted in hypertension and diabetes mellitus (14), and it has been proposed that screening such pregnancies for the amount of fetal breathing movement will be of prognostic value in identifying fetuses at especially high risk of intrauterine demise; however, the wide range of breathing movement frequency in normal fetuses and the effects of maternal glucose and drug ingestion on breathing frequency make the standardization of normal frequency difficult (43). It is possible that evaluation of breathing frequency may be useful to discriminate between a diagnosis of fetal well-being and fetal danger when results of other tests are confusing or contradictory (51).

The measurement of the production rate of fetal urine is also possible with ultrasonography. By measuring bladder size and rate of emptying, urine volume per unit time is calculated. At 30 postmenstrual weeks, a rate of 9.6 ml/hr is seen. This rises to 27.3 ml/hr at term. An abnormally low rate is correlated with intrauterine growth retardation (82).

To date, exposure of the fetus or mother to ultrasonography has not been found to be harmful; however, the absorption of sound energy by developing tissues is a cause for concern about as yet undiscovered risks of this technique. For this reason, the indiscriminate use of ultrasonography is avoided, and the technique used only when clinically indicated.

## X-Ray

The use of X-ray for the detection of major morphological abnormalities in the fetus has been supplanted to a great extent by ultrasonography. Injection of radio-opaque contrast material into the amniotic fluid, however, may provide additional information. This technique, called amniography, will outline the fetus and thereby indicate soft tissue features in contrast to the bony skeleton. In addition, a delayed film permits fetal swallowing of the contrast material with subsequent identification of the fetal gastrointestinal tract. Amniography has been of use in the detection of hydrops fetalis, intestinal obstruction, conjoined twinning, diaphragmatic hernia, and in confirmation of fetal demise (absence of fetal swallowing) (12).

## Fetal Electrocardiography

The electrical activity of the fetal heart may yield information about cardiac disease similar to the information obtained in electrocardiography after birth. Direct electrode contact with the fetal scalp produces the most satisfactory electrocardiograms and has been used during labor in the diagnosis of rhythm disturbances in the unborn infant (71). Prior to rupture of the fetal membranes, an electrocardiogram may be obtained using electrodes applied to the maternal abdomen. This has the disadvantage of producing a tracing with poor P and T wave readability, and the maternal electrocardiogram will be superimposed on the fetal, further increasing the difficulties in interpretation (70).

In spite of the difficulties, antenatal electrocardiography has been used in the diagnosis of fetal rhythm disturbances (78). Combination of electrocardiography and phonocardiography yields additional information about congenital heart disease in the unborn (30).

The period of time between the initiation of ventricular depolarization (the Q wave of the electrocardiogram) and the opening of the semilunar valves (identifiable on phonocardiography) is the preejection period (PEP). It has been found in animal models (54) that the PEP is prolonged by acidosis. Investigation into the usefulness of the PEP in identifying fetuses with impaired placental respiratory function is encouraging, although normal values appear to vary with gestational age and fetal body weight (53,55). There is no known maternal or fetal risk from fetal electro-cardiography.

## Evaluation of Placental Function

The placenta is a complex organ that not only serves to transport nutrients and respiratory gases but also is active in hormone elaboration. Tests of several of these functions are used in an attempt to gain information concerning overall placental integrity.

Maternal urinary estrogen excretion has been known to correlate with evidence of fetal undernutrition (40). More specifically, the major estrogen of pregnancy, estriol, has shown some value in predicting fetuses with chronically impaired placental function (39). Virtually all of the maternal estriol is of placental origin, arising from aromatization of fetal 16-hydroxydehydroepiandrosterone sulfate (47). Estriol measurements have not shown usefulness in acute placental insufficiency, since the drop in hormone level is measurable too long after the time at which intervention would be indicated (45). In addition, wide fluctuations in values during serial collections and the failure of placental hormonal function to exactly parallel respiratory function have caused estriol measurement to be regarded as at best an adjunct in the following of high-risk pregnancy (2,39).

Another placental hormone, human placental lactogen (HPL), has been found to correlate with placental size and birth weight (85). Its measurement may lead to identification of the growth-retarded baby or the postmature baby with failing placental function (84,26). Used in a prospective study, HPL measurements were found to be valuable in reducing perinatal mortality by identifying the fetus at high risk (74).

Both estriol and HPL are present in widely varying amounts for a given gestational age, and unless levels are very low, their usefulness in managing a pregnancy is limited. Some value has been found for the measurement of the placental conversion of exogenously administered dehydroepiandrosterone sulfate (61,76) to estriol. This test has not gained widespread clinical acceptance because of the cumbersome method of the technique.

The evaluation of placental respiratory function consists of observation of the fetal heart rate in the face of an induced challenge to placental perfusion. The challenge that has been used is the induction of uterine contractions that diminish perfusion of the placental intervillous space. The occurrence of three mild contractions within 10 min is accepted as the standard challenge, and a positive test, suggesting impaired placental reserve, is indicated by the deceleration of the fetal heart rate following the onset of the contraction (20,63). This oxytocin challenge test (OCT) has been found to be most reliable when it is negative (79); a negative test has greater than a 98% predictive value for at least 1 week of continued fetal life *in utero* (4). The false positive rate, however, may be as high as 33% (4), although, generally, positive OCTs are associated with impaired perinatal survival (2) and poorer initial neurological function in surviving infants (67).

The observation that actively moving fetuses are rarely in danger from placental insufficiency has led to the development of the nonstress test (NST) in which accelerations of the fetal heart rate associated with fetal movement are interpreted as a reactive pattern. Nonreactive patterns may indicate impaired placental function or may merely reflect fetal sleep; in such cases, an OCT may be expected to discriminate between the presence or absence of respiratory difficulties. A reactive NST predicts adequate placental function with 99.9% accuracy (42,68). The finding that positive OCTs are always predicted by nonreactive NSTs (3,41) has led most centers to perform the NST initially as a screening procedure to determine whether an OCT is indicated.

When properly performed, the OCT and NST are safe for the mother and the fetus. The dose of oxytocin used is controlled by a constant-infusion pump and titration of this drug begins at a low level to avoid uterine hyperstimulation. Occasionally, labor is noted shortly after an OCT is performed; however, this is generally seen in term gestations and is not considered an adverse development.

## Evaluation of Fetal Maturity

In caring for pregnancies at high risk, decisions must frequently be made regarding the optimal time for delivery. The risks of prematurity must be weighed against the risk of continuing the pregnancy. Information regarding the maturity of the fetus, and particularly of the fetal lung, is often of prime importance.

X-ray evaluation of long-bone epiphyseal calcification has been used in estimating fetal age (60). No information about lung maturity is thus gained, however, and the procedure involves exposure to ionizing radiation. Ultrasonographic measurement of the biparietal diameter has been thought to show a correlation between values of 9.0 cm and fetal maturity (25), but more recently this method has not been considered reliable enough for clinical usefulness in predicting maturity of the lung (75).

The evaluation of amniotic fluid obtained by amniocentesis has been the most important method of determining fetal maturity. Measurements of fluid creatinine (58) and the percentage of fetal cells stainable for fat (7,8) have been used in the past to predict maturity and are now used chiefly to confirm direct measurement of pulmonary surface-active materials. These materials which are related to or part of pulmonary surfactant, provide very reliable indicators of fetal lung maturity.

The measurement of lecithin and its comparison with sphingomyelin levels (to standardize the dilutional factor of the amniotic fluid) have been the standard determination of fetal maturity (21). The major drawback of this test is its controversial usefulness in diabetic pregnancies where amniotic fluid lipids may be elevated in the absence of fetal lung maturity (44). Other phospholipids in amniotic fluid have been noted to be correlated with fetal lung maturity (29), and one of these, phosphatidyl glycerol, appears especially valuable in predicting adequate fetal pulmonary surfactant. Newborns who developed respiratory distress syndrome were noted never to have had detectable pulmonary phosphatidyl glycerol (28), and, conversely, no pregnancy in which any phosphatidyl glycerol was found in the amniotic fluid resulted in delivery of an infant with respiratory distress syndrome (9). It appears likely that this measurement will provide obstetricians with the most reliable indicator of when the high-risk fetus may be delivered without fear of pulmonary immaturity.

## SUMMARY

There is a new emphasis in obstetrics on the detection of the fetus at risk for developmental abnormalities and for impaired *in utero* survival. Methods to detect the former have permitted affected pregnancies to be terminated in the second trimester. The latter pregnancies are followed closely with a battery of tests of placental integrity, hopefully until tests of fetal maturity indicate that the fetus may be safely delivered from the high-risk intrauterine environment.

## REFERENCES

1. Aubrey, R. H., and Pennington, J. C. (1973): Identification and evaluation of high risk pregnancy: The perinatal concept. *Clin. Obstet. Gynecol.*, 16:3–27.
2. Barrada, M. I., Edwards, L. E., and Hakanson, E. Y. (1979): Antepartum fetal testing: I. The oxytocin challenge test. *Am. J. Obstet. Gynecol.*, 134:532–537.
3. Barrada, M. I., Edwards, L. E., and Hakanson, E. Y. (1979): Antepartum fetal testing: II. The acceleration/constant ratio: A nonstress test. *Am. J. Obstet. Gynecol.*, 134:538–543.
4. Baskett, T. F., and Sandy, E. A. (1977): The oxytocin challenge test and antepartum fetal assessment. *Br. J. Obstet. Gynaecol.*, 84:39–43.
5. Boddy, K., and Robinson, J. S. (1971): External method for detection of fetal breathing *in utero*. *Lancet*, 2:1231–1233.
6. Brock, D. J. H. (1976): Alphafetoprotein and neural tube defects. *J. Clin. Pathol. [Suppl.]*, 10:157–164.
7. Brosens, I. A. (1966): Cytological study of amniotic fluid with Nile blue sulfate staining. *Acta Cytol. (Baltimore)*, 10:159–160.
8. Brosens, I., and Gordon, H. (1966): The estimation of maturity by cytologic examination of the liquor amnii. *J. Obstet. Gynecol. Br. Commonw.*, 73:88–90.
9. Bustos, R., Kulovich, M. V., Gluck, L., Gabbe, S. G., Evertson, L., Vargas, C., and Lowenberg, E. (1979): Significance of phosphatidylglycerol in amniotic fluid in complicated pregnancies. *Am. J. Obstet. Gynecol.*, 133:899–903.
10. Campbell, S. (1974): Fetal growth. *Clin. Obstet. Gynecol.*, 1:41–65.
11. Campbell, S., and Wilkin, D. (1975): Ultrasonic measurement of fetal abdomen circumference in the estimation of fetal weight. *Br. J. Obstet. Gynaecol.*, 82:689–697.

12. Caterini, H., Sama, J., Iffy, L., Harrington, J., Pelosi, M., and Tiku, J. (1976): A re-evaluation of amniography. *Obstet. Gynecol.,* 47:373–377.
13. Davies, P. A. (1974): Maternal and fetal infection. *Clin. Obstet. Gynecol.,* 1:17–39.
14. Dawes, G. S. (1974): Fetal circulation and breathing. *Clin. Obstet. Gynecol.,* 1:139–149.
15. Eriksson, M., Catz, C. S., and Yaffe, S. J. (1973): Drugs and pregnancy. *Clin. Obstet. Gynecol.,* 16:199–224.
16. Ferguson-Smith, M. A., and Ferguson-Smith, M. E. (1976): Screening for fetal chromosome aberrations in early pregnancy. *J. Clin. Pathol. [Suppl.],* 10:165–176.
17. Firshein, S. I., Hoyer, L. W., Lazarchick, J., Forget, B. J., Hobbins, J. C., Clyne, L. P., Pitlick, F. A., Muir, W. A., Merkatz, I. R., and Mahoney, M. J. (1979):Prenatal diagnosis of classic hemophilia. *N. Engl. J. Med.,* 300:938–941.
18. Fox, H. E., Inglis, J., and Steinbrecher, M. (1979): Fetal breathing movements in uncomplicated pregnancies. *Am. J. Obstet. Gynecol.,* 134:544–546.
19. Fox, H. E., Steinbrecher, M., Pessel, D., Inglis, J., Medvid, L., and Angel, E. (1978): Maternal ethanol ingestion and the occurrence of human fetal breathing movements. *Am. J. Obstet. Gynecol.,* 132:354–358.
20. Freeman, R. K., Goebelsman, U., Nochimson, D., and Cetrulo, C. (1976): An evaluation of the significance of a positive oxytocin challenge test. *Obstet. Gynecol.,* 47:8–13.
21. Gluck, L., Kulovich, M. V., Borer, R. C., Brenner, P. H., Anderson, G. G., and Spellacy, W. N. (1971): Diagnosis of the respiratory distress syndrome by amniocentesis. *Am. J. Obstet. Gynecol.,* 109:440–445.
22. Gohari, P., Berkowitz, R. L., and Hobbins, J. C. (1977): Prediction of intrauterine growth retardation by determination of total intrauterine volume. *Am. J. Obstet. Gynecol.,* 127:255–260.
23. Golbus, M. S., Laughman, W. D., Epstein, J., Halbasch, G., Stephens, J. D., and Hall, B. D. (1979): Prenatal genetic diagnosis in 3000 amniocenteses. *N. Engl. J. Med.,* 300:157–163.
24. Golbus, M. S., Stephens, J. D., Mahoney, M. J., Hobbins, J. C., Haseltine, F. P., Caskey, C. T., and Banker, B. Q. (1979): Failure of fetal creatinine phosphokinase as a diagnostic indicator of Duchenne muscular dystrophy. *N. Engl. J. Med.,* 300:860–861.
25. Goldstein, P., Gershenson, D., and Hobbins, J. C. (1976): Fetal biparietal diameter as a predictor of a mature lecithin/sphingomyelin ratio. *Obstet. Gynecol.,* 48:667–669.
26. Granat, M., Sharf, M., Dengott, D., Spindel, A., Kahana, L., and Elrad, H. (1977): Further investigation on the predictive value of human placental lactogen in high risk pregnancies. *Am. J. Obstet. Gynecol.,* 129:647–654.
27. Grebner, E. E., and Jackson, L. G. (1979): Prenatal diagnosis of Tay-Sachs disease. *Am. J. Obstet. Gynecol.,* 134:547–550.
28. Hallman, M., Feldman, B. H., Kirkpatrick, E., and Gluck, L. (1977): Absence of phosphatidyl-glycerol (PG) in respiratory distress syndrome in the newborn. *Pediatr. Res.,* 11:714–720.
29. Hallman, M., Kulovich, M., Kirkpatrick, E., Sugarman, R. G., and Gluck, L. (1976): Phosphatidylinositol and phosphatidylglycerol in amniotic fluid. *Am. J. Obstet. Gynecol.,* 125:613–617.
30. Hamilton, L. A., Fisher, E., Horn, C., DuBrow, I., and Vidyasagar, D. (1977): A new prenatal cardiac diagnostic device for congenital heart disease. *Obstet. Gynecol.,* 50:491–494.
31. Higginbottom, J., Slater, J., Porter, G., and Whitfield, C. R. (1975): Estimation of fetal weight from ultrasonic measurement of trunk circumference. *Br. J. Obstet. Gynaecol.,* 82:698–701.
32. Hobbins, J. C., Grannum, P. A. T., Berkowitz, R. L., Silverman, R., and Mahoney, M. J. (1979): Ultrasound in the diagnosis of congenital anomalies. *Am. J. Obstet. Gynecol.,* 134:331–345.
33. Hobbins, J. C., and Mahoney, M. J. (1974): *In utero* diagnosis of hemoglobinopathies: Technique for obtaining fetal blood. *N. Engl. J. Med.,* 290:1065–1067.
34. Hobbins, J. C., and Mahoney, M. J. (1977): Fetoscopy in continuing pregnancies. *Am. J. Obstet. Gynecol.,* 129:440–443.
35. Hobel, C. J., Hyvarinen, M. A., Okada, D. M., and Oh, W. (1973): Prenatal and intrapartum high risk screening: Prediction of the high risk neonate. *Am. J. Obstet. Gynecol.,* 117:1–9.
36. Jeppsson, J. O., Franzen, B., Sveger, T., Cordesius, E., Stromberg, P., and Gustavii, B. (1979): Prenatal exclusion of alpha-1-antitrypsin deficiency in a high risk fetus. *N. Engl. J. Med.,* 300:1441.
37. Kjessler, B., and Johansson, S. G. O. (1977): Monitoring of the development of early pregnancy by determination of alpha-fetoprotein in maternal serum and amniotic fluid samples. *Acta Obstet. Gynecol. Scand. [Suppl.],* 69:5–14.

38. Kjessler, B., Johansson, S. G. O., Lidbjork, G., and Sherman, M. S. (1977): Alphafetoprotein (AFP) levels in maternal serum in relation to pregnancy outcome in 7158 pregnant women prospectively investigated during their 14th–20th week post last menstrual period. *Acta Obstet. Gynecol. Scand. [Suppl.]*, 69:25–44.
39. Klopper, A. (1972): The assessment of fetoplacental function by estriol assay. *Obstet. Gynecol. Surv.*, 23:813–838.
40. Law, J. A., Galbraith, R. S., and Boston, R. W. (1973): Maternal urinary estrogen patterns in intrauterine growth retardation. *Obstet. Gynecol.*, 42:325–329.
41. Lee, C. Y., DiLoreto, P. C., and Logrand, B. (1976): Fetal activity acceleration determination for the evaluation of fetal reserve. *Obstet. Gynecol.*, 48:19–26.
42. Lee, C. Y., and Drukker, B. (1979): The non-stress test for the antepartum assessment of fetal reserve. *Am. J. Obstet. Gynecol.*, 134:460–470.
43. Lewis, P., and Boylan, P. (1979): Fetal breathing: A review. *Am. J. Obstet. Gynecol.*, 134:587–598.
44. Lowensohn, R. I., and Gabbe, S. G. (1979): The value of lecithin/sphingomyelin ratios in diabetes. *Am. J. Obstet. Gynecol.*, 134:702–704.
45. Lundy, E. L., Chung-Shiu, W., and Lee, S. G. (1973): Estrogen assessment in the high risk pregnancy. *Clin. Obstet. Gynecol.*, 16:279–297.
46. Macri, J. N., Haddow, J. E., and Weiss, R. R. (1979): Screening for neural tube defects in the United States. *Am. J. Obstet. Gynecol.*, 133:119–125.
47. Madden, J. D., Gant, N. F., and MacDonald, P. C. (1978): Study of the kinetics of conversion of maternal plasma dehydroisoandrosterone sulfate to 16-alpha-hydroxydehydroisoandrosterone sulfate, estradiol, and estriol. *Am. J. Obstet. Gynecol.*, 132:392–395.
48. Magenis, R. E., Overton, K. M., Chamberlin, J., Brady, T., and Lovrien, E. (1977): Parental origin of the extra chromosome in Down's syndrome. *Hum. Genet.*, 37:7–16.
49. Mahoney, M. J., Haseltine, F. P., Hobbins, J. C., Banker, B. Q., Caskey, C. T., and Golbus, M. S. (1977): Prenatal diagnosis of Duchenne's muscular dystrophy. *N. Engl. J. Med.*, 247:968–973.
50. Manganiello, P. D., Byrd, J. R., Tho, P. T., and McDonaugh, P. G. (1979): A report of the safety and accuracy of mid-trimester amniocentesis at the Medical College of Georgia. *Am. J. Obstet. Gynecol.*, 134:911–916.
51. Manning, F. A., and Platt, L. D. (1979): Fetal breathing movements and the abnormal contraction stress test. *Am. J. Obstet. Gynecol.*, 135:590–593.
52. Milunsky, A., and Atkins, L. (1974): Prenatal diagnosis of genetic disorders. *J.A.M.A.*, 230:232–235.
53. Murata, Y., Martin, C. B., Ikenoue, T., and Lu, P. S. (1978): Antepartum evaluation of the pre-ejection period of the fetal cardiac cycle. *Am. J. Obstet. Gynecol.*, 132:278–284.
54. Murata, Y., Miyake, K., and Quilligan, E. J. (1979): Pre-ejection period of cardiac cycles in fetal lamb. *Am. J. Obstet. Gynecol.*, 133:509–514.
55. Murata, Y., Pijls, N., Miyake, K., Schmidt, P., Martin, C. B., and Singer, J. (1979): Antepartum determination of pre-ejection period of fetal cardiac cycle. *Am. J. Obstet. Gynecol.*, 133:515–518.
56. Newburger, P. E., Cohen, J. J., Rothchild, S. B., Hobbins, J. C., Malawista, S. E., and Mahoney, M. J. (1979): Prenatal diagnosis of chronic granulomatous disease. *N. Eng. J. Med.*, 300:178–181.
57. NICHD National Registry for Amniocentesis Study Group (1976): Midtrimester amniocentesis for genetic diagnosis: Safety and accuracy. *J.A.M.A.*, 236:1471–1476.
58. Pitkin, R. M., and Zwirek, S. J. (1967): Amniotic fluid creatinine. *Am. J. Obstet. Gynecol.*, 98:1135–1139.
59. Pritchard, J. A., and MacDonald, P. C. (1976): *Williams Obstetrics*, 15th Edition, pp. 1–8. Appleton-Century-Crofts, New York.
60. Pritchard, J. A., and MacDonald, P. C. (1976): *Williams Obstetrics*, 15th Edition, pp. 276–277. Appleton-Century-Crofts, New York.
61. Pupkin, M. J., Nagey, D. A., Schomberg, D. W., MacKenna, J. M., and Crenshaw, C. (1979): The dehydroepiandrosterone loading test. *Am. J. Obstet. Gynecol.*, 134:281–288.
62. Queenan, J. T., Kubarych, S. F., Cook, L. N., Anderson, G. D., and Griffin, L. P. (1976): Diagnostic ultrasound for detection of intrauterine growth retardation. *Am. J. Obstet. Gynecol.*, 124:865–873.
63. Ray, M., Freeman, R. K., Pine, S., and Hesselgesser, R. (1972): Clinical experience with the oxytocin challenge test. *Am. J. Obstet. Gynecol.*, 114:1–9.

64. Robinson, H. P., and Fleming, J. E. E. (1975): A critical evaluation of sonar "crown–rump length" measurements. *Br. J. Obstet. Gynaecol.*, 82:702–710.
65. Rodeck, C. H., and Campbell, S. (1978): Sampling pure fetal blood by fetoscopy in second trimester of pregnancy. *Br. Med. J.*, 2:728.
66. Sadovsky, E., Yaffe, H., and Polishuk, W. Z. (1974): Fetal movement monitoring in normal and pathologic pregnancy. *Int. J. Gynecol. Obstet.*, 12:75.
67. Scanlon, J. W., Suzuki, U., Shea, E., and Tronick, E. (1979): A prospective study of the oxytocin challenge test and newborn neurobehavioral outcome. *Obstet. Gynecol.*, 54:6–11.
68. Schifrin, B. S., Foye, G., Amato, J., Kates, R., and MacKenna, J. (1979): Routine fetal heart rate monitoring in the antepartum period. *Obstet. Gynecol.*, 54:21–25.
69. Sever, J. L. (1973): Effects of infections on pregnancy risk. *Clin. Obstet. Gynecol.*, 16:225–234.
70. Shenker, L. (1966): Fetal electrocardiography. *Obstet. Gynecol. Surv.*, 21:367–388.
71. Shenker, L. (1979): Fetal cardiac arrhythmias. *Obstet. Gynecol. Surv.*, 34:561–572.
72. Simmons, S. C. (1974): Organisation of fetal intensive care. *Clin. Obstet. Gynaecol. (Lond.)*, 1:139–149.
73. Simpson, N. E., Dallaire, L., Miller, J. R., Siminovich, L., Hamerton, J. L., Miller, J., and McKeen, C. (1976): Prenatal diagnosis of genetic disease in Canada. *Can. Med. Assoc. J.*, 115:739–748.
74. Spellacy, W. N., Buhi, W. C., and Birk, S. A. (1975): The effectiveness of human placental lactogen measurements as an adjunct in decreasing perinatal mortality. *Am. J. Obstet. Gynecol.*, 121:835–843.
75. Spellacy, W. N., Gelman, S. R., Wood, S. D., Birk, S. A., and Buhi, W. C. (1978): Comparison of fetal maturity evaluation with ultrasound biparietal diameter and amniotic fluid lecithin/sphingomyelin ratio. *Obstet. Gynecol.*, 51:109–111.
76. Stembara, Z. K., and Herzmann, J. (1973): Evaluation of the DHEA-S test as an index of fetoplacental insufficiency. *J. Perinat. Med.*, 1:192–197.
77. Sternberg, J. (1973): Radiation risk in pregnancy. *Clin. Obstet. Gynecol.*, 16:235–278.
78. Teteris, N. J., Chishold, J. W., and Ullery, J. C. (1968): Antenatal diagnosis of congenital heart block. *Obstet. Gynecol.*, 32:851–853.
79. Weingold, A. B., DeJesus, T. P. S., and O'Kieffe, J. (1975): Oxytocin challenge test. *Am. J. Obstet. Gynecol.*, 123:466–472.
80. Whitfield, C. R. (1974): The diagnostic value of amniocentesis. *Clin. Obstet. Gynaecol. (Lond.)*, 1:67–84.
81. Winick, M., Brasel, J. A., and Velasco, E. G. (1973): Effects of prenatal nutrition upon pregnancy risk. *Clin. Obstet. Gynecol.*, 16:184–198.
82. Wladimiroff, J. W., and Campbell, S. (1974): Fetal urine production rates in normal and complicated pregnancy. *Lancet*, 1:151–154.
83. Yamaguchi, D. T., and Lee, F. Y. L. (1979): Ultrasonic evaluation of the fetal heart. *Am. J. Obstet. Gynecol.*, 134:422–430.
84. Zlatnik, F. J., Varner, M. W., and Hauser, K. S. (1979): Human placental lactogen: A predictor of perinatal outcome? *Obstet. Gynecol.*, 54:205–210.
85. Zlatnik, F. J., Varner, M. W., Hauser, K. S., and Lee, S. S. (1979): HPL: Physiologic and pathophysiologic observations. *Obstet. Gynecol.*, 54:314–317.

*Developmental Toxicology*, edited by
C. A. Kimmel and J. Buelke-Sam. Raven Press,
New York © 1981.

# Biochemical Disturbances Associated with Developmental Toxicity

## F. D. Andrew and P. S. Lytz

*Biology Department, Pacific Northwest Laboratory, Richland,
Washington 99352*

Theoretical considerations and recent experience have led us to propose (5) that evaluation of perinatal enzymology represents one approach for improved testing of postnatal functional development. The general assumption is made that detectable changes in developmental profiles of key enzymes in the main metabolic pathways may account for postnatal growth inhibition, mental retardation, or decreased viability. Only recently has this concept begun to receive consideration in experimental teratology (5,40,41,87,90). Quantifiable deviations in the activity of organ-characteristic enzyme systems may be sensitive and reliable indicators for estimating threshold levels for deleterious effects.

Considerable attention has been given to basic studies of the developmental profiles of enzymes that catalyze essential steps in various metabolic processes (18,38,39,41,44,47,51,57,67,76,85,112,113,124). In this respect, temporal and/or quantitative deviations of individual enzyme profiles, as well as related evaluations of specific target tissues, may be of practical predictive value. Enzymes are one of the largest and most varied classes of specific chemical constituents of cells. Therefore, detection of metabolic lesions, particularly in the absence of morphological abnormalities, would greatly extend the sensitivity of standard teratological procedures.

Quantitative analysis of enzyme patterns in developing tissues should provide valid and objective criteria for maturational and functional comparisons. Thus, alterations of enzyme activity ontogenic profiles, changes in key regulatory enzyme activity, modifications of isoenzyme patterns, or other enzymic changes may reflect perturbation of fundamental biochemical processes such as those essential for energy production and utilization (11). In addition, organ-specific enzyme profiles continue to evolve and undergo drastic changes long after these organs have become morphologically distinct. This allows for evaluation of maturational status of organ function (112). This chapter will attempt to demonstrate that quantification of even a small battery of enzymes in a limited group of tissues could provide a baseline for distinguishing differences in degree of developmental toxicity.

*145*

## BACKGROUND

Several physical, chemical, and nutritional insults incurred during gestation have been shown to modify enzyme ontogeny (Tables 1 and 2). In the preparation of these tables, we focused on: (a) the apparent relationship between specific agents and their associated target tissues; (b) the number of different tissues possessing the same enzyme activity; (c) our knowledge of the ages of onset of enzyme activity; and (d) the inclusion of several major metabolic pathways. The following discussion is not intended as a comprehensive review of all perinatal enzymology literature. It is a survey of pertinent sources that provide a general overview to those who are unfamiliar with this topic.

### Effects of Physical Agents

It is well documented that irradiation (e.g., γ- or X-ray) of rats at levels of 100 to 150 rad or greater induces some degree of developmental toxicity if administered during the embryonic or fetal periods (16). Classic effects of prenatal irradiation of mammalian embryos are intrauterine and postnatal growth retardation and mortality (16,96,100) and structural and functional malformations (15,64).

Radiation-induced alterations in tissue enzyme activity during development have also been found. Rats exposed to 180 rad at 15 days of gestation (dg) and sacrificed at 1 day postnatally (pn) show a decrease in liver glucose-6-phosphatase (EC 3.1.3.9), glycerophosphate dehydrogenase (EC 1.1.99.5), and lactic dehydrogenase (EC 1.1.1.27) activities as well as growth retardation and increased postnatal mortality (104). Garner et al. (33) exposed rats to 140 rad on 14 dg and reported elevated liver serine dehydratase (EC 4.2.1.13/14) at 3 pn and decreased liver and brain nonspecific esterase (EC 3.1.1.1) at 9 pn.

Responses to pre- and postnatal irradiation vary because of differential sensitivity during these two periods; i.e., a much greater dose is required postnatally than prenatally (15,16). For example, postnatal exposure of rats to 280 rad at 10 pn with sacrifice at 18 pn caused an increase in tryptophan oxygenase (EC 1.13.1.12) and ornithine aminotransferase (EC 2.6.1.13) activities with no other apparent effects (60).

Collectively, these data suggest that perinatal irradiation during late organogenesis in rats may alter enzyme ontogeny. Unfortunately, the cited studies generally failed to report whether other manifestations of exposure also were detected. Thus, the relative sensitivity of this approach cannot be determined from these studies.

### Effects of Chemical Agents

Recent studies have shown that exposure to certain environmental chemicals can affect a number of enzymes in adults and occasionally in immature individuals. Exposure of pregnant guinea pigs to triethylene-tetramine has been shown to alter γ-glutamyl transpeptidase (EC 2.3.2.2), cholinesterase (EC 3.1.1.8), and alanine and aspartate aminotransferase (EC 2.6.1.2/1) activities in maternal kidney, brain,

TABLE 1. *Toxicity-related modifications of rat tissue enzyme ontogeny*

| Enzyme name | EC No.[a] | Tissue | Agent | Dose | Age[b] | Effect | References |
|---|---|---|---|---|---|---|---|
| Lactic dehydrogenase | 1.1.1.27 | Liver | X-ray | 180 rad | pn 1 | ↓ | 104 |
| Glycerophosphate dehydrogenase | 1.1.99.5 | Liver | X-ray | 180 rad | pn 1 | ↓ | 104 |
| Glucose-6-phosphatase | 3.1.3.9 | Liver | X-ray | 180 rad | pn 1 | ↓ | 104 |
| Serine dehydratase | 4.2.1.13/14 | Liver | γ-ray | 140 rad | pn 3 | ↑ | 33 |
| Carboxylesterase | 3.1.1.1 | Liver | γ-ray | 140 rad | pn 9/pn 40 | ↓/↑ | 33 |
| Carboxylesterase | 3.1.1.1 | Brain | γ-ray | 140 rad | pn 9/pn 40 | ↓/↑ | 33 |
| Glutathione S-transferase | 2.5.1.18 | Liver | PCB (isomers) | 3,10,30 mg/kg | pn 6,21 | ↑ | 78 |
| Benzo(a)pyrene hydroxylase | 1.14.14.1 | Liver | PCB (Aroclor) | 25 mg/kg | dg 20 | ↑ | 3 |
| Benzo(a)pyrene hydroxylase | 1.14.14.1 | Placenta | PCB (Aroclor) | 25 mg/kg | dg 20 | ↑ | 3 |
| Glucose-6-phosphatase | 3.1.3.9 | Liver | Methylmercury | 4,8 ppm | dg 20 pn 16 | ↑ | 106 |
| Monoamine oxidase | 1.4.3.4 | Liver | Methylmercury | 5,10 ppm | dg 19 | ↓ | 30 |
| Cytochrome oxidase | 1.9.3.1 | Liver | Methylmercury | 5,10 ppm | dg 19 | ↓ | 30 |
| Lactase | 3.2.1.23 | Intestine[c] | Hydrazine | 150, 260 mg/kg | pn 3,4 | ↑ | 97 |
| Invertase | 3.2.1.26 | Intestine[c] | Hydrazine | 150, 260 mg/kg | pn 24,25 | ↑ | 97 |
| Alkaline phosphatase | 3.1.3.1 | Intestine[c] | Hydrazine | 150, 260 mg/kg | pn 3,4,24,25 | ↑ | 97 |
| Succinate dehydrogenase | 1.3.99.1 | Brain | Low protein diet | 8% Casein | pn 14,21 | ↓ | 22,121 |
| Glucose-6-phosphate dehydrogenase | 1.1.1.49 | Brain | Low protein diet | 8% Casein | pn 21/pn 42 | ↓/↑ | 22,121 |
| Fructose diphosphate aldolase | 4.1.2.13 | Brain | Low protein diet | 8% Casein | pn 14,21,42 | ↑ | 22,121 |
| Acetylcholinesterase | 3.1.1.7 | Brain | Low protein diet | 8% Casein | pn 14/42 | ↓/↑ | 22,121 |
| Succinate dehydrogenase | 1.3.99.1 | Brain | Undernourishment | 10 g/rat per day | pn 21 | ↓ | 1 |
| Fructose diphospate aldolase | 4.1.2.13 | Brain | Undernourishment | 10 g/rat per day | pn 21 | ↓ | 1 |
| Acetylcholinesterase | 3.1.1.7 | Brain | Undernourishment | 10 g/rat per day | pn 21 | → | 1 |

[a]Enzyme Commission number (70).
[b]Age at sacrifice.
[c]Experiments were with hamsters.

TABLE 2. Endocrine regulation of rat tissue enzyme ontogeny

| Enzyme name | EC No.[a] | Tissue | Agent[b] | Dose[c] | Age[d] | References |
|---|---|---|---|---|---|---|
| Tyrosine aminotransferase | 2.6.1.5 | Liver | Glucagon | 0.05 mg(F)/0.25 mg (P) | dg 19–21/pn 2–5 | 37,45,66 |
| Glucose-6-phosphatase | 3.1.3.9 | Liver | Glucagon | 0.05 mg(F) | dg 18–21 | 37,45 |
| Serine dehydratase | 4.2.1.13 | Liver | Glucagon | 0.05 mg(F)/0.25 mg(P) | dg 22/pn 4 | 45,108 |
| Phosphoenolpyruvate carboxykinase | 4.1.1.32 | Liver | Glucagon | 0.05, 0.5 mg(F) | dg 17–21 | 53 |
| L-Serine-pyruvate aminotransferase | 2.6.1.51 | Liver | Glucagon | 0.05 mg(F) | dg 21 | 108 |
| Tyrosine aminotransferase | 2.6.1.5 | Liver | Hydrocortisone | 2.5 mg(P) | pn 3–21, 50 | 31,37,45 |
| Tyrosine aminotransferase | 2.6.1.5 | Liver | Dexamethasone | 3 mg(P) | pn 1,2,4,11,42 | 20 |
| Tyrosine aminotransferase | 2.6.1.5 | Liver | Triamcinolone | 0.5 mg (F) | dg 17–21 | 130 |
| Serine dehydratase | 4.2.1.13 | Liver | Cortisol | 2.5 mg (F) | pn 4,10,11,21,26 | 108 |
| Ornithine aminotransferase | 2.6.1.13 | Liver | Hydrocortisone | 0.05, 0.5 mg (P) | pn 8 | 58 |
| Ornithine aminotransferase | 2.6.1.13 | Liver | Triamcinolone | 5 mg(P) | Birth–pn 12 | 58,92 |
| Tryptophan oxygenase | 1.13.11.11 | Liver | Hydrocortisone | 2.5 mg(P) | pn 7–21 | 31 |
| Phosphoserine phosphatase | 3.1.3.3 | Liver | Hydrocortisone | 0.125 mg(F) | dg 19–21 | 71 |
| Arginine synthetase system[e] | 6.3.4.5/4.3.2.1 | Liver | Triamcinolone | 0.5 mg(M) | pn 4 | 94 |
| Glucokinase | 2.7.1.2 | Liver | Hydrocortisone | 0.05 mg(M) | pn 15 | 72 |
| Glucose-6-phosphatase | 3.1.3.9 | Kidney | Cortisol | 5, 12.5 mg(P) | pn 5–8 | 42 |
| Aspartate aminotransferase | 2.6.1.1 | Kidney | Cortisol | 12.5 mg(P) | pn 7 | 42 |
| Aspartate aminotransferase | 2.6.1.1 | Heart | Cortisol | 12.5 mg(P) | pn 7 | 42 |
| Aspartate aminotransferase | 2.6.1.1 | Liver | Cortisol | 12.5 mg(P) | pn 7 | 42 |
| Glucose-6-phosphatase | 3.1.3.9 | Liver | Thyroxine | 0.003 mg(F) | dg 20–21 | 37 |
| NADP dehydrogenase | 1.6.99.1 | Liver | Thyroxine | 0.003 mg(F) | dg 20–21 | 37 |
| Malate:NADP oxidoreductase | 1.1.1.40 | Liver | Thyroxine | 0.025 mg(M) | pn 7 | 48 |
| Pyruvate kinase | 2.7.1.40 | Liver | Thyroxine | 0.025 mg(M) | pn 7 | 48 |
| Ornithine aminotransferase | 2.6.1.13 | Kidney | Estrogen | 0.5 mg(P) | pn 21 | 58 |
| Ornithine aminotransferase | 2.6.1.13 | Kidney | Estrogen | 0.5 mg(M) | pn 11 | 58 |
| Tyrosine aminotransferase | 2.6.1.5 | Liver | Cyclic AMP | 0.125, 0.5 mg(F)/2.5 mg(P) | dg 18–21/pn 2,50 | 37 |
| Glucose-6-phosphatase | 3.1.39 | Liver | Cyclic AMP | 0.125 mg(F) | dg 18–21 | 37 |
| Phosphoenolpyruvate carboxykinase | 4.1.1.32 | Liver | Cyclic AMP | 0.1–1.0 μmol(F) | dg 17–21 | 53 |
| L-Serine-pyruvate aminotransferase | 2.6.1.51 | Liver | Cyclic AMP | 0.5 mg(F) | dg 21 | 108 |

[a]Enzyme Commission number (70).
[b]Examples listed are those where the agent accelerates enzyme development.
[c]All substances were administered intraperitoneally 2–48 hr before assay, except reference 42, where dosing was 7 days before assay. Fetal doses (F) were per fetus, postnatal doses (P) were per 100 g body weight, and multiple doses (M) were per day for 3–6 days.
[d]Age at sacrifice.
[e]Argininosuccinate synthetase (EC 6.3.4.5) and argininosuccinase (EC 4.3.2.1).

and liver homogenates, respectively (27). Transplacental exposure of mammalian embryos to polychlorinated hydrocarbons (e.g., PCBs) induces a broad spectrum of toxic manifestations including enzymatic effects (74,80,123).

Another organochlorine compound suspected of altering enzyme ontogeny is 2,3,7,8-tetrachlorodibenzo-*p*-dioxin (TCDD), a potent contaminant of numerous polychlorinated hydrocarbons, which induces a variety of toxic effects (81). Prenatal exposure to subteratogenic doses of TCDD increased the activity of nonsteroidal UDP glucuronyl transferase (EC 2.4.1.17) in several tissues of neonatal and weanling rats but not in those of fetal rats (81). Thus, polychlorinated hydrocarbon toxicity may include disturbances of enzyme maturation if intoxication occurs during pregnancy (see also G. W. Lucier, *this volume*).

The environmental hazards of organomercury compounds are well known, and manifestations of intoxication include neurological dysfunction and hepatotoxicity in humans and rodents. Methylmercury induces ultrastructural changes and depression of enzymatic function of fetal rat liver mitochondria following exposure before and throughout gestation (30). Altered levels of glucose-6-phosphatase (EC 3.1.3.9) activity in neonatal rat livers, together with postnatal hypoglycemia and depressed carbohydrate metabolism, have been demonstrated following a single exposure at 9 dg (106). Thus, organomercurials also may perturb enzyme development.

Hydrazine is a widely used industrial chemical, a contaminant of malic hydrazide herbicides, and a missile propellant (97,109). Toxic effects on brain, liver, and intestine include teratogenicity, carcinogenicity, and alterations of polyamine synthesis in rats and/or hamsters (97,109). In particular, hydrazine inhibits several pyridoxal-requiring enzymes and stimulates adult rat liver ornithine decarboxylase (EC 4.1.1.17) which is involved in polyamine regulation (109). In addition, it alters the development of three key brush border enzymes of hamster intestine which possess different metabolic functions and different ontogenic profiles (97). Thus, these effects on intestinal enzymes may compromise the ability of neonatal hamsters to accomodate the nutritional changes associated with postnatal life.

Although the effects of ethanol on enzyme development are less spectacular than those produced by the organochlorines or organomercurials, the number of pregnant individuals exposed to ethanol is undoubtedly much larger. There is some suggestive evidence that prenatal exposure to ethanol alters perinatal development of rat brain tyrosine 3-monooxygenase (EC 1.14.16.2) (14) and ornithine decarboxylase activity in rat brain and heart (117).

Again, as was the case for irradiation, most of the investigations cited in Table 1 and/or in the text focused on only one aspect of the effects associated with chemical intoxication, i.e., altered enzyme activity. These examples do provide comprehensive information concerning the susceptibility of many enzyme systems and chemical-induced interference during various stages of development. In a few instances, these investigators were able to provide some understanding of the factors responsible for variations in developmental activity. However, there were insufficient cases of comparative evaluations to clearly demonstrate the relative sensitivity of enzymatic evaluations as compared to morphological or physiological indicators of altered functional capacity. Nevertheless, these data strongly support a case for direct chemical effects on fetal tissues and suggest that the early enzymatic changes resulting from exposure *in utero* may be the first step in pathogenesis of dysfunction and/or dysmorphology.

### Effects of Nutritional Deficiency

It is well documented that maternal dietary protein deprivation in rats results in severe intrauterine growth retardation, postnatal depression of organ weights relative to body weight, and altered functional capacity (54,69,99). Immature brain and kidney are often the most severely retarded organs (2,35,103,121). For instance, body and brain weights were reduced, and brain acetylcholinesterase (EC 3.1.1.7) activity was elevated in pups with restricted protein intake (22).

Nutritional factors play a very important role in regulating the activity of many enzyme systems during neonatal life. This aspect of developmental biochemistry of liver has been investigated extensively with special regard to carbohydrate metabolism (69,99,122,124). For example, hepatic glucokinase develops very rapidly during the late suckling period, and the nature of the diet determines its ontogeny (125). Markedly diminished glucokinase levels at weaning would severely restrict the ability of individuals to maintain adequate blood glucose levels and thereby maintain metabolic homeostasis. The abrupt shift from milk to standard diet for laboratory animals at weaning represents a dramatic nutritional transition from a high-fat and high-protein diet to one that is relatively low in these nutrients but rich in carbohydrates. Thus, continued growth and development may be limited by an individual animal's capability to adapt to the altered diet. Any prenatal insult that significantly depresses the development of adaptive processes, such as prolonged protein deficiency, would compromise survival.

### Effects of Hormones

Alterations in endocrine function or hormone levels may also be regarded as a perturbation of developmental processes. It is conceivable that toxic agents might exert their effects via the endocrine system rather than directly on a developmental or metabolic process as suggested in the preceding section. More details on the interaction of toxic agents and endocrinology are found elsewhere in this volume (see chapters by G. L. Kimmel and J. A. McLachlan et al., *this volume* ).

Hormones are also the natural stimuli for evoking the synthesis of many enzymes, especially those required for adaptation to extrauterine life (40,42,43). Consequently, premature acquisition of the enzyme compliment characteristic of adult tissues may be manipulated by the administration of exogenous hormones (41). All of the examples listed in Table 2 represent accelerated maturation, whereby enzyme activities are prematurely induced to adult levels as a result of hormone or intermediate (cyclic AMP) administration. In addition, hormone administration may accelerate the maturation of enzymes whose profiles are decreased during development. For example, hydrocortisone administered to fetal and neonatal rats prematurely decreased the level of thymidine kinase in liver and spleen, respectively, within 24 to 48 hr (49).

There are two major implications of such hormone-evoked alterations in developmental processes. First, much of our current knowledge regarding endocrine regulation of protein synthesis derives from such experiments in enzyme ontogeny. Second, major perinatal disorders may result from impairments or imbalances in developmental endocrinology if they occur at critical stages when hormones normally exert discrete maturational effects.

It is important to note that during development the same hormone does not necessarily influence a given enzyme the same way in all tissues. Ornithine aminotransferase (EC 2.6.1.13) is a good example (58). In the liver, corticosteroids induce development of this enzyme, whereas estrogens inhibit it. The opposite is true in the kidneys where estrogens induce a precocious development of ornithine aminotransferase activity, and glucocorticoids inhibit this effect.

## GENERAL DESIGN CONSIDERATIONS

### Species Selection

Because of the large amount of information available, examples presented in Table 3 and Fig. 1 have been limited to hepatic enzyme ontogeny in the rat. However, similar listings may be prepared for most organs (39) and various species (52,110), including rabbits (111,112), mice (118), hamsters (97), and guinea pigs (10). Rats, guinea pigs, and hamsters might offer interesting comparisons due to marked variations in length of gestation, degree of maturity of the offspring at term, and differences in metabolic regulatory mechanisms. Some investigators recommend consideration of species phylogenetically closer to man (77,86). But, according to Smyth and Hottendorf (105), experimental evidence indicates that the degree of similarity among species in pharmacokinetics and biotransformation varies from one test substance to another. Thus, routine use of nonrodent species cannot be justified at this time.

A number of characteristics are considered important in selecting a species as the experimental model for studies to explore the validity of perinatal enzyme studies. One necessary characteristic is that the near-term conceptus be of sufficient size so it can be easily manipulated experimentally. Another is the display of immature characteristics during early postnatal life (44). Also of importance is that the animal be a convenient source of a number of organs at different stages of development.

Rats are a suitable choice for several reasons. For example, perinatal rat liver lacks the versatile metabolic capability of mature liver (24,115), and it does not acquire full competence until some weeks following weaning (39,113). Not only are rats a convenient source for liver samples, but they are also a reliable source for brain (1,32,65,102), kidney (2,34,35,55), and intestine (56,62,131). However, data on most immature rat tissues, other than liver, are still limited (47,113). In

TABLE 3. *Established ontogenic periods for some rat liver enzymes*

| Enzyme name | EC No. [a] | Major metabolic process | Developmental period [b] | References |
|---|---|---|---|---|
| Alcohol dehydrogenase | 1.1.1.1 | Alcohol metabolism | Weaning | 93 |
| Lactate dehydrogenase | 1.1.1.27 | Glycolysis | Fetal | 18 |
| Glycerol-3-phosphate dehydrogenase | 1.1.99.5 | Glycolysis | Neonatal | 18 |
| Tryptophan 2,3-dioxygenase | 1.13.11.11 | Amino acid metabolism | Weaning | 31,46 |
| Malate dehydrogenase (NADP) | 1.1.1.40 | Glycolysis | Weaning | 8,48,88,122 |
| Malate dehydrogenase (NAD) | 1.1.1.37 | Gluconeogenesis | Neonatal | 122 |
| Isocitrate dehydrogenase (NADP) | 1.1.1.42 | TCA cycle (glycolysis) | Fetal | 122 |
| Glycogen synthetase | 2.4.1.11 | Glycogen synthesis | Fetal | 9 |
| Aspartate aminotransferase | 2.6.1.1 | Gluconeogenesis | Neonatal | 129 |
| Alanine aminotransferase | 2.6.1.2 | Gluconeogenesis | Postweaning | 129 |
| Tyrosine aminotransferase | 2.6.1.5 | Amino acid metabolism | Postweaning | 31,36 |
| Ornithine aminotransferase | 2.6.1.13 | Urea cycle | Weaning | 61,92 |
| Glucokinase | 2.7.1.2 | Glycolysis | Weaning | 48,126 |
| Phosphorylase | 2.4.1.1 | Glycolysis | Fetal | 9,18 |
| Phosphoglucomutase | 2.7.5.1 | Glycogen synthesis | Fetal | 9 |
| Pyruvate kinase | 2.7.1.40 | Glycolysis | Weaning | 48,122 |
| Ornithine carbamoyltransferase | 2.1.3.3 | Urea cycle | Neonatal | 91,98 |
| Glucose-6-phosphatase | 3.1.3.9 | Gluconeogenesis | Neonatal | 18,122,130 |
| Asparaginase | 3.5.1.1 | Amino acid metabolism | Neo/Wean [c] | 84 |
| Hexosediphosphatase | 3.1.3.11 | Gluconeogenesis | Neonatal | 130 |
| Serine dehydratase | 4.2.1.13 | Amino acid metabolism | Weaning | 36 |
| Phosphoenolpyruvate carboxykinase | 4.1.1.32 | Gluconeogenesis | Neonatal | 88,130 |
| Fumarate hydratase | 4.2.1.2 | TCA cycle | Weaning | 122 |
| Pyruvate carboxykinase | 6.4.1.1 | Gluconeogenesis | Neonatal | 88,130 |

[a] Enzyme Commission number (see reference 70).
[b] The period during which offspring enzyme activity reaches adult level. Only enzymes that increase to adult level are included.
[c] Female/male.

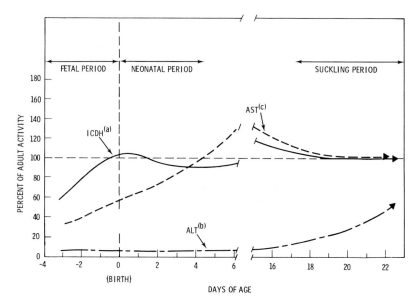

**FIG. 1.** Typical rat liver enzyme ontogenic profiles. (a) Isocitrate dehydrogenase (EC 1.1.1.42); references: 7,122. (b) Alanine aminotransferase (EC 2.6.1.2); references: 63,107,129. (c) Aspartate aminotransferase (EC 2.6.1.1); references: 59,129.

addition to the developmental information available for rats, there is a broad background of toxicologic and metabolic data for rats at all ages. Therefore, rats appear to be an appropriate and acceptable species for exploring the effects of toxicants on functional competence and ontogenic enzyme profiles.

In addition, young and/or immature animals offer several advantages in predictive toxicity testing. Mammalian embryonic and fetal tissues often exhibit a higher degree of sensitivity to the adverse actions of a variety of agents than do corresponding adult tissues. The ultimate indicator of such interference with normal processes may be manifestations of developmental toxicity such as those described above (87).

## Enzyme Selection

Ideally, one aspect in selecting biochemical indicators of developmental toxicity would be consideration of known actions of the agent in question. In particular, any demonstrated or hypothetical relationship concerning the specific toxic agent would aid in selection of organ-specific enzymes. While such knowledge of the developmental toxicity of proposed test agents would be helpful, it is not requisite to the selection of the best biochemical indicators. Additional criteria that should be considered in enzyme selection are presented in Table 4. After a preliminary list of enzymes is prepared for a particular agent, initial range-finding studies are conducted, then the list is reevaluated and modified if necessary. For instance, the time of initial appearance of activity in various tissues for some of these potential

TABLE 4. *Enzyme selection criteria*

---
Constituent in a major metabolic pathway
Exhibits regulatory properties
Localized in intracellular organelle(s)
Distributed in more than one tissue
Developmental pattern known for at least one tissue
Developmental pattern perturbed by physicochemical insult
Altered enzyme activity level associated with pathophysiology
Isoenyzme patterns known and associated with development
Relative ease of assay in crude preparations using standard methods

---

indicator enzymes may be uncertain. Once actual measurement of the selected enzymes is initiated, the results may validate their selection or replacement.

Thus, there are a number of factors in the selection of the specific test battery, and there are pros and cons for each consideration. Relatively important factors include inducibility of temporal shifts in ontogenic profiles, measurement of key regulatory enzymes, determination of isoenzyme patterns, and a demonstrated relationship between enzyme deficiency in humans and/or animals and specific disorders. A brief discussion of some of these factors as well as characteristics of a few well-defined enzyme ontogenic profiles follows.

Readily detectable deviations in activity may not necessarily reflect enzyme deficiency (79). Since the total activity of many enzymes present in a pathway or tissue may greatly exceed the requirement of that specific catalytic process, deviations may reflect only minor fluctuations in reserve capacity. It may be necessary to measure precursor metabolite levels in order to distinguish between transient alterations of reserve capacity and relatively permanent adverse effects on enzyme levels (10,17,25).

Some investigators strongly favor limiting the selection to regulatory or key enzymes in essential metabolic sequences. According to Weber (127), focusing on key enzymes precludes the necessity of assaying a larger portion of the enzyme complement of a tissue. He maintains that a quartet of key gluconeogenic enzymes and a trio of key glycolytic enzymes may adequately evaluate effects on carbohydrate metabolism (128). Similar groups of enzymes operating in purine, pyrimidine, DNA, ornithine, and cyclic AMP metabolism have been identified as key enzymes (128).

Table 3 represents examples of rat liver enzymes with clearly defined enzyme ontogenic profiles that may be potentially useful in evaluating toxicants. Included in Table 3 are enzymes that attain or even temporarily exceed adult levels during the perinatal period. These examples are integral parts of essential metabolic pathways of synthesis or degradation. These pathways either provide energy for growth and differentiation or are specific for a physiological process common to all tissues. Greater detail on their specific biochemical role may be found in references cited in the table as well as in various reviews (18,39,113,124).

Schematic representations of three typical ontogenic profiles are presented in Fig. 1. Some enzyme ontogenic profiles are multiphasic, with activity increasing during two or more perinatal periods (39). Not all enzyme profiles show accumulation of enzyme activity. For example, thymidine kinase (EC 2.7.1.21) activity in rat liver peaks at 17 to 19 dg and decreases to about 1% of this value by adulthood (75,82). This decline in activity during the perinatal period presumably reflects the concomitant decrease in hepatic hematopoietic activity.

Other rat liver enzymes that exhibit decreasing activity profiles with increasing age include phosphofructokinase (EC 2.7.1.11), glucose-6-phosphate dehydrogenase (EC 1.1.1.49), fructose-1-6-disphosphate aldolase (EC 4.1.2.13), and triose phosphate isomerase (EC 5.3.1.1) (18). These profiles reflect maturational changes in carbohydrate metabolism. Clearly, the simultaneous decline in hexokinase and the rise in glucokinase (EC 2.7.1.1/2) activity is such a case (72,126).

In summary, enzymes should be selected on the basis of their overall suitability as markers for detecting early changes in appropriate target tissues following insult. However, until the validity of this approach has been established as a valuable predictive screening test, we favor application of rigid selection criteria based on a prior knowledge of the effects expected from a specific agent.

## Range Finding

Range-finding studies are recommended to select appropriate dose levels of the agent under study as well as enzymes for evaluation and target tissues to be sampled for a specific stock of animals. There often can be quantitative differences between laboratories and between animal strains. Often only a crude estimate of dosage levels can be obtained from data in the published literature (or other appropriate sources). Therefore, pilot studies are needed to define the highest dosage level of each agent that does not cause significant feto–neonatal mortality. A 10 to 20% increase above control values in the frequency of embryolethality may represent the highest dosage level acceptable for prenatal exposures. A similar relative reduction in the rate of weight gain in neonatal and suckling rats may be used as the dosage limit for postnatal exposures. This may require testing a wide range of dosage levels to define the upper and lower limits of exposure, with the latter being a "no apparent effect level."

An effective dosage range for each agent is considered the ultimate goal of such preliminary studies. Subsequent definitive studies can then establish whether or not dose-related effects are produced. Low prevalence of nonrelated effects in the absence of an apparent dose–response relationship should be attributed to the agent only with extreme caution. Spontaneous occurrence of effects of variable severity are inherent in all populations and represent background incidence.

Indications of marked effects on the progeny during the pilot study may justify extending the observations to later postnatal times to determine the duration and/ or the latency of manifestations. Results of such range-finding studies can significantly modify not only enzyme and tissue selections but also the age span for analysis. Such preliminary studies may also suggest additional measures to be considered for incorporation into an evaluation, for example: (a) radiolabeled precursor incorporation into macromolecules of appropriate target organs of progeny; (b) abbreviated screening of typical indicators of clinical pathology in 21- and 50- to 60-day-old rats; (c) histopathologic evaluations of suspected target tissues of near-term fetuses and juvenile rats; and (d) evaluations of various indices of maturation between birth and 7 to 9 weeks of age.

## Tissue Selection

Ideally, determinations could use tissues of most organs or systems, depending on the nature of the agent and its distribution in the test subjects. Consequently, representation of the cardiovascular, pulmonary, hepatorenal, gastrointestinal, central nervous, and endocrine systems is important. The rationale for selecting brain, liver, kidney, and intestine is obvious; they are key to survival, and the last three facilitate elimination of agents. Placenta is a unique tissue both structurally and functionally, and its growth and development are essential for a normal pregnancy outcome (26,50,54). Amniotic fluid may prove to be a natural reservoir for indicators of developmental pathology as well as being a logical target for clinical testing (19,95,116). The same reasoning supports the assay of blood (serum) in weanlings. For neonatal or weanling animals, lung might replace placenta and amniotic fluid as an appropriate material. Connective tissue, myocardium, or specific portions of the reproductive tract of one or both sexes might have special significance for certain agents, e.g., heart for cardioactive agents or gonads for sex hormones.

An obvious criterion for tissue selection is that the organ be of adequate size at the intended time of analysis. Based on the neonatal rat tissue weight data of Sikov and Thomas (101), weights of only brain, liver, and intestine are sufficiently large for individual analysis in this species. Therefore, pooling of fetal and neonatal tissues may be necessary depending on size of individual tissues and volume of tissue samples required for analyses. To evaluate analytical precision, values per litter should represent the mean of duplicate or triplicate determinations of the same tissue pool. For statistical validity, 6 to 10 litters for each developmental age and exposure group should be adequate. If rats are used, fetal and neonatal samples are generally pooled, e.g., 5 to 8 pups, and sexes combined. Because of their larger size, 3 to 5 weanling rats may be combined, by sex, for a tissue pool.

## Sample Preparation

In most laboratories, enzyme activity measurements are made in homogenates after centrifugation to eliminate cellular debris (39,111). Extensive extraction and fractionation of tissues for isolation and separation of discrete cellular components do not seem practical and in general are avoided because of the considerable time required for enzyme purification. The efficiency of cell disruption, choice of diluents, and the force of gravity applied for the sedimentation of particulates influence the amount of enzyme activity present in the supernatant fluid (cytosol) (12,111). We recommend that each investigator optimize the procedures for his or her operations.

Fluid samples, such as blood, urine, and amniotic fluid, may require some form of separation, dilution, or concentration prior to assaying enzyme activities. Although tissue preparations may, in some cases, be frozen and stored for future use, there is a marked hazard of diminished activity due to enzyme inactivation when storage is at $-20$ to $-190°C$ for any period of time (23,68). Thus, use of fresh tissue preparations is recommended whenever possible.

## Enzyme Analysis

There are a number of factors that can cause age-dependent changes in the kinetic properties of an enzyme. Maturational changes in the following factors may alter enzyme activity *in vivo* and *in vitro*: (a) isoenzyme distribution; (b) substrate affinity; (c) subcellular localization; (d) conversion of apoenzyme to holoenzyme; and (e) cofactor requirements. Consequently, many enzymes require individual adjustments of their reaction mixture in order to fully determine potential activity *in vitro* (44,111). This may be achieved by determining the optimal substrate concentration for each enzyme, tissue, and age combination under investigation.

Generally, enzymes are quantified in assay systems supplemented with saturating amounts of the appropriate substrates and cofactors so that the catalytic rate is limited only by the amount of enzyme in the tissue extracts. Often standard spectrophotometric enzyme methods may be used with few modifications (12,28,83). Expressions of catalytic activity traditionally serve as reliable indicators of the concentration of enzymes in the samples; however, in some cases, additional measurements may be required to rule out the presence of activators or inhibitors (111).

Enzyme activities are generally expressed in units (U), e.g., μmoles of converted substrate per min; International Units, or, alternatively, moles/sec; katal (13,29). Activity also may be calculated per gram of tissue wet weight or per gram of soluble protein and expressed as a proportion of comparable adult activity or as an activity quotient (44). Care must be taken with this latter approach, since adult activity is not constant and may be influenced by the experimental regime and/or pregnancy. Thus, if identically exposed maternal tissues are analyzed for the same enzyme indicators at the same sacrifice times to provide adult values, they may not be comparable. For example, ornithine carbamoyltransferase (EC 2.1.3.3) activity in adult rat liver decreases throughout the course of pregnancy and returns to pregravid levels 3 to 5 days postpartum (98). Thus, "adult activity" must be defined for each enzyme, tissue, and agent with respect to age, sex, and reproductive status.

## Pragmatic Approach

Since methodology for the enzyme approach is too new for adequate description in the literature, we consider it to be of value to briefly describe the methodology we and others have evolved for the performance of such studies. For the present, testing in this laboratory has been restricted to the late fetal, early neonatal, and late suckling periods, based on the presumption that biochemical lesions precede other manifestations of pathophysiology (89). Theoretically, functional tests in animal subjects with a short life-span, e.g., rodents, should be conducted for an extended period, from conception through gestation and perinatal development until maturity or even old age (21). As it is not possible to predict the type and severity of all functional or structural changes, a variety of tests may be needed over the entire observation and analysis period. In conjunction with the validation of biochemical procedures, both anatomical and physiological indicators of maturation can often be measured on the same animals.

Evaluations of offspring in our laboratory include the following: physical characteristics (e.g., general appearance, posture, and malformations), maturational landmarks (eye opening and incisor eruption), growth (weight gain), specific reflexes (surface and air righting), swimming development, neuromuscular coordination and endurance, sensory perception (vibrissal and visual placing), CNS excitability (audiogenic seizure), and ontogeny of cellular and humoral immunity.

Organs and tissues for all experiments dealing with enzyme ontogeny in our laboratory are taken from CD rats (Charles River). Adult rats (3–6 months old) are deprived of food for approximately 15 hr (overnight) prior to sacrifice. Neonatal and suckling animals are allowed to nurse. Our standard procedure for tissue preparation is to sacrifice rats by decapitation via guillotine (facilitating blood collection), open the abdomen and thorax, and remove the viscera. The tissues are prepared for analysis within 1 hr following decapitation. Tissues are blotted, weighed, and homogenized (Tissuemizer®, Tekmar) for 15 sec × 3 in four volumes of ice-cold 0.15 M-sucrose–0.25M-KCl. Livers of neonatal, suckling, and adult rats are perfused with cold sucrose–KCl prior to excision and removal of the organs. Crude homogenates are centrifuged at 550 × $g$ for 10 min at approximately 5°C. The resulting supernatants are recentrifuged at 40,000 × $g$ for 20 min at approximately 5°C. The remaining cytosol is assayed for activity after preparing appropriate dilutions in 0.9% NaCl. The preceding conditions were selected because they gave maximum activity when used for control tissues.

In our laboratory, spectrophotometric measurements are made with a centrifugal fast analyzer (GEMSAEC®; Electro Nucleonics, Inc.). This instrumentation enhances our capability to apply a comprehensive battery of indicators to a number of relatively small tissue pools, since it combines microtechniques (e.g., 5–50 μl of samples and 250–500 μl of reagents), large-scale sample methods (up to 15 samples/10 min per procedure), and automated assay programs [minicomputer functions (4,119,120)]. Adjustments of standard methods for compatibility with our instrumentation pose few problems (114) but are necessary in order to adapt the procedures for rat tissue extracts at various ages.

To date, we have tested the effect of various substrate concentrations in the reaction mixture for four enzymes: aspartate aminotransferase, alanine aminotransferase, alkaline phosphatase (EC 3.1.3.1), and isocitrate dehydrogenase (EC

1.1.1.42). Baseline values for these enzymes are being established for brain, liver, kidney, small intestine, placenta, and blood in immature and adult rats (6).

## CONCLUSIONS

The validity and applicability of the approach presented in this chapter are still hypothetical. Significant dose-related alterations in enzyme activity in any tissue at any age, however, should be considered a meaningful measure of toxicity. But whether our approach is the most sensitive measure of developmental toxicity will remain uncertain until more comparative studies are reported. Validation and general acceptance of this proposed approach will depend on a clear demonstration that deviations in enzyme activity ontogenic profiles are more sensitive indicators of developmental toxicity than other alternative measures. The interpretation of enzyme ontogenic profiles is limited, since enzyme activity as measured at "optimized conditions" *in vitro* may not be considered equivalent to catalytic capability *in vivo*. The data may, however, be considered as a measure of enzyme concentrations and may therefore also be regarded as a relative measure of metabolic capacities in comparative studies.

A modification of this approach has already been extended to consider the effects of trace metals on human placental enzymes (73) as a screening procedure for identifying populations at risk to metal-induced toxicity. Thus, the proposed methodology appears to be applicable beyond the scope of experimental teratology in laboratory animals. However, a major limitation is that samples must be obtained by noninvasive or by currently acceptable clinical procedures. This is difficult for most tissues other than placenta, amniotic fluid, and blood.

In summary, systematic enzymological studies of developing tissues make it possible to characterize major differences in enzyme activity patterns of essential metabolic processes. In comparative analyses, aberrations of ontogenic profiles may be regarded as "biochemical malformations." Altered ontogenic profiles may be considered estimates of altered enzyme concentrations and, as such, indicators of age-dependent differences in enzyme properties. Numerous examples of quantitative shifts in developmental enzyme patterns following chemical intoxication *in utero* are available. Other examples demonstrate marked temporal shifts of some enzyme activity ontogenic profiles following premature gestational exposure to hormones. A brief description of appropriate methodology is provided to facilitate the application of this proposed approach in other laboratories. In addition, we stress the importance of correlating changes in enzyme activity profiles in immature animals with appropriate morphological and functional indicators at various developmental periods to facilitate evaluation of the relative sensitivity of this approach.

## NOTE ADDED IN PROOF

A related application of this approach is being incorporated into a mutagenesis test system by R. J. Feuers et al. (*Anal. Biochem.*, 101:123–130, 1980). They are attempting to detect chemically induced mutations as alterations of activity in approximately 30 liver or brain enzymes of mice.

## ACKNOWLEDGMENTS

We thank Drs. M. R. Sikov, D. D. Mahlum, D. L. Springer, and B. J. Kelman for their helpful comments. This work was supported by the United States Department of Energy, Contract No. DE-AC06-76RLO-1830.

## REFERENCES

1. Adlard, B. P. F., and Dobbing, J. (1971): Vulnerability of developing brain. III. Development of four enzymes in the brains of normal and undernourished rats. *Brain Res.*, 28:97–107.
2. Allen, L. H., and Zeman, F. J. (1973): Kidney function in the progeny of protein-deficient rats. *J. Nutr.*, 103:1467–1478.
3. Alvares, A. P., and Kappas, A. (1975): Induction of aryl hydrocarbon hydroxylase by polychlorinated biphenyls in the foeto–placental unit and neonatal livers during lactation. *FEBS Lett.*, 50:172–174.
4. Anderson, N. G. (1970): Basic principles of fast analyzers. *Am. J. Clin. Pathol.*, 53:778–785.
5. Andrew, F. D. (1976): Techniques for assessment of teratogenic effects: Developmental enzyme patterns. *Environ. Health Perspect.*, 18:111–116.
6. Andrew, F. D. (1980): Application of perinatal enzyme patterns as biochemical indicators of developmental toxicity. In: *Pacific Northwest Laboratory Annual Report for 1979 to DOE, Part 1, Biomedical Sciences.* PNL-3300, pp. 61–63. National Technical Information Service, Springfield, Virginia.
7. Ballard, F. J., and Hanson, R. W. (1967): Changes in lipid synthesis in rat liver during development. *Biochem. J.*, 102:952–958.
8. Ballard, F. J., and Hanson, R. W. (1967): Phosphoenolpyruvate carboxykinase and pyruvate carboxylase in developing rat liver. *Biochem. J.*, 104:866–871.
9. Ballard, F. J., and Oliver, I. T. (1963): Glycogen metabolism in embryonic chick and neonatal rat liver. *Biochim. Biophys. Acta*, 71:578–588.
10. Bartels, H. (1974): Metabolite levels reflecting changes in liver energy metabolism during the neonatal period. *Biol. Neonate*, 24:32–40.
11. Battaglia, F. C., and Meschia, G. (1978): Principal substrates of fetal metabolism. *Physiol. Rev.*, 58:499–527.
12. Bergmeyer, H. U. (1974): *Methods of Enzymatic Analysis, Vol. 1, Second Edition.* Academic Press, New York.
13. Bowers, G. N., Bergmeyer, H. U., and Moss, D. W. (1976): Provisional recommendation (1974) on IFCC methods for the measurement of catalytic concentrations of enzymes. *Clin. Chem.*, 22:384–391.
14. Branchy, L., and Friedhoff, A. J. (1976): Biochemical and behavioral changes in rats exposed to ethanol *in utero. Ann. N.Y. Acad. Sci.*, 273:328–330.
15. Brent, R. L. (1976): Environmental factors: Radiation. In: *Prevention of Embryonic, Fetal, and Perinatal Disease*, edited by R. L. Brent and M. I. Harris, pp. 179–197. DHEW Publication No. (NIH) 76-853, United States Government Printing Office, Washington.
16. Brent, R. L. (1980): Radiation teratogenesis. *Teratology*, 21:281–298.
17. Burch, H. B. (1965–66): Metabolite levels as indicators of changes during growth and development. *Biol. Neonate*, 9:176–186.
18. Burch, H. B., Lowry, O. H., Kuhlman, A. M., Skerjance, J., Diamant, E. J., Lowry, S. R., and Von Dippe, P. (1963): Changes in patterns of enzymes of carbohydrate metabolism in the developing rat liver. *J. Biol. Chem.*, 238:2267–2273.
19. Butterworth, J., Broadhead, D. M., Sutherland, G. R., and Bain, A. D. (1974): Lysosomal enzymes of amniotic fluid in relation to gestational age. *Am. J. Obstet. Gynecol.*, 9:821–828.
20. Cake, M. H., Ghisalberti, A. V., and Oliver, I. T. (1973): Cytoplasmic binding of dexamethasone and induction of tyrosine aminotransferase in neonatal rat liver. *Biochem. Biophys. Res. Commun.*, 54:983–990.

21. Collins, T. F. X., and Collins, E. V. (1976): Current methodology in teratology research. In: *Advances in Modern Toxicology, Vol. 1*, edited by M. A. Mehlman, R. Schapiro, and H. Blumenthal, pp. 155–175. Hemisphere Publishing Corporation, Washington.
22. Coupain, J. G., Tyzbir, R. S., and Beecher, G. R. (1977): Influence of altering dietary protein levels during early development of the rat on the activity of several brain enzymes. *J. Nutr.*, 107:1102–1113.
23. Cryer, A., and Bartley, W. (1974): The effect of storage on enzyme activities in tissues. *Biochem. J.*, 144:433–434.
24. Cutler, M. G. (1974): The sensitivity of function tests in detecting liver damage in the rat. *Toxicol. Appl. Pharmacol.*, 28:349–357.
25. DeMeyer, R., Verellen, G., and Gerard, P. (1972): Study of carbohydrate metabolism in the newborn rat as a tool for evaluating effects of drugs administered during pregnancy. In: *Drugs and Fetal Development*, edited by M. A. Klingberg, A. Abramovici, and J. Chemke, pp. 83–96. Plenum Press, New York.
26. Diamant, Y. Z., Beyth, Y., Neuman, S., and Shafrir, E. (1975): Activity of placental enzymes of carbohydrate and lipid metabolism in normal, toxemic and small-for-date pregnancies. *Isr. J. Med. Sci.*, 12:243–247.
27. Dobryszycka, W., Kulpa, J., Woyton, A., Woyton, J., Szacki, J., and Dzioba, A. (1975): Influence of industrial toxic compounds on pregnancy. *Arch. Immunol. Ther. Exp. (Warsz.)*, 23:867–870.
28. Dooley, J. F. (1979): The role of clinical chemistry in chemical and drug safety evaluation by use of laboratory animals. *Clin. Chem.*, 25:345–347.
29. Dybkaer, R. (1975): Problems of quantities and units in enzymology. *Enzyme*, 20:46–64.
30. Fowler, B. A., and Woods, J. S. (1977): The transplacental toxicity of methylmercury to fetal liver mitochondria. *Lab. Invest.*, 36:122–130.
31. Franz, J. M., and Knox, W. E. (1967): The effect of development and hydrocortisone on tryptophan oxygenase, formamidase, and tyrosine aminotransferase in the livers of young rats. *Biochemistry*, 6:3464–3471.
32. Furchtgott, E. (1975): Ionizing radiations and the nervous system. In: *Biology of Brain Dysfunction*, edited by G. E. Gaull, pp. 343–379. Plenum Press, New York.
33. Garner, R. J., Graves, J. P., and Lane, C. E. (1969): Irradiation and enzyme ontogenesis in the rat and beagle. In: *Radiation Biology of the Fetal and Juvenile Mammal*, edited by M. R. Sikov and D. D. Mahlum, pp. 975–984. Publication AS; CONF-690501, National Technical Information Service, Springfield, Virginia.
34. Gibson, J. E. (1976): Perinatal nephropathies. *Environ. Health Perspect.*, 15:121–130.
35. Goldstein, R. S., Hook, J. B., and Bond, J. T. (1979): The effects of maternal protein deprivation on renal development and function in neonatal rats. *J. Nutr.*, 109:949–957.
36. Goswami, M. N. D., Boulekbache, H., and Meury, F. (1972): Age-correlated variations of rat liver serine dehydratase and tyrosine aminotransferase activities—A comparative analysis. *Comp. Biochem. Physiol.*, 41B:323–330.
37. Greengard. O. (1969): The hormonal regulation of enzymes in prenatal and postnatal rat liver. *Biochem. J.*, 115:19–24.
38. Greengard, O. (1970): The developmental formation of enzymes in rat liver. In: *Biochemical Actions of Hormones, Vol. 1*, edited by G. Litwack, pp. 53–85. Academic Press, New York.
39. Greengard, O. (1971): Enzymic differentiation in mammalian tissues. *Essays Biochem.*, 7:159–205.
40. Greengard, O. (1973): Effects of hormones on development of fetal enzymes. *Clin. Pharmacol. Ther.*, 14:721–726.
41. Greengard, O. (1974): Enzymic and morphological differentiation of rat liver. In: *Perinatal Pharmacology: Problems and Priorities*, edited by J. Dancis and J. C. Hwang, pp. 15–26. Raven Press, New York.
42. Greengard, O. (1975): Cortisol treatment of neonatal rats: Effects on enzymes in kidney, liver and heart. *Biol. Neonate*, 27:352–360.
43. Greengard, O. (1975): Steroids and the maturation of rat tissues. *J. Steroid Biochem.*, 6:639–642.
44. Greengard, O. (1977): Enzymic differentiation of human liver: Comparison with the rat model. *Pediatr. Res.*, 11:669–676.
45. Greengard,O., and Dewey, H. K. (1967): Initiation by glucagon of the premature development of tyrosine aminotransferase, serine dehydratase, and glucose 6-phosphatase in fetal rat liver. *J. Biol. Chem.*, 242:2986–2991.

46. Greengard, O., and Dewey, H. K. (1971): The prematurely evoked synthesis of liver tryptophan oxygenase. *Proc. Natl. Acad. Sci. U.S.A.*, 68:1698–1701.
47. Greengard, O., and Herzfeld, A. (1977): The undifferentiated enzymic composition of human fetal lung and pulmonary tumors. *Cancer Res.*, 3:884–891.
48. Greengard, O., and Jamdar, S. C. (1971): The prematurely promoted formations of liver enzymes in suckling rats. *Biochim. Biophys. Acta*, 237:476–483.
49. Greengard, O., and Machovich, R. (1972): Hydrocortisone regulation of thymidine kinase in thymus involution and hematopoietic tissues. *Biochim. Biophys. Acta*, 286:382–388.
50. Hagerman, D. D. (1969): Enzymology of the placenta. In: *Foetus and Placenta*, edited by A. Klopper and E. Diczfalusy, pp. 413–469. Blackwell Scientific Publications, Oxford.
51. Hahn, P., and Skala, J. (1971): Development of enzyme systems. *Clin. Obstet. Gynecol.*, 14:655–668.
52. Hanson, R. W. (1974): The choice of animal species for studies of metabolic regulations. *Nutr. Rev.*, 32:1–8.
53. Hanson, R. W., Fisher, L., Ballard, F. J., and Reshef, L. (1973): The regulation of phosphoenolpyruvate carboxykinase in fetal rat liver. *Enzyme*, 15:97–110.
54. Hastings-Roberts, M. M., and Zeman, F. J. (1977): Effects of protein deficiency, pair-feeding, or diet supplementation on maternal, fetal and placental growth in rats. *J. Nutr.*, 107:973–982.
55. Hauser, C. A., and Bailey, E. (1975): Changes in the activities of enzymes of kidney gluconeogenesis during development of the rat. *Int. J. Biochem.*, 6:61–64.
56. Herbst, J. J., and Sunshine, P. (1969): Postnatal development of the small intestine of the rat. *Pediatr. Res.*, 3:27–33.
57. Herrmann, H., and Tootle, M. L. (1964): Specific and general aspects of the development of enzymes and metabolic pathways. *Physiol. Rev.*, 44:289–371.
58. Herzfeld, A., and Greengard, O. (1969): Endocrine modification of the developmental formation of ornithine aminotransferase in rat tissues. *J. Biol. Chem.*, 244:4894–4898.
59. Herzfeld, A., and Greengard, O. (1971): Aspartate aminotransferase in rat tissues: Changes with growth and hormones. *Biochim. Biophys. Acta*, 237:88–98.
60. Herzfeld, A., and Greengard, O. (1972): The dedifferentiated pattern of enzymes in livers of tumor-bearing rats. *Cancer Res.*, 32:1826–1832.
61. Herzfeld, A., and Knox, W. E. (1968): The properties, developmental formation, and estrogen induction of ornithine aminotransferase in rat tissues. *J. Biol. Chem.*, 243:3327–3332.
62. Herzfeld, A., and Raper, S. M. (1976): Enzymes of ornithine metabolism in adult and developing rat intestine. *Biochim. Biophys. Acta*, 428:600–610.
63. Herzfeld, A., Rosenoer, V. M., and Raper, S. M. (1976): Glutamate dehydrogenase, alanine aminotransferase, thymidine kinase, and arginase in fetal and adult human and rat liver. *Pediatr. Res.*, 10:960–964.
64. Hicks, S. P., and D'Amato, C. J. (1966): Effects of ionizing radiations on mammalian development. In: *Advances in Teratology*, Vol. 1, edited by D. H. M. Woollam, pp. 195–250. Logos Press, London.
65. Hicks, S. P., and D'Amato, C. J. (1978): Effects of ionizing radiation on developing brain and behavior. In: *Studies on the Development of Behavior and the Nervous System*, edited by G. Gottlieb, pp. 35–72. Academic Press, New York.
66. Holt, P. G., and Oliver, I. T. (1968): Factors affecting the premature induction of tyrosine aminotransferase in foetal rat liver. *Biochem. J.*, 108:333–338.
67. Hommes, F. A., and Wilmink, C. W. (1968): Developmental changes of glycolytic enzymes in rat brain, liver and skeletal muscle. *Biol. Neonate*, 12:181–193.
68. Hopgood, M. F., and Ballard, F. J. (1974): The relative stability of liver cytosol enzymes incubated *in vitro. Biochem. J.*, 144:371–376.
69. Hsueh, A. M., Simonson, M., Kellum, M. J., and Chow, B. F. (1973): Perinatal undernutrition and the metabolic and behavioral development of the offspring. *Nutr. Rep. Int.*, 7:437–445.
70. IUPAC–IUB Commission on Biochemical Nomenclature (1978): *Enzyme Nomenclature*. Academic Press, New York.
71. Jamdar, S. C., and Greengard, O. (1969): Phosphoserine phosphatase: Development, formation and hormonal regulation in rat tissues. *Arch. Biochem. Biophys.*, 134:228–232.
72. Jamdar, S. C., and Greengard, O. (1970): Premature formation of glucokinase in developing rat liver. *J. Biol. Chem.*, 245:2779–2783.

73. Karp, W. B., and Robertson, A. F. (1977): Correlation of human placental enzymatic activity with trace metal concentration in placentas from three geographical locations. *Environ. Res.*, 13:470–477.

74. Kimbrough, R., Buckley, J., Fishbein, L., Flamm, G., Kasza, L., Marcus, W., Shibko, S., and Teske, R. (1978): Animal toxicology. *Environ. Health Perspect.*, 24:173–184.

75. Klemperer, H. G., and Haynes, G. R. (1968): Thymidine kinase in rat liver during development. *Biochem. J.*, 108:541–546.

76. Knox, W. E. (1972): *Enzyme Patterns in Fetal, Adult and Neoplastic Rat Tissues.* S. Karger, New York.

77. LaLonde, M., LeClair, M., and Johnson, A. W. (1973): *The Testing of Chemicals for Carcinogenicity, Mutagenicity and Teratogenicity.* Ministry of Health and Welfare, Ottawa.

78. Lamartiniere, C. A., Dieringer, C. S., and Lucier, G. W. (1979): Altered ontogeny of glutathione *S*-transferase by 2,4,5-2′,4′,5′-hexachlorobiphenyl. *Toxicol. Appl. Pharmacol.*, 51:233–238.

79. Lehninger, A. L. (1975): *Biochemistry, Second Edition.* Worth Publishers, New York.

80. Lucier, G. W., Davis, G. J., and McLachlan, J. A. (1978): Transplacental toxicology of the polychlorinated and polybrominated biphenyls. In: *Developmental Toxicity of Energy-Related Pollutants*, edited by D. D. Mahlum, M. R. Sikov, P. L. Hackett, and F. D. Andrew, pp. 188–203. Publication As; CONF-771017, National Technical Information Service, Springfield, Virginia.

81. Lucier, G. W., and McDaniel, O. S. (1979): Developmental toxicology of the halogenated aromatics: Effects on enzyme development. *Ann. N.Y. Acad. Sci.*, 320:449–457.

82. Machovich, R., and Greengard, O. (1972): Thymidine kinase in rat tissues during growth and differentiation. *Biochim. Biophys. Acta*, 286:375–381.

83. Mattenheimer, H. (1971): *Mattenheimer's Clinical Enzymology: Principles and Applications.* Ann Arbor Science Publishers, Ann Arbor, Michigan.

84. McGee, M., Greengard, O., and Knox, W. E. (1971): The developmental formation of asparaginase in liver and its distribution in rat tissues. *Enzyme*, 12:1–12.

85. Moog, F. (1971): The control of enzyme activity in mammals in early development and in old age. In: *Enzyme Synthesis and Degradation in Mammalian Systems*, edited by M. Rechcigl, pp. 47–76. S. Karger, Basel.

86. Nelson, N. (1975): *Principles for Evaluating Chemicals in the Environment.* National Academy of Sciences, Washington.

87. Neubert, D., Merker, H. J., Kohler, E., Krowke, R., and Barrach, H. J. (1971): Biochemical aspects of teratology. *Adv. Biosci.*, 6:575–622.

88. Palkovic, M., Macho, L., Skottova, N., and Hestacka, A. (1976): Influence of early weaning on the activity of several enzymes in the liver of rat. *Biol. Neonate*, 29:41–47.

89. Peters, R. A. (1969): The biochemical lesion and its historical development. *Br. Med. Bull.*, 25:223–226.

90. Petrova-Vergieva, T. (1976): Survey of international requirements for testing environmental pollutants on prenatal toxicity. In: *Advances in the Detection of Congenital Malformation*, edited by E. B. Van Julsingha, J. M. Tesh, and G. M. Fara, pp. 126–134. The European Teratology Society, Michael Roblin, Printers, Chelmsford, England.

91. Raiha, N. C. R. (1971): Development of arginine and ornithine metabolism in the mammal. In: *Biochemistry of Development*, edited by P. Benson, pp. 141–160. Lippincott, New York.

92. Raiha, N. C. R., and Kekomaki, M. P. (1968): Studies on the development of ornithine-keto acid amino-transferase activity in rat liver. *Biochem. J.*, 108:521–525.

93. Raiha, N. C. R., Koskinen, M., and Pikkarainen, P. (1967): Development changes in alcohol-dehydrogenase activity in rat and guinea pig liver. *Biochem. J.*, 103:623–626.

94. Raiha, N. C. R., and Suihkonen, J. (1968): Factors influencing the development of urea-synthesizing enzymes in rat liver. *Biochem. J.*, 107:793–797.

95. Ressler, N. (1974): Enzymes and principles of their assay in the prenatal diagnosis of inherited diseases. In: *Amniotic Fluid*, edited by S. Natelson, A. Schommegna, and M. B. Epstein, pp. 317–326. John Wiley & Sons, New York.

96. Rugh, R., Duhamel, L., Osborne, A. W., and Varma, A. (1964): Persistent stunting following X-irradiation of the fetus. *Am. J. Anat.*, 115:185–198.

97. Schiller, C. M., Walden, R., and Kee, T. E., Jr. (1979): Effects of hydrazine and its derivatives on the development of intestinal brush border enzymes. *Toxicol. Appl. Pharmacol.*, 49:305–311.

98. Schuit, K. E., and Dickie, M. W. (1973): Induction of enzyme activity during fetal development. *Biol. Neonate*, 23:171–179.

99. Shrader, R. E., and Zeman, F. J. (1969): Effect of maternal protein deprivation on morphological and enzymatic development of neonatal rat tissue. *J. Nutr.*, 99:401–421.
100. Sikov, M. R., Resta, C. F., and Lofstrom, J. E. (1969): The effects of prenatal X-irradiation of the rat on postnatal growth and mortality. *Radiat. Res.*, 40:133–148.
101. Sikov, M. R., and Thomas, J. M. (1970): Prenatal growth of the rat. *Growth*, 34:1–14.
102. Smart, J. L., and Dobbing, J. (1971): Vulnerability of developing brain. II. Effects of early nutritional deprivation on reflex ontogeny and development of behaviour in the rat. *Brain Res.*, 28:85–95.
103. Smart, J. L., Dobbing, J., Adlard, B. P. F., Lynch, A., and Sands, J. (1973): Vulnerability of developing brain: Relative effects of growth restriction during the fetal and suckling periods on behavior and brain composition of adult rats. *J. Nutr.*, 103:1327–1338.
104. Smith, C. H., and Shore, M. L. (1966): Impaired development of rat liver enzyme activities at birth after irradiation *in utero*. *Radiat. Res.*, 29:499–504.
105. Smyth, R. D., and Hottendorf, G. H. (1980): Application of pharmacokinetics and biopharmaceutics in the design of toxicological studies. *Toxicol. Appl. Pharmacol.*, 53:179–195.
106. Snell, K., Ashby, S. L., and Barton, S. J. (1977): Disturbances of perinatal carbohydrate metabolism in rats exposed to methylmercury in utero. *Toxicology*, 8:277–283.
107. Snell, K., and Walker, D. G. (1972): The adaptive behaviour of isoenzyme forms of rat liver alanine aminotransferases during development. *Biochem. J.*, 123:403–413.
108. Snell, K., and Walker, D. G. (1974): Regulation of hepatic L-serinedehydrate and L-serine-pyruvate aminotransferase in the developing neonatal rat. *Biochem. J.*, 144:519–531.
109. Springer, D. L., Broderick, D. J., and Dost, F. N. (1980): Effects of hydrazine and its derivatives on ornithine decarboxylase synthesis, activity and inactivation. *Toxicol. Appl. Pharmacol.*, 53:365–372.
110. Stanton, H. C. (1978): Factors to consider when selecting animal models for postnatal teratology studies. *J. Environ. Pathol. Toxicol.*, 2:201–210.
111. Stave, U. (1967): Importance of proper substrate concentration for enzyme assays in tissue homogenates for developmental studies. *Enzymol. Biol. Clin.*, 8:21–32.
112. Stave, U. (1975): Perinatal changes of interorgan differences in cell metabolism. *Biol. Neonate*, 26:318–332.
113. Stave, U. (1978): Liver enzymes. In: *Perinatal Physiology, Second Edition*, edited by U. Stave, pp. 499–521. Plenum Press, New York.
114. Stewart, T. C., and Farrell, B. A. (1976): Adaptation of manual test reagents to centrifugal fast analyzer system. *Lab. Med.*, 7:29–30.
115. Street, A. E. (1970): Biochemical tests in toxicology. In: *Methods in Toxicology*, edited by G. E. Paget, pp. 313–337. Blackwell Scientific Publications, Oxford.
116. Sutcliffe, R. G., Brock, D. J. H., Robertson, J. G., Scrimgeour, J. B., and Monaghan, J. M. (1972): Enzymes in amniotic fluid: A study of specific activity patterns during pregnancy. *J. Obstet. Gynecol.*, 79:895–901.
117. Thadani, P. V., Slotkin, T. A., and Schanberg, S. M. (1977): Effects of late prenatal or early postnatal ethanol exposure on ornithine decarboxylase activity in brain and heart of developing rats. *Neuropharmacology*, 16:289–293.
118. Thorndike, J. (1972): Comparison of the levels of three enzymes in developing livers of rats and mice. *Enzyme*, 13:252–256.
119. Tiffany, T. O., Chilcote, D. D., and Burtis, C. A. (1973): Evaluation of kinetic enzyme parameters by use of a small computer interfaced "fast analyzer"—an addition to automated clinical enzymology. *Clin. Chem.*, 19:908–918.
120. Tiffany, T. O., Johnson, G. F., and Chilcote, M. E. (1971): Feasibility of multiple simultaneous enzyme assays, for diagnostic purposes, with the GeMSAEC fast analyzer. *Clin. Chem.*, 17:715–720.
121. Tyzbir, R. S., Coupain, J. G., and Beecher, G. R. (1977): Influence of dietary protein levels on rat brain enzyme activities during early development. *J. Nutr.*, 107:1094–1101.
122. Vernon, R. G., and Walker, D. G. (1968): Changes in activity of some enzymes involved in glucose utilization and formation in developing rat liver. *Biochem. J.*, 106:321–329.
123. Villeneuve, D. C., Grant, D. L., Khera, K., Clegg, D. J., Baer, H., and Phillips, W. E. J. (1971): The fetotoxicity of a polychlorinated biphenyl mixture (Aroclor 1254) in the rabbit and in the rat. *Environ. Physiol.*, 1:67–71.

124. Walker, D. G. (1971): Development of enzymes for carbohydrate metabolism. In: *Biochemistry of Development*, edited by P. Benson, pp. 77–95. Lippincott, New York.
125. Walker, D. G., and Eaton, S. W. (1967): Regulation of development of hepatic glucokinase in the neonatal rat by diet. *Biochem. J.*, 105:771–777.
126. Walker, D. G., and Holland, G. (1965): The development of hepatic glucokinase in the neonatal rat. *Biochem. J.*, 97:845–854.
127. Weber, G. (1975): Role of key enzymes in metabolic regulation. In: *Mechanism of Action and Regulation of Enzymes*, edited by T. Keleti, pp. 237–251. Elsevier North-Holland, Amsterdam.
128. Weber, G., Queener, S. F., and Ferdinandus, J. A. (1971): Control of gene expression in carbohydrate, pyrimidine and DNA metabolism. *Adv. Enzyme Regul.*, 9:63–95.
129. Yeung, D., and Oliver, I. T. (1967): Gluconeogenesis from amino acids in neonatal rat liver. *Biochem. J.*, 103:744–748.
130. Yeung, D., Stanley, R. S., and Oliver, I. T. (1967): Development of gluconeogenesis in neonatal rat liver. *Biochem. J.*, 105:1219–1227.
131. Younoszai, M. K., and Ranshaw, J. (1973): Gastrointestinal growth in the fetus and suckling rat pups: Effects of maternal dietary protein. *J. Nutr.*, 103:454–461.

*Developmental Toxicology*, edited by
C. A. Kimmel and J. Buelke-Sam. Raven Press,
New York © 1981.

# Concepts Essential to the Assessment of Toxicity to the Developing Immune System

## Dean W. Roberts and John R. Chapman

*Immunotoxicology Branch, Division of Molecular Biology, National Center for Toxicological Research, Food and Drug Administration, Jefferson, Arkansas 72079*

The production of healthy offspring able to adapt to postnatal life requires the normal development and function of immunologic systems. The detection and characterization of chemical compounds that affect immune ontogeny are important within the context that exposure to such substances may either suppress the development of beneficial immune responses vital to host defense against bacterial, viral, parasitic, and neoplastic disease or may predispose to adverse immune reactions such as hypersensitivity and autoimmune disease. These defects potentially range from lethal suppression of components of the immune system, as seen in congenital primary immunodeficiency disease (2), to suppressed or improperly regulated responses that diminish the quality of life. The former would be obvious and apparent through lethal postnatal infection. The latter manifestation, however, is insidious and could result in increased seriousness and frequency of infectious disease, chronic hypersensitivity, or development of one of many disease states of autoimmune etiology (13).

It should be stressed that, in concept, the detection of defects in immune development differs from the detection of many classical parameters of developmental toxicity. In contrast to vital systems in which continuous function is important or necessary, the immune system may be considered a potential system, many vital aspects of which remain dormant when the host is unchallenged. However, survival frequently depends on host capacity to mount a rapid, amplified, specific immune response on pathogen challenge. Lesions in specific immunity can only be detected by evaluating the response to an appropriate antigenic challenge.

The magnitude and frequency of adverse health effects resulting from fetal and neonatal exposure of the developing immune system to chemicals are unknown. However, the serious potential of such defects is clear. It is also evident that the human conceptus is being exposed to a complex variety of xenobiotics, including over-the-counter medications, social poisons including alcohol, tobacco, and caffeine, prescribed therapeutics, food additives, pesticide residues, environmental pollutants, and ionizing radiation. This intentional and inadvertent exposure of the developing conceptus, its susceptibility to toxic chemicals, and the range of relevant parameters of toxicity present a special challenge in risk detection and estimation to the toxicologist. These factors dictate the need for coordinated, multidisciplinary efforts by immunologists and teratologists to assess adverse health effects due to chemical toxicity to the developing immune system. The timeliness and propriety of such joint studies are suggested by several considerations.

1. Complexity of the developing immune system: the development of functional immune systems involves complex interaction, directed and sequential migration, and subsequent organization of diverse cell types throughout an extended but temporally ordered period of fetal and neonatal development (67,75).

2. Enhanced sensitivity of the immune system during development: compounds that interfere with adult immune systems have more profound effects on developing immune systems and are more likely to be identified through a protocol in which exposure is concurrent with the ontogenesis of the immune system (112).

3. Improvements in interpretation and study design: measurement of immunologic functions vital to host resistance to infectious agents emphasizes those parameters of immunity that are similar in laboratory animals and in man and have importance in the clearly interpretable context of morbidity and mortality. The correlation of immunologic deficits with other functional (e.g., behavioral) and morphologic changes is greatly improved when animals are part of the same study and exposure regimen. This approach will result in more economic use of animals and resources, improve interpretation of functional deficits, and further define the dose–response curve to reveal the comparative sensitivity of these measures.

4. Improved methodology: traditional procedures used to test toxic substances underestimate the importance of the immune system. Knowledge from the highly sophisticated and growing discipline of immunology can significantly contribute to and should be incorporated into the field of toxicology (66,112).

The specific intent of this chapter is to focus on the eclectic nature of developmental toxicology, drawing relevant features from each of the component areas of toxicology, developmental biology, and immunology as they apply to testing for toxicity to the developing immune system. Emphasis will be placed on relating concepts and principles to experimental design. Hopefully, this will provide a more systematic approach to identifying environmental factors and circumstances of exposure that contribute to pathologic immune development and related adverse effects on health and the quality of life.

## BACKGROUND

### Immunocompetence

Immunocompetence is a term used to describe the capacity of the host to defend itself against bacterial, viral, parasitic, and neoplastic disease. Implicit in the concept of immunocompetence is the ability to make an appropriate immune response against antigenic challenge and to avoid aberrant immune responses and subsequent immunologic injury. Successful resolution of infection and the development of protective immunity involves a delicate balance and appropriate interaction of many factors including both nonspecific resistance mechanisms and the development of specific acquired immunity. Nonspecific mechanisms include simple physiologic barriers at the portal of entry, such as skin and mucous membranes, substances with antimicrobial properties such as the lysozymes in tears, and the low pH of the stomach, and complex interactive mechanisms such as the complement cascade and effective phagocytosis. Deficiencies in protective immunity may involve these nonspecific factors or defects in acquisition and/or expression of specific acquired immunity.

## Dichotomy of the Immune System

Available evidence indicates that the lymphocytes responsible for specific acquired immunity comprise two developmentally distinct lines of immunocompetent cells. This dichotomy (depicted in Fig. 1) consists of thymus-derived (T) cells, lymphocytes that differentiate under the influence of thymic epithelium and later are responsible for cell-mediated immunity (CMI) and the regulation of certain antibody responses; and bursa of Fabricius equivalent-derived (B) lymphocytes that differentiate to become plasma cells that secrete one of the five separate classes of immunoglobulin (Ig) responsible for various specific antibody (Ab) responses. The progenitors of T cells and B cells are derived from a common lymphoid stem cell thought to be an early descendent of multipotent stem cells (75). A third cell population, composed of macrophages and monocytes, is derived from another lineage of hematopoietic stem cells, and functions to enhance interactions among B cells, T cells, and antigen, to phagocytize and kill bacteria and some viruses, and to synthesize elements of the complement cascade.

The qualitative and quantitative nature of a specific immune response (either beneficial or deleterious) depends on the regulation and interaction of three essential events: (a) initial recognition of the invading pathogen or other immunogenic substance, hereafter referred to as antigen (Ag); (b) activation, which involves the subsequent proliferation and differentiation of antigen-specific reactive clones of either B or T lymphocytes; and (c) the expression of immunity. The evaluation of B-cell and T-cell expression involves assessment of these different functional effector mechanisms.

T lymphocytes are responsible for the expression of cell-mediated immune responses (those transferable by immune cells but not by immune sera) such as graft-versus-host (GVH) reaction, delayed hypersensitivity, and the rejection of antigenic tumors and allografts. T-effector mechanisms include the release of a variety of chemical mediators of immunity, termed lymphokines. Lymphokines are released as a consequence of a sensitized T cell encountering the antigen that initially induced proliferation and differentiation and to which that T cell is now programmed to react. Some of the identified lymphokines include cytotoxic factors, chemotactic

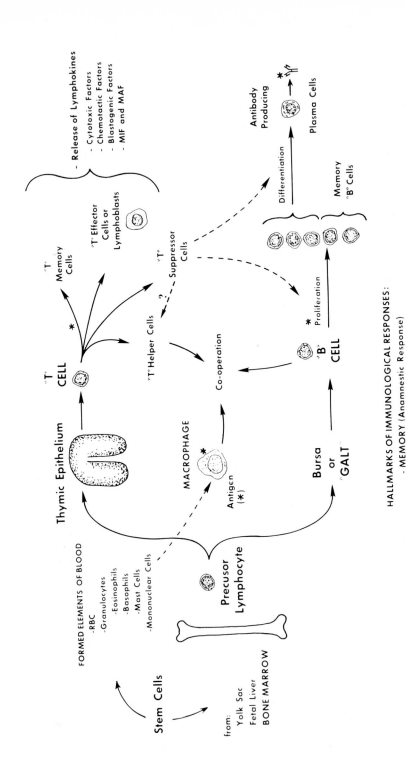

**FIG. 1.** Thymus-dependent and bursa of Fabriclus equivalent aspects of immune system.

factors, macrophage activation factor (MAF), and macrophage inhibitory factor (MIF) (114). The role of lymphokines in recruiting various leukocytes as well as the direct effects of lymphokines on target cells are essential aspects of the amplified sequence of inflammatory events subsequent to sensitized T cells encountering antigen. The biologic relevance of cell-mediated immunity includes its vital role in host resistance to many (primarily intracellular) bacterial, viral, fungal, and protozoan infections, and possibly surveillance against neoplastic clones of cells. Adverse effects of CMI include, but are not limited to, contact allergy, aspects of autoimmune disease, and unwanted rejection of organ transplants (2,120).

B-lymphocyte effector mechanisms are mediated not by cells but by specific antibody. Subsequent to antigen exposure, e.g., intentional immunization with tetanus toxoid or killed pertussis organisms, antigen-sensitized B cells proliferate to form an expanded clone of antigen-reactive B cells, some of which differentiate to become plasma cells that secrete antibody belonging to one of the five classes of immunoglobulin, while others differentiate to become memory cells. Depending on the chemical nature of the antigen, T cell help may be required for the inductive (antigen recognition and proliferation) phase of the humoral response. T-independent antigens are usually polymers that have repeating identical antigenic determinants which induce an IgM response and no immunologic memory. Examples of T-cell-independent antigens include Type III pneumococcal polysaccharide, polymerized flagellin, and lipopolysaccharide. Examples of T-cell-dependent antigens include substances such as sheep red blood cells, tetanus toxoid, and most proteins. T-cell-dependent antigens elicit immunologic memory or anamnesis. The special biologic and chemical properties of the different classes of immunoglobulin (Ig), IgM, IgG, IgA, IgE, and IgD, may be found in any immunology text. It should be of special significance to the developmental immunotoxicologist that toxicant exposure may selectively affect classes of Ig; only IgG crosses the placenta in humans and laboratory rodents (99), and IgA has a special tropism and protective function in secretions such as colostrum and at mucosal surfaces including those of the reproductive system (47). Specific antibody is responsible for protective reactions such as the inactivation of pathogenic bacteria, bacterial toxins, and viruses, and the inhibition of protozoan pathogens. Deleterious roles include immediate type hypersensitivity and anaphylaxis, maternal–fetal Rh incompatibilities, immune complex diseases such as the sequelae of streptococcal infection, and autoimmune diseases such as rheumatoid arthritis (9,32). In-depth discussion of interactions and functions of immune cell populations from a toxicology perspective are given by Vos (112), Koller (45), and Silkworth and Loose (97).

## Immune Ontogenesis

The morphologic and functional development of the immune system has been thoroughly studied in both mice and man. Although the following discussion of temporal sequences of immune ontogenesis uses the mouse as an example, similar sequences occur in other laboratory animals and in man, the major difference being the stage of development relative to parturition and, therefore, the degree of immunocompetence at birth. The ontogeny of the immune system can be divided arbitrarily into four phases: (a) the development of embryonic and fetal stem cells; (b) organogenesis of primary lymphoid organs (thymus and bursa equivalent); (c) maturation and peripheralization of lymphocytes to secondary lymphoid tissues; and (d) maturation of functional capabilities. Delayed maturation or malfunction of primary lymphoid tissue may arrest, delay, or otherwise prevent the development of specific populations of immunocompetent cells. Because of the interdependent and temporally important nature of these events, chemicals that alter immune function in the adult, even in a transient way, may produce similar, more profound or permanent defects in developing systems (67).

The earliest progenitors of lymphocytes in mice and other species are the hematopoietic stem cells formed initially in the area vasculosa and subsequently in the yolk sac (75). By day 9 of gestation in the mouse, stem cells from the yolk sac have migrated and seeded other sites of early hematopoiesis. The liver initiates its hematopoietic activity on the 10th day of gestation, and bone marrow begins hematopoiesis around day 12 of gestation (75,99). These embryonic and fetal stem cells seed the developing thymus where they mature into thymocytes (75).

In the mouse as in man, the thymus is the first lymphoid organ to develop and appears to be a master organ essential to immune development and the orchestration of events in lymphoid organs throughout life (9). In normal mice, the thymus is a bilobular midline structure which in the adult lies anteriorily in the superior mediastinum (see R. M. Hoar and I. W. Monie, *this volume*). The primary anlage of this organ arises from a ventral outpocketing of the third and, to a lesser degree, the fourth pharyngeal pouches (89). While it is generally known that the thymus arises from epithelial tissue, there are differing views as to whether this prethymic epithelium is entirely endodermal (pharyngeal pouch) or if both pharyngeal pouch endoderm and brachial cleft ectoderm contribute to the forming thymus (30). At 9 to 10 days of fetal development, the paired thymus precursors are evident, positioned lateral to the pharynx, and by days 13 and 14 of gestation, their migration toward the superior mediastinum has begun, and the cranial aspect of the thymus precursor, which will become the parathyroid, is demarcated by a constriction. Days 10,11, and 12 of gestation have been shown to be a critical period of heightened susceptibility to the induction of immunologic defects (80). During days 14, 15, and 16 of gestation, the mouse thymus grows rapidly, becomes vascularized, and shows histogenic changes. On days 17 and 18, intense mitotic activity is apparent in the peripheral regions of the thymic cortex. Postnatally, the thymus continues to grow until about 8 to 10 weeks of age without undergoing major morphologic changes (60). The reader is directed to the following references for further details on thymic organogenesis (68,98,117).

Many of the functionally consequential events in differentiation occur prior to the migration of lymphocytes from central to peripheral lymphoid tissues. Goldschneider (29) has surmised that these events include: (a) the generation of immunological diversity; (b) the expression of an antigen receptor repertoire; (c) the establishment of self-tolerance by T cells; (d) the acquisition of future migratory patterns; and (e) the development of functional heterogeneity. As an in-depth review of the above-mentioned aspects of lymphocyte development is beyond the scope of this chapter, the reader is referred to several reviews (29,43,70). The discussion here will be limited to a brief and by no means complete introduction to the development of B-cell and T-cell functional activities as they correlate with the expression of cell surface markers.

Lymphocyte surface markers may be separated into two general categories: surface receptors and surface antigens. Receptors may be recognized by their ability to bind labeled or identifiable substances. For lymphocytes, these may include crystallizable fragment (Fc) receptors for various Igs, receptors for heterologous erythrocytes, receptors for mitogens, and receptors for elements of the complement cascade. Surface antigens are recognized and demonstrated by their reaction with specific, often fluorochrome-labeled, antisera. Confusion may be avoided if one recognizes that membrane-bound immunoglobulins both are immunogenic (and therefore recognizable as cell surface antigens by specific antisera) and function as antigen-specific receptors that may be demonstrated by virtue of either a function (i.e., reduction of substrate in the case of an enzyme antigen), or a fluorochrome or radioisotope marker on the bound antigen/ligand.

Insight into the ontogeny of lymphocyte differentiation in the thymus to form T-cell subpopulations has been achieved through the use of highly specific antisera. Three T-cell subsets, designated as Ly 1,2,3 + , Ly 1 + , and Ly 2,3 + , have been defined through the use of antisera prepared against the murine Ly alloantigen. Additional useful T-cell markers include Thy 1 + (formerly theta alloantigen); and TL, an early differentiation antigen found only on T cells within the thymus (70).

The Thy 1 + , Ly 2,3 + cells are the earliest functional T cells to appear in ontogeny. This subset of T cells appears at 17 to 18 days of gestation and has the corresponding functional attribute of being able to respond to allogeneic cells in mixed lymphocyte cultures and to the plant mitogen phytohemagglutinin. Cells of phenotype Thy 1 + , Ly 1,2,3 + appear soon after birth and are characterized by responsiveness to the mitogen conconavalin A and suppressor cell function in the regulation of the immune response. A third subpopulation, Ly 1 + , does not express appreciable function until 4 weeks post-partum and has helper cell function necessary in the response to T-dependent antigens (39,70). Cell-mediated immunity as measured by the parameter of capacity to reject skin allografts is intact at birth (11).

The anatomic site of central lymphoid organ processing of future B lymphocytes is known to be the bursa of Fabricius in avian species (76) and was thought to be the gut-associated lymphoid tissue (GALT) in mammalian species. Evidence obtained in the rabbit indicated that stem cells of hematopoietic origin migrate to the GALT where they mature and are induced to differentiate along the B-cell line (79). An alternative view is that initially fetal liver and subsequently bone marrow serve not only as sources of stem cells but also as sites of B-cell differentiation (75). Removal of the bursa at various times during perinatal development and/or the administration of heterologous antisera specific for the heavy chain of IgM (anti-μ) have convincingly demonstrated that IgM-bearing progenitor B cells give rise in a sequential manner to cells bearing IgG and IgA on their cell surface (15). Similar studies in which heterologous antiimmunoglobulin antiserum was administered either prenatally or during early postnatal life have demonstrated similar murine susceptibility and B-cell developmental sequences. The development of IgM-bearing (precursor) cells is anti-μ sensitive and an apparent prerequisite for the ontogeny of B lymphocytes bearing the later developing immunoglobulins IgG, IgA, and IgE. Cooper and co-workers (15) have presented a model of B-cell differentiation which is based on experimental evidence and evidence obtained from the human immune system. Stem cells differentiate within the bone marrow primary lymphoid tissue to cells bearing surface IgM. The subsequent states of development to subsets of cells bearing IgM and IgD, IgM, IgD and IgG, or IgM, IgD, and IgA correspond to a mitogen-inducible/antigen-independent stage. This stage is antecedent to an antigen- and T-cell-driven stage when these subsets respectively differentiate to become IgM-, IgG-, and IgA-producing plasma cells. Several points are noteworthy: (a) the IgM-to-IgG or IgA developmental sequence is similar in chicken, mouse, and man and parallels the sequence of developed specific antibody subsequent to primary immunization; (b) the suppression of humoral immunity is both more efficient and less subject to recovery the earlier precursor cells are blocked; (c) the biologic relevance of B-cell suppression, in terms of host resistance to infection even in the presence of intact T-cell immunity, has been demonstrated in neonatally bursectomized chickens (78), anti-μ-suppressed mice (88), and congenitally dysgammaglobulinemic humans (10,120).

In the mouse, small numbers of B cells bearing IgM and IgG or IgM and IgA may be detected within 2 weeks of birth. Soon afterwards, B cells bearing only IgG or IgA are found. The mouse equivalent of IgD appears on large numbers of splenic lymphocytes at about 4 weeks of age, and cells bearing both IgM and IgD-like determinants are the predominant subclass of B cells in the adult (71). Receptors for elements of the complement cascade and for the Fc determinants of immunoglobulin molecules are first observed at around 2 weeks of age (27). The ability to make an lgM response to T-independent antigens develops before the ability to make IgG, IgA, or IgE responses to T-dependent antigens. In general, mice respond to T-independent antigens at adult levels by 3 to 4 weeks of age (69). Details and exceptions regarding the ontogeny of murine responses to T-independent antigens were elucidated by Lindstein (51) using mice that bear a genetically determined B-cell maturation defect. Murine responses to T-dependent antigens may be achieved in mice immunized at 4 weeks of age but generally do not reach adult levels until 6 weeks of age (71).

Perhaps the best way to illustrate both the consequences of developmental failure in a primary lymphoid organ and the structure–function relationships is to present as an example the congenitally athymic nude mouse. Mice homozygous (genotype nu/nu) for the autosomal recessive trait (nu) are phenotypically hairless and fail to develop a functional thymus. Mice heterozygous for this trait (nu/+) are phenotypically normal and immunologically intact. The nude mouse has an epithelial thymic rudiment located in the same anatomic position as a normal thymus. Unlike the normal thymus, the nude thymic equivalent does not grow rapidly after birth and does not become populated with future T-lymphoid cells.

The immunologic consequences of the homozygous nu/nu condition are summarized below and depicted in Fig. 2. As a result of their developmental defect, nude mice lack a functional thymus, T cells, and all thymus-dependent immune functions. These animals are unable to distinguish "self" from foreign antigens and are unable to reject tumors or skin grafts of wide phylogenetic disparity. They are also unable to make specific antibody responses to thymus-dependent antigens because of the absence of T-helper cells. As would be expected, they respond normally with specific IgM antibodies to T-independent antigens. Another reflection of thymic dysgenesis in the nude mouse is an abnormal depletion of thymic-dependent areas of peripheral lymphoid organs (18,19). Further evidence of their T-cell deficit is the relative absence of lymphocytes bearing the T-cell marker, Thy 1 + (formerly theta alloantigen) (82). However, the relevant legacy of this developmental defect in thymic epithelium is that these animals are exquisitely sensitive, as are T-cell deficient humans (120), to lethal infection with normally avirulent organisms (84) and opportunistic pathogens (24), and they survive only if housed in specific pathogen-free, laminar flow or other protective environments (24,81).

As a result of their "compartmentalized" defect and because of the ease with which their developmental defect can be manipulated, the clear relationship of developmental defect/functional immunologic deficit has been demonstrated by thymic reconstitution. All of the described defects in the immune system of nude mice that are the consequences of thymic dysgenesis, including susceptibility to infection, are remedied by a histocompatible thymus graft (87,91). A series of elegant experiments has definitively proven that nude mice have precursor cells capable of becoming T lymphocytes and that the defect results from a blockage in the pathway by which stem cells differentiate in the thymus to become immuno-competent T cells (44,53,121).

In addition to the temporal considerations of immune development, it is especially important that the non-immunology-oriented developmental toxicologist appreciate certain hallmarks and unique characteristics of immunologic systems. These hallmarks are specificity, amplification, and memory. It should be evident that a compound may be immunotoxic by virtue of its effect on (a) the development of an intact immune system or (b) the capacity of an intact animal to mount a protective immune response. The former describes effects on a developing immune system, the latter on a developing immune response. These are conceptually quite different, but evaluation of the former depends on the latter for all measures of specific acquired immunity. In contrast to vital systems, in which continuous function is important or necessary, specific aspects of immune function remain dormant when the host is unchallenged. Frequently, lesions in this potential system can only be detected by evaluating the response to an appropriate antigenic challenge.

It was in this context that earlier mention of the insidious nature of immune dysfunction was intended. In human pathology and toxicology studies, it is fre-

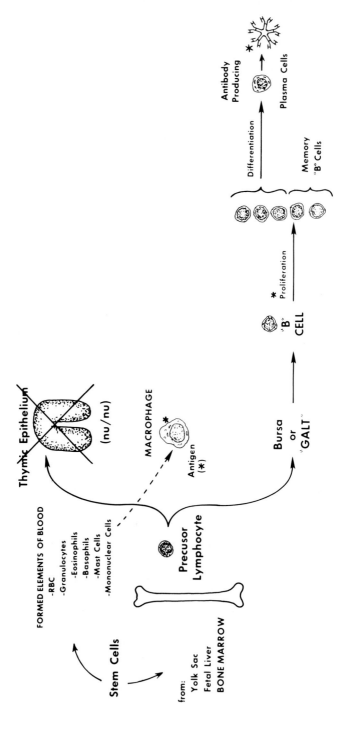

**FIG. 2.** Immunologic consequences of homozygous (nu/nu) condition. Congenitally athymic (nude) mice lack T-cell-dependent cell-mediated immune function and are unable to make antibodies specific for T-cell-dependent antigens. The immunologic consequences of their developmental defect may be reversed by thymus grafting.

quently difficult to determine the underlying predisposing factors in the development of a disease that eventually leads to death. A substance that caused minimal classic manifestations of toxicity but caused immune dysfunction would be particularly insidious as it would be difficult or impossible to attribute death or susceptibility to infection to the causative (immuno) toxicant. In this context, one wonders if housing toxicant-treated animals under protective conditions such as a specific pathogen-free barrier may conceal immunologic deficits that would be manifested as increased susceptibility to opportunistic pathogens if the animals were housed in conventional animal facilities.

## EXPERIMENTAL DESIGN CONSIDERATIONS

A number of experimental design considerations are of great practical importance because they involve decisions that are made early in the design of an experiment and carry with them a set of logistical and biological limitations. The eventual impact of these early critical decisions on the inherent assumptions, reliability, reproducibility, and possible regulatory value of the resultant data must be considered. Some of the critical design components of particular importance to the immunologist include, but are not limited to, species selection, antigen selection, route and dose of immunization, and the timing of immunization and assay relative to toxicant exposure. Similarly, the functional teratologist is concerned with such design components as exposure duration, exposure range and level, stage of development at time of exposure, route of exposure, number of control and experimental litters, placental transport, and fetal and maternal metabolism of the test substance. In experiments designed to assess toxicity to developing immune systems, many of the critical components of experimental design listed above have special implications and consequences for both the immunologist and the functional teratologist. The requirement is for joint input and eclectic experimental design in collaborative studies.

### Selection of Experimental Animals

The first of many problems arising from the use of animals to assess the potential of a test substance to alter immune development in man is selection of the appropriate animal species. This decision is in part determined by those animals that are well characterized immunologically. These include laboratory rodents such as the mouse, guinea pig, rabbit, and rat, and to a much lesser degree, larger animals such as the dog, pig, and monkey. The choice of species in most developmental toxicology studies has been essentially limited to the mouse and rat. Both species, but especially the mouse, are well suited for developmental immunotoxicology studies because of: (a) the availability of methods and reagents for quantitating their immune responses; (b) the extensive data base concerning the morphologic and functional maturation of their immune system; (c) their widespread use in developmental toxicology studies which provides both the opportunity for joint studies and preliminary information on optimum dosage, route of administration, vehicle, and many other aspects of experimental design; and (d) the practical considerations of availability, relatively low cost, and ease of maintaining high-quality animal husbandry. These factors allow the use of sufficiently large numbers of mice per experimental point to allow the detection of statistically significant differences even with subtle defects in the immune system. The investigator should be aware that animals treated *in utero* may be considered as independent units only if litter effects are demonstrated not to be present (33,103). The statistical unit in developmental immunotoxicity studies is usually considered to be the litter.

A disadvantage of using mice and nearly all common laboratory animals including rats, rabbits, and hamsters, for developmental immunotoxicology studies are the differences, as compared to man, in the schedule of development of the immune system relative to parturition. Typical of animals with short gestation periods, the immune system of mice is relatively immature at birth, and significant development occurs postnatally. In contrast, humans, cows, guinea pigs, and sheep have relatively long gestation periods and are essentially immunocompetent at birth (99). This observation has important implications with regard to time and duration of exposure as well as extrapolation of the experimental findings to man. It is essential that the investigator be familiar with developmental sequences of the immune system in the selected test species. An excellent text by Solomon (99) reviews immune ontogenesis in detail for numerous species. An additional consideration is the type of placenta in the species selected, as placentation profoundly affects the transmission of maternal antibody and potentially the distribution and metabolism of the toxicant (see also F. Beck, *this volume*). Finally, both male and female animals should be evaluated, as a significant interaction between sex and altered immunocompetence has been observed in some developmental immunotoxicology studies (17,22,55).

## Toxicant Exposure and Immunologic Assessment

The outcome of developmental toxicology studies is critically dependent both on the temporal relationship of toxicant exposure to events in immune ontogenesis and on the temporal relationship between toxicant exposure and assessment of immunologic function. Critical events in immune ontogenesis that could conceivably be altered by environmental chemicals include: (a) the generation of stem cells; (b) thymic and bursa-equivalent organogenesis; (c) the processing of stem cells to mature T and B lymphocytes with concomitant generation of an antigen recognition repertoire and functional diversity; (d) the establishment of self tolerance; and (e) the seeding of peripheral lymphoid organs. Toxicant exposure should span these milestones of immune ontogenesis. In the mouse, this would, at minimum, include dosing on day 9 of gestation through postnatal day 21. The selection of a dosing schedule should be considered carefully, particularly for those compounds that elicit an adaptive response such as enzyme induction by the maternal or neonatal animal leading to qualitative or quantitative changes in toxicant exposure during treatment. The use of multiple dose levels ranging from the maximum tolerated dose (producing a 10% weight loss as compared to vehicle control animals over the duration of exposure) down to a dose at which "no effect" can be detected in any of the parameters measured will aid in determining the specificity of the toxicant for particular organs or functional systems. The assessment of immunocompetence should begin shortly after exposure to the test substance is completed and sufficient time allowed for the parent compound and its metabolites to be essentially eliminated or sequestered. An interval, during which no compound is administered, allows the investigator to focus on damage to the developing immune system rather than effects on a developing immune response.

## Evaluation of Immune Function

An unfortunate legacy of our multiple and complex immune defense mechanisms is the absence of a single test that is adequate to assess the possible effects of toxic substances on developing immune systems. The approach recommended here is to employ a battery of antigens selected for their capacity to qualitatively and quantitatively test specific T-cell- and B-cell-dependent immune responses, as well as nonspecific measures of immune function. The assay systems should be capable of demonstrating specifically altered immune function as a consequence of toxicant exposure during immune ontogenesis.

Selection of specific immune function assays is complicated by the immense number of assay systems available and the lack of widespread agreement among immunologists as to which assay system should be employed, each tending to prefer the system with which he has had personal experience. Despite this problem, there is general agreement as to which parameters of immune function should be tested in the evaluation of chemically induced immune dysfunction. By general category, immunologic evaluation should include the parameters listed in Table 1. Some animals should be immunologically evaluated both as adolescents and again as adults with the same battery of antigens. This group will test the development and maintenance of immunologic memory as well as the relative immunocompetence of the animal at each time of evaluation. Another group of animals should have their primary exposure to the battery of antigens as adults in order to detect the persistence of an immune aberration detected in the adolescent animal and/or the expression of a latent immune dysfunction. Fortunately, many of the procedures available for evaluating the specific acquisition of humoral and cell-mediated immunity are relatively noninvasive, so that repeated testing over an individual animal's lifetime is possible.

Once a compound is found to be a developmental immunotoxicant, a second phase involves identification of the critical temporal circumstances of exposure and the site and mechanism of the toxicant-induced lesion. In those situations where preliminary studies involved prolonged exposure, replicate studies utilizing smaller increments of exposure and/or appropriate cross-fostering paradigms may be required. In instances where the putative developmental toxicant is persistent or present as depots in the adult, follow-up studies may require simulating the same tissue levels in adult animals as persist in neonatally-exposed animals exhibiting

TABLE 1. *Methods of evaluating immunocompetence*

|  | Reference |
|---|---|
| 1. Measures of specific acquired immunity | |
|    a. Antibody responses to a T-dependent antigen (e.g., heterologous erythrocytes, tetanus toxoid) | 38,65 |
|    b. Antibody responses to a T-independent antigen (e.g., lipopolysaccharide, Type III pneumococcal polysaccharide) | 6,12,94,100 |
|    c. Cell-mediated immunity (e.g., delayed type hypersensitivity to a contact allergen, rejection of incompatible skin or tumor graft, mixed lymphocyte response) | 3–5,11,23,86, 108 |
| 2. Nonspecific indicators of immunocompetence | |
|    a. Capacity of (B and T) lymphocytes to be activated by mitogen (e.g., phytohemagglutinin, pokeweed mitogen, concanavalin A or *Staph.* enterotoxin A) | 37,74,108 |
|    b. Macrophage function (e.g., *in vivo* phagocytosis of colloidal carbon, intracellular killing of bacteria, chemiluminescence) | 35,96,104, 111 |
|    c. Total immunoglobulin levels | 59 |
|    d. Actual and relative lymphoid organ weights (e.g., thymus and spleen) | |
|    e. Histopathology of lymphoid organs (e.g., thymus, spleen, peripheral lymph nodes, and Peyer's patches) | 1 |
| 3. Host resistance to selected pathogens (may involve nonspecific mechanism as well as B and T compartments for specific immunity) | |
|    a. *Listeria monocytogenes* | 58,109 |
|    b. *Salmonella species* | 105,106 |
|    c. *Plasmodium* species | 83,87,88 |
|    d. Endotoxin challenge | 14,54 |
|    e. Viruses | 46,62 |

immunosuppression. As a further aid in pinpointing toxicant-induced lesions, nude mice with their well-defined T-cell deficiency as well as immunologically intact animals may be used either as recipients in cell transfer studies or as a source of defined cells for: (a) cell transfer to or from toxicant-treated neonatal animals; (b) *in vitro* sensitization studies; or (c) flow cytometric analysis of specific cell populations (36).

The interpretation of developmental immunotoxicity data should be approached from the functional/protective perspective that immune responses are important in host defense against disease. Although a substance may cause deflections in various tests of immune function, these changes must be related to adverse health effects to be considered deleterious. Furthermore, an impairment in one aspect of immunity may be transient or it may be accompanied by a compensatory increase in another protective immune parameter.

### Developmental Immunotoxicology

Compounds with diverse chemical and biologic properties have been shown to alter the normal development of the immune system (see Table 2). Rather than review the experimental literature on each of these compounds, examples will be

TABLE 2. *Developmental immunotoxicants*

|  | References |
| --- | --- |
| Heavy metals | |
| Methylmercury | 73,101,102 |
| Lead acetate | 22,55 |
| Hormones | |
| Estrogen | 41–43,57, 85,107,116 |
| Testosterone | 63,72,84,115 |
| Cortisone | 21,37,41,49, 90,92,93,95, 116,119 |
| Epinephrine | 118 |
| Diethylstilbestrol | 40–42,56 |
| Organochlorines | |
| 2,3,7,8-tetrachlorodibenzo-*p*-dioxin (TCDD) | 23,106,113 |
| Polychlorinated biphenyls (PCBs) | 25 |
| Alkylating agents | |
| Busulfan | 80 |
| Cyclophosphamide | 28,50,52 |
| Carcinogens | |
| Urethan | 31,48,61,77 |
| 7,12-Dimethyl-benz(*a*)anthracene (DMBA) | 7,8 |
| Methylcholanthrene (MC) | 20 |
| Benz(*a*)pyrene | 110 |
| Pesticides | |
| Diazinon | 17 |
| Carbofuran | 17 |
| Chlordane | 16 |
| Nutrition | |
| Protein deficiency | 26 |
| Irradiation | |
| X-rays | 110 |

cited to illustrate concepts in the field of developmental immunotoxicology that relate to risk detection and estimation. These concepts will undoubtedly be expanded and refined as developmental immunotoxicology continues to grow as an area of developmental toxicology. The relationship of toxicant and immunotoxicant, and of effects on the developing immune system versus other aspects of immunotoxicology are depicted in Fig. 3. Since testing for toxicity to the developing immune system involves the eventual challenge and expression of immunocompetence, it is important to recognize that this evaluation may be influenced by toxicant-induced direct or indirect effects on antigen recognition, memory, or effector mechanisms. These indirect effects may be the result of toxicant-induced alterations in a variety of host physiologic and pathologic conditions including alterations in nutritional status, malignant disease, and hormonal balance. Further, toxic chemicals may affect the development of immunoregulatory mechanisms, altering the development of the immune system by shifting the qualitative nature of immune responses away from protective/beneficial responses towards potentially harmful responses. Effects

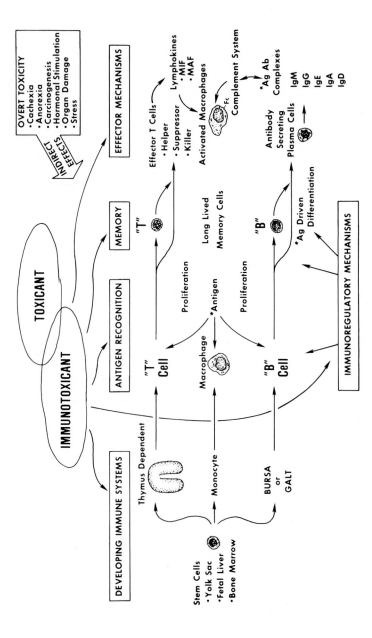

**FIG. 3.** Toxic compounds may act either directly or indirectly on the development of lymphoid organs and/or the subsequent acquisition and expression of specific immunity.

on the development of regulatory mechanisms may be especially important in the etiology of hypersensitivity and autoimmune disease.

An important goal of toxicology in general is the development of the capability to predict a compound's toxicity from its known biological and chemical properties. In regard to developmental immunotoxicology, those chemicals that are capable of altering adult immunocompetence are highly suspect of also being developmental immunotoxicants. Chemically induced immune dysfunction is often irreversible and of greater magnitude when exposure occurs during immune development. Compounds known to alter adult immunocompetence and profoundly affect development of the immune system include tetrachlorodibenzo-*p*-dioxin (TCDD), estradiol, cortisone, busulfan, and cyclophosphamide (see Table 2). It is important to note, however, that chemicals that do not significantly alter adult immunocompetence may disrupt the normal development of the immune system. This concept is exemplified by 19-nortestosterone (63). Whereas testosterone essentially lacks an immunosuppressive action in mature animals (1,34), treatment with this steroid is an extremely effective means of chemically bursectomizing embryonic chickens resulting in the depression of the humoral arm of the immune system. Highest priority for developmental immunotoxicity testing should be given to those compounds with high exposure indices during pregnancy and infancy with special emphasis on those compounds that are immunotoxic in adults.

As stated earlier, the stage of immune development at the time of toxicant exposure may affect the nature, magnitude, and the persistence of a chemically induced immune defect. This has been demonstrated by Pinto-Machado (80) who treated maternal mice on one of the first 18 days of pregnancy with a single injection of the alkylating agent busulfan. Only those animals treated on gestation days 10,11, or 12 developed thymic hypoplasia. Another alkylating agent, cyclophosphamide, has been shown to preferentially delete the humoral (B-cell dependent) arm of the immune system of developing chickens exposed during the first 3 days of extraembryonic life. The selective nature of cyclophosphamide suppression on the ontogeny of the humoral response was evidenced by intact graft-versus-host reactivity in the treated chicks (50,52). The persistence of the immune defect can also be dependent on the time of exposure; for example, Kalland (42), using diethylstilbestrol, reported that long-term effects on mitogen reactivity were observed only when mice were exposed prior to the sixth day of postnatal life. It should also be noted that toxicant exposure during immune ontogenesis may produce defects that remain dormant and are not manifested until adulthood, as reported by Spyker (102) for methylmercury. Evaluation of mice treated prenatally with methylmercury revealed a susceptibility to eye infections and a highly significant depression of the humoral response to a T-independent antigen in adult animals but not adolescents, thus indicating the latent expression of a prenatally acquired immune defect (18,19). It should be emphasized that longitudinal experimental designs are required to detect such latent defects. It is the potential nature of the immune system discussed earlier in the chapter that allows immunologic abnormalities to exist in apparently normal animals. For example, Faith and Moore (23) treated mice prenatally and postnatally with TCDD and observed persistent depression of cell-mediated immune responses to a contact allergen despite normal body weight and appearance of animals as well as normal thymus weight and thymic morphology. These observations support the contention that the most sensitive measure of immunocompetence is the quantification of specific immune responses to antigens.

A runting syndrome characterized by progressive weight loss, ruffling of the fur, diarrhea, and premature death has been observed with several but not all developmental immunotoxicants. Tetrachlorodibenzo-*p*-dioxin (113), estradiol (107), cortisone (95), and busulfan (80), have all been associated with such a runting syndrome as well as causing a general disruption of thymic architecture. The possibility that "chemical thymectomy" is responsible for the runting syndrome is supported by the fact that a similar syndrome is seen in mice that are neonatally thymectomized (64) and in nude mice which are congenitally athymic (91). Caution should be exercised, however, in assuming that all cases of runting syndrome are associated with thymic dysfunction (67). For example, neonatal exposure of mice to high doses of epinephrine induces a comparable runting syndrome despite no significant alterations in thymic morphology (118). It has been suggested that effects may be produced by either endogenous or exogenous adrenal hormones and that when corticosteroid-mediated indirect effects are suspected, adrenal function and corticosteroid levels should be monitored (1,23,112).

## SUMMARY

Public and scientific anxiety stemming from our inadvertent exposure to an increasing variety of environmental chemicals has underscored the requirement for reliable means to identify hazardous substances. As toxicologists endeavor to identify compounds and circumstances of exposure that are deleterious to health, well-being, and quality of life, they should remain attentive to the vulnerability of developing systems and to our vital requirement for an intact immune system. Infectious disease, immune disorders, and cancers of the immune system (lymphomas/leukemias) are among the leading health problems in the early years of life, and it is probable that environmental factors are partially responsible for each of these states by adversely affecting the normal development of the immune system.

Although developmental immunotoxicology is a relative newcomer to the field of toxicology, many chemicals already known to be mutagenic, teratogenic, or carcinogenic also have clear potential to affect developing immune systems. This should be viewed from the perspective that toxic compounds may produce a constellation of adverse effects and that common mechanisms may be involved which can be better elucidated by multidisciplinary studies. Such studies should include the eclectic coupling of teratology and immunology and must be conceived and implemented in such a way that dosing and toxicological events are well controlled and documented and do not confound the interpretation of the immunologic data.

It is important that toxicologists integrate the "worst case scenarios" put forth to exemplify the potential hazards of polluting our environment with our somewhat belated realization that immune ontogenesis is a labile process that can be disrupted by chemicals introduced and controlled by man. It is also apparent that the human conceptus is currently being exposed to a multitude of chemicals without particular regard for their effect on the developing immune system. For proper balance of the risk–benefit equation for chemicals, it is of vital importance to include testing for effects on the development and subsequent expression of functional immunity.

## REFERENCES

1. Ahlqvist, J. (1976): *Endocrine Influence of Lymphatic Organs, Immune Responses, Inflammation, and Autoimmunity.* Almqvist and Wiksell International, Stockholm.
2. Allen, J. C. (1971): Recurrent infections in man associated with immunologic or phagocytic deficiencies. *Postgrad. Med.,* 50:88–94.
3. Asherson, G. L., Zembala, M., and Wood, P. J. (1974): Proceedings: Control mechanisms in cell-mediated immunity. The separate control of net DNA synthesis and of contact sensitivity skin reactions and the role of thymus-derived cells. *Monogr. Allergy,* 8:154–167.
4. Bach, F. H., and Voynow, N. K. (1966): One-way stimulation in mixed leukocyte cultures. *Science,* 153:545–547.
5. Bain, B., and Lowenstein, L. (1964): Genetic studies on the mixed leukocyte reaction. *Science,* 145:1315–1316.
6. Baker, P. J., Stashak, P. W., Amsbaugh, D. F., and Prescott, B. (1971): Characterization of the antibody response to type III pneumococcal polysaccharide at the cellular level. I. Dose–response studies and the effect of prior immunization on the magnitude of the antibody response. *Immunology,* 20:469–480.
7. Ball, J., and Dawson, D. (1969): Biological effects of the neonatal injection of 7,12-dimethyl-benz(a)anthracene. *J. Natl. Cancer Inst.,* 42:579–591.
8. Ball, J., Sinclair, N., and McCarter, J. (1966): Prolonged immunosuppression and tumor induction by a chemical carcinogen injected at birth. *Science,* 152:650–651.
9. Bellanti, J. A. (1978): *Immunology II.* W. B. Saunders, Philadelphia.
10. Biggar, W. D. (1976): Analysis and treatment of immunodeficiency diseases. In: *Infection and the Compromised Host,* edited by J. C. Allen, pp. 1–27. Williams & Wilkins, Baltimore.
11. Boraker, D. K., and Hildemann, W. H. (1965): Maturation of alloimmune responsiveness in mice. *Transplantation,* 3:202–203.
12. Britton, S. (1969): Regulation of antibody synthesis against *Escherichia coli* endotoxin. *Immunology,* 16:527–536.
13. Cohen, A. S. (1979): *Rheumatology and Immunology,* Grune and Stratton, New York.
14. Cook, J. A., DiLuzio, N. R., and Hoffman, E. O. (1975): Factors modifying susceptibility to bacterial endotoxin: The effect of lead and cadmium. *CRC Crit. Rev. Toxicol.,* 3(2):201–229.
15. Cooper, M. D., and Seligmann, M. (1977): *Development of Host Defenses.* Raven Press, New York.
16. Cranmer, J. S., Avery, D. L., and Barnett, J. B. (1979): Altered immune competence of offspring exposed during development to the chlorinated hydrocarbon pesticide chlordane. *Teratology,* 19:23A.
17. Cranmer, J. S., Avery, D. L., and Barnett, J. B. (1979): Persistent postnatal effects on the immune system following prenatal exposure to the anticholinesterase pesticides diazinon or carbofuran. *Toxicol. Appl. Pharmacol.,* 48:A88.
18. DeSousa, M., Parrott, D., and Pantelouris, E. (1969): The lymphoid tissues in mice with congenital aplasia of the thymus. *Clin. Exp. Immunol.,* 4:637–644.
19. De Sousa, M., Pritchard, H., and Parrott, D. (1974): An analysis of some morphological features of the lymphoid system in nude mice. In: *Proceedings of the First International Workshop on Nude Mice,* edited by J. Rygaard and C. Povlsen, pp. 119–126. Gustav Fischer Verlag, Stuttgart.
20. Doell, R., De Vaux St. Cyr, C., and Grabar, P. (1967): Immune reactivity prior to development of thymic lymphoma in C57BL. *Int. J. Cancer,* 2:103–108.
21. Fachet, J., Palkovits, M., Vallent, K., and Stark, E. (1966): Effect of a single glycocorticoid injection on the first day of life in rats. *Acta Endocrinol. (Kbh.),* 51:71–76.
22. Faith, R., Luster, M., and Kimmel, C. (1979): Effect of chronic developmental lead exposure on cell-mediated immune functions. *Clin. Exp. Immunol.,* 35:413–420.

23. Faith, R., and Moore, J. (1977): Impairment of thymus-dependent immune functions by exposure of the developing immune system to 2,3,7,8-tetrachlorodibenzo-p-dioxin (TCDD). *J. Toxicol. Environ. Health*, 3:451–464.

24 Festing, M., and King, D. (1974): Large scale production of nude mice. In: *Proceedings of the First International Workshop on Nude Mice*, edited by J. Rygaard and C. Povlsen, pp. 189–202. Gustav Fischer Verlag, Stuttgart.

25. Friend, M., and Trainer, D. (1970): Polychlorinated biphenyl: Interaction with duck hepatitis virus. *Science*, 170:1314–1316.

26. Gebhardt, B. M., and Newberne, P. M. (1974): Nutrition and immunological responsiveness. T-cell function in the offspring of lipotrope and protein-deficient rats. *Immunology*, 26:489–495.

27. Gelfland, M. C., Elfenbein, G. J., Frank, M. M., and Paul, W. E. (1974): Ontogeny of B lymphocytes. II. Relative rates of appearance of lymphocytes bearing surface immunoglobulin and complement receptors. *J. Exp. Med.*, 139:1125–1141.

28. Glick, B. (1971): Morphologic changes and humoral immunity in cyclophosphamide-treated chicks. *Transplantation*, 11:433–439.

29. Goldschneider, I. (1980): Early stages of lymphocyte development. *Cur. Top. Dev. Biol.*, 14:33–96.

30. Hair, J. (1974): The morphogenesis of thymus in nude and normal mice. In: *Proceedings of the First International Workshop on Nude Mice*, edited by J. Rygaard and C. Povlsen, pp. 23–30. Gustav Fischer Verlag, Stuttgart.

31. Haran-Ghera, N., and Kaplan, H. (1964): Significance of thymus and marrow injury in urethan leukemogenesis. *Cancer Res.*, 24:1926–1931.

32. Harris, E. D., Jr., (1979): Rheumatoid arthritis: Epidemiology, etiology, pathogenesis, and pathology. In: *Rheumatology and Immunology*, edited by A. S. Cohen, pp. 168–179. Grune and Stratton, New York.

33. Haseman, J. K., and Hogan, M. D. (1975): Selection of the experimental unit in teratology studies. *Teratology*, 12:165–172.

34. Hellman, A., and Weislow, O. S. (1979): Potential biohazards associated with depressed cellular and humoral immunity. In: *Naturally Occurring Biological Immunosuppressive Factors and Their Relationship to Disease*, edited by R. H. Neubauer, pp. 259–281. CRC Press, Boca Raton, Florida.

35. Herbert, W. J. (1973): Laboratory animal techniques for immunology. In: *Handbook of Experimental Immunology*, edited by D. M. Weiss, pp. A3.1–3.27. Blackwell Scientific Publications, London.

36. Hudson, J. L. (1978): *In Vitro* assessment methods in immunotoxicology. In: *Inadvertent Modification of the Immune Responses*, edited by I. M. Asher, pp. 88–93. United States Government Printing Office, Washington.

37. Ioachim, H. (1971): The cortisone-induced wasting disease of newborn rats: Histopathological and autoradiographic studies. *J. Pathol.*, 104:201–205.

38. Ipsen, J. (1953): Bioassay of 4 tetanus toxoids (aluminum precipitated) in mice, guinea pigs and humans. *J. Immunol.*, 70:426–434.

39. Janeway, C. A. (1971): The child with recurrent infections. *Postgrad. Med.*, 49:158–163.

40. Kalland, T. (1980): Alterations of antibody response in female mice after neonatal exposure to diethylstilbestrol. *J. Immunol.*, 124:194–198.

41. Kalland, T., Fossberg, T., and Fossberg, J. (1978): Effect of estrogen and corticosterone on the lymphoid system in neonatal mice. *Exp. Mol. Pathol.*, 28:76–95.

42. Kalland, T., Strand, O., and Forsberg, J. (1979): Long-term effects of neonatal estrogen treatment on mitogen responsiveness of mouse spleen lymphocytes. *J. Natl. Cancer Inst.*, 63:413–421.

43. Katz, D. H. (1977): *Lymphocyte Differentiation, Recognition and Regulation*. Academic Press, New York.

44. Kindred, B., and Loor, F. (1974): Immune responses in nude mice injected with thymus cell suspensions or grafted with neonatal thymus. In: *Proceedings of the First International Workshop on Nude Mice*, edited by J. Rygaard and C. Povlsen, pp. 149–164. Gustav Fischer Verlag, Stuttgart.

45. Koller, L. D. (1978): Effects of environmental contaminants on the immune system. *Adv. Vet. Sci. Comp. Med.*, 27:267–295.

46. Koller, L. D., and Thigpen, J. E. (1973): Reduction of antibody to pseudorabies virus in polychlorinated biphenyl exposed rabbits. *Am. J. Vet. Res.*, 34:1605–1606.

47. Lamm, M. E. (1976): Cellular aspects of immunoglobulin A. *Adv. Immunol.*, 22:223–290.

48. Lappe, M. A., and Steinmuller, D. S. (1970): Depression of weak allograft immunity in the mouse by neonatal or adult exposure to urethan. *Cancer Res.*, 30:674–678.
49. Lee, J., R. E., and Domm, L. V. (1967): A histological and histochemical study on the effects of adrenal cortical steroids in the fetal and neonatal rat thymus. *Anat. Rec.*, 157:105–116.
50. Lerman, S. P., and Weindanz, W. P. (1970): The effect of cyclophosphamide on the ontogeny of the humoral response in chickens. *J. Immunol.*, 105:614–619.
51. Lindstein, T., and Andersson, B. (1979): Ontogeny of B cells in CBA/N mice. *J. Exp. Med.*, 150:1285–1292.
52. Linna, T. J., Frommel, D., and Good, R. A. (1972): Effects of early cyclophosphamide treatment on the development of lymphoid organs and immunological functions in the chicken. *Int. Arch. Allergy Appl. Immunol.*, 42:20–39.
53. Loor, F., and Kindred, B. (1973): Differentiation of T-cell precursors in nude mice demonstrated by immunofluorescence of T-cell membrane markers. *J. Exp. Med.*, 138:1044–1045.
54. Loose, L. D., Pittman, K. A., Benitz, K. F., Silkworth, J. B., Mueller, W., and Coulston, F. (1978): Environmental chemically-induced immune dysfunction. *Ecotoxicol. Environ. Safety*, 2:173–198.
55. Luster, M., Faith, R., and Kimmel, C. (1978): Depression of humoral immunity in rats following chronic developmental lead exposure. *J. Environ. Pathol. Toxicol.*, 1:397–402.
56. Luster, M., Faith, R., McLachlan, J., and Clark, G. (1979): Effect of *in utero* exposure to diethylstilbestrol on the immune response in mice. *Toxicol. App. Pharmacol.*, 47:279–285.
57. Luz, N., Margues, M., Ayub, A., and Correa, P. (1969): Effects of estradiol upon the thymus and lymphoid organs of immature female rats. *Am. J. Obstet. Gynecol.*, 105:525–528.
58. Mackaness, G. B., and Hill, W. C. (1968): The effect of anti-lymphocyte globulin on cell-mediated resistance to infection. *J. Exp. Med.*, 129:993–1012.
59. Mancini, G., Carbonara, A. O., and Heremans, J. F. (1965): Immunochemical quantification of antigens by single radial immunodiffusion. *Int. J. Immunochem.*, 2:235–254.
60. Mandel, T. (1970): Differentiation of epithelial cells in the mouse thymus. *Z. Zellforsch.*, 106:498–515.
61. Menard, S., Colnaghi, M., and Cornabla, G. (1973): Immunogenicity and immunosensitivity of urethane-induced murine lung adenomata, in relation to the immunological impairment of the primary tumor host. *Br. J. Cancer*, 27:345–350.
62. Menna, J. H., Moses, E. G., and Barron, A. L. (1980): Influenza type A virus infection of suckling mice pre-exposed to insecticide carrier. *Toxicol. Lett.*, 6:357–363.
63. Meyer, R. K., Rao, M. A., and Aspinall, R. L. (1959): Inhibition of the development of the bursa of Fabricius in the embryos of common fowl by 19-nortestosterone. *Endocrinology*, 64:890–897.
64. Miller, J. F. A. P. (1962): Effect of neonatal thymectomy on the immunological responsiveness of the mouse. *Proc. R. Soc. Lond. [Biol.]*, 156:415–428.
65. Mishell, R. I., and Dutton, R. W. (1967): Immunization of dissociated spleen cell cultures from normal mice. *J. Exp. Med.*, 126:423–442.
66. Moore, J. A. (1979): The immunotoxicology phenomenon. *Drug Chem. Toxicol.*, 2:1–4.
67. Moore, J. A., and Faith, R. E. (1976): Immunologic response and factors affecting its assessment. *Environ. Health Perspect.*, 18:125–131.
68. Moore, M., and Owen, J. (1967): Experimental studies on the development of the thymus. *J. Exp. Med.*, 126:715–726.
69. Morse, H. C. III, Prescott, B., Cross, S., Stashak, P., and Baker, P. (1976): Regulation of the antibody response to type III pneumococcal polysaccharide. *J. Immunol.*, 116:279–287.
70. Mosier, D. (1977): Ontogeny of T-cell function in the neonatal mouse. In: *Development of Host Defenses*, edited by M. Cooper and D. Dayton, pp. 115–124. Raven Press, New York.
71. Mosier, D., Zaldivar, N., Goldings, E., Mond, J., Scher, I., and Paul, W. (1977): Formation of antibody in the newborn mouse: Study of T-cell independent antibody response. *J. Infect. Dis.*, 136:S14–S19.
72. Mueller, A. P., Wolfe, H. R., and Meyer, R. K. (1960): Precipitin production in chickens. XXI. Antibody production in bursectomized chickens with 19-nortestosterone on the fifth day of incubation. *J. Immunol.*, 85:172–179.
73. Ohi, G., Fukada, M., Seto, H., and Yagyu, H. (1976): Effect of methylmercury on humoral immune responses in mice under conditions simulated to practical situations. *Bull. Environ. Contam. Toxicol.*, 15:175–180.

74. Oppenheim, J. J., and Rosenstreich, D. L. (1975): *Mitogens in Immunobiology*. Academic Press, New York.
75. Owen, J. J. T. (1972): The origins and development of lymphocyte populations. In: *Ontogeny of Acquired Immunity, A Ciba Foundation Symposium*, edited by R. Porter and J. Knight, pp. 35–54. Elsevier, New York.
76. Papermaster, B. W., Friedman, D. I., and Good, R. A. (1962): Relationship of the bursa of Fabricius to immunological responsiveness and homograft immunity in the chicken. *Proc. Soc. Exp. Biol. Med.*, 110:62–64.
77. Parmiani, G., Golnaghi, M., and Porta, G. (1968): Immunodepressive and leukemogenic effects of urethan in C3Hf and SWR mice. *Proc. Soc. Exp. Biol. Med.*, 130:828–830.
78. Perek, M., and Drill, A. E. (1962): The role of the bursa of Fabricius in developing immunity in chickens treated with *Salmonella typhimurium* and *Spirochaeta gallinarum*. *Br. Vet. J.*, 118:390–393.
79. Perey, D. Y., Cooper, M. D., and Good, R. A. (1968): The mammalian homologue of the avian bursa of Fabricius. I. Neonatal extirpation of Peyer's patch-type lymphoepithelial tissues in rabbits: Methods and inhibition of humoral immunity. *Surgery*, 64:614–621.
80. Pinto-Machado, J. (1970): Influence of prenatal administration of busulfan on the postnatal development of mice. Production of a syndrome including hypoplasia of the thymus. *Teratology*, 3:363–370.
81. Poiley, S., Ovejera, A., Otis, A., and Reeder, C. (1974): Reproductive behavior of athymic nude (nu/nu-BALB/c/A/BOM Cr) mice in a variety of environments. In: *Proceedings of the First International Workshop on Nude Mice*, edited by J. Rygaard and C. Povlsen, pp. 189–202. Gustav Fischer Verlag, Stuttgart.
82. Raff, M. (1973): Theta-bearing lymphocytes in nude mice. *Nature*, 246:350–351.
83. Rank, R. G., and Weidanz, W. P. (1976): Non-sterilizing immunity in avian malaria: An antibody-independent phenomenon. *Proc. Soc. Exp. Biol. Med.*, 151:257–259.
84. Rao, M., Aspinall, R., and Meyer, R. (1962): Effect of dose and time of administration of 19-nortestosterone on the differentiation of lymphoid tissue in the bursa Fabricii of chick embryos. *Endocrinology*, 70:159–166.
85. Reilly, R. W., Thompson, J. A., Bielski, R. K., and Severson, C. D. (1967): Estradiol-induced wasting syndrome in neonatal mice. *J. Immunol.*, 98:321–330.
86. Roberts, D. W. (1978): Important aspects of immunotoxicity testing. In: *Inadvertent Modification of the Immune Response*, edited by I. M. Asher, pp. 60–69. United States Government Printing Office, Washington.
87. Roberts, D. W., Rank, R. G., Weidanz, W. P., and Finerty, J. F. (1977): Prevention of recrudescent malaria in nude mice by thymic grafting or by treatment with hyperimmune serum. *Infect. Immunol.*, 16:821–826.
88. Roberts, D. W., and Weidanz, W. P. (1979): T-cell immunity to malaria in the B-cell deficient mouse. *Am. J. Trop. Med. Hyg.*, 18:1–3.
89. Rugh, R. (1968): *The Mouse: Its Reproduction and Development*, Burgess Publishing, Minneapolis.
90. Russel, A., Ornoy, A., Ritchie, J., Golenser, J., Fein, A., and Nebel, L. (1972): Transplacental and neonatal effects of hypercortisonism in the rat on thymo–lymphatic system differentiation and serum immunoglobulin levels. *Adv. Exp. Med. Biol.*, 27:257–271.
91. Rygaard, J., and Povlsen, C. (1974): *Proceedings of the First International Workshop on Nude Mice*, Gustav Fischer Verlag, Stuttgart.
92. Schapiro, S. (1965): Neonatal cortisol administration: Effect on growth, the adrenal gland, and pituitary–adrenal response to stress. *Proc. Soc. Exp. Biol. Med.*, 120:771–774.
93. Schapiro, S., and Huppert, M. (1967): Neonatal cortisol administration and immunological impairment in the adult rat. *Proc. Soc. Exp. Biol. Med.*, 124:744–746.
94. Schiffman, G., and Austrian, R. (1971): A radioimmunoassay for the measurement of pneumococcal capsular antigens and of antibodies thereto. *Fed. Proc.*, 30:658.
95. Schlesinger, M., and Mary, R. (1964): Wasting disease induced in young mice by administration of cortisol acetate. *Science*, 11:965–966.
96. Schleupner, C. J., and Glasgow, L. A. (1978): Peritoneal macrophage activation indicated by enhanced chemiluminescence. *Infect. Immun.*, 21:886–895.

97. Silkworth, J. B., and Loose, L. D. (1980): Environmental chemical-induced modification of cell-mediated immune responses. In: *Macrophages and Lymphocytes, Part A*, edited by M. R. Escobar and H. Friedman, pp. 499–522. Plenum Press, New York.

98. Smith, C. (1965): Studies on the thymus of the mammal. XIV. Histology and histochemistry of embryonic and early postnatal thymuses of C57BL/6 and AKR strain mice. *Am. J. Anat.*, 116:611–630.

99. Solomon, J. B. (1971): *Foetal and Neonatal Immunology*, North-Holland, Amsterdam.

100. Speirs, R. S., Benson, R. W., and Roberts, D. W. (1979): Modification of antibody response to type III pneumopolysaccharide by route of injection of pertussis vaccine. *Infect. Immun.*, 23:675–680.

101. Spyker, J. M. (1975): Assessing the impact of low level chemicals on development: Behavioral and latent effects. *Fed. Proc.*, 34:1835–1844.

102. Spyker, J. M., and Fernandes, G. (1973): Impaired immune function in offspring from methylmercury-treated mice. *Teratology*, 7:A28.

103. Staples, R. E., and Haseman, J. K. (1974): Commentary: Selection of appropriate experimental units in teratology. *Teratology*, 9:259–260.

104. Stuart, A. E., Habeshan, J. A., and Davidson, A. E. (1973): Phagocytes *in vitro*. In: *Handbook of Experimental Immunology*, edited by D. M. Weir, pp. 24.1–24.26. Blackwell Scientific Publications, London.

105. Thigpen, J. E., Faith, R. E., McConnell, E. B., and Moore, J. A. (1975): Increased susceptibility to bacterial infection as a sequela of exposure to 2,3,7,8-tetrachlorodibenzo-*p*-dioxin. *Infect. Immun.*, 12:1319–1324.

106. Thomas, P. T., and Hinsdill, R. D. (1979): The effect of perinatal exposure to tetrachlorodibenzo-*p*-dioxin on the immune response of young mice. *Drug Chem. Toxicol.*, 2:77–98.

107. Thompson, J., and Russe, H. (1965): Estradiol induced wasting syndrome in newborn mice. *Fed. Proc.*, 24:A161.

108. Thorpe, P. E., and Knight, S. C. (1974): Microplate culture of mouse lymph node cells. I. Quantitation of responses of allogeneic lymphocytes, endotoxins and phytomitogens. *J. Immunol. Meth.*, 5:387–404.

109. Tripathy, S. P., and MacKaness, M. B. (1969): The effect of cytotoxic agents on the primary immune response to *Listeria monocytogenes*. *J. Exp. Med.*, 130:1–16.

110. Urso, P., and Gengozian, N. (1980): Depressed humoral immunity and increased tumor incidence in mice following *in utero* exposure to benzo(a)pyrene. *J. Toxicol. Environ. Health*, 6:569–576.

111. Van Furth, R., and Zwet, T. (1973): *In vitro* determination of phagocytosis and intracellular killing by polymorphonuclear and mononuclear phagocytes. In: *Handbook of Experimental Immunology*, edited by D. M. Weir, pp. 31.1–36.24. Blackwell Scientific Publications, London.

112. Vos, J. (1977): Immune suppression as related to toxicology. *CRC Crit. Rev. Toxicol.*, 5:67–107.

113. Vos, J., and Moore, J. (1974): Suppression of cellular immunity in mice by maternal treatment with 2,3,7,8-tetrachlorodibenzo-*p*-dioxin. *Int. Arch. Allergy Appl. Immunol.*, 47:777–794.

114. Waksman, B. H. (1976): On soluble mediators of immunologic regulation. *Cell. Immunol.*, 21:161–176.

115. Warner, N. L., Uhr, J. W., Thorbecke, G. J., and Ovary, Z. (1969): Immunoglobulins, antibodies, and the bursa of Fabricius: Induction of agammaglobulinemia and the loss of all antibody-forming capacity by hormonal bursectomy. *J. Immunol.*, 103:1317–1330.

116. Ways, S. C., and Bern, H. A. (1979): Long-term effects of neonatal treatment with cortisol and/or estrogen in the female BALB/c mouse. *Proc. Soc. Exp. Biol. Med.*, 160:94–98.

117. Weissman, I., Small, M., Fatham, C., and Herzenberg, L. (1975): Differentiation of thymus cells. *Fed. Proc.*, 34:141–144.

118. Wilkes, T., Imrie, S., and Brunson, J. (1964): Effects of epinephrine on newborn rabbits. *Am. J. Pathol.*, 43:825–836.

119. Winick, M., and Coscia, A. (1968): Cortisone-induced growth failure in neonatal rats. *Pediatr. Res.*, 2:451–455.

120. World Health Organization Technical Report Series (1978): *Immunodeficiency*. World Health Organization, Geneva.

121. Wortis, H. H., Nehlsen, S., and Owen, J. J. (1971): Abnormal development of the thymus in "nude" mice. *Clin. Exp. Immunol.*, 8:305–317.

*Developmental Toxicology*, edited by
C. A. Kimmel and J. Buelke-Sam. Raven Press,
New York © 1981.

# Effects of Prenatal Exposure to Chemical Carcinogens and Methods for Their Detection

### Jerry M. Rice

*Perinatal Carcinogenesis Section, Laboratory of Experimental Pathology, National Cancer Institute, Bethesda, Maryland 20205*

Chemical carcinogens ingested by or administered to a pregnant female may induce tumors in her offspring. This phenomenon is known as transplacental carcinogenesis. No known substance is carcinogenic only during the prenatal phase of mammalian development; rather, any agent that is carcinogenic during postnatal life and that is physically capable of reaching the fetus by way of the placenta (perhaps in the form of metabolites) can be expected to act as a transplacental carcinogen. Whether it will affect the same organ systems in both mother and offspring and whether mother or offspring will be more vulnerable depend on many factors including the metabolic fate of the substance and the stage of pregnancy during which exposure occurs. Fetal tissues differentiate rapidly, especially in rodents, and profound changes in susceptibility to carcinogens accompany this process.

During transplacental exposure to carcinogens, the fetus is subjected to the carcinogen itself and to any metabolites formed in its own tissues; it may also be exposed to the same or different metabolites formed in maternal or placental tissues. For a given agent, the relative importance of fetal versus maternal metabolism depends to a great extent on how stable the carcinogenic metabolites of maternal origin are and whether they may survive in the maternal environment long enough to reach and traverse the placenta. Fetal tissues themselves are intrinsically highly vulnerable to carcinogens because of their high rate of cellular proliferation; dividing cells are more susceptible to chemical carcinogens (12). In many cases, the outcome of transplacental exposure to carcinogens appears to constitute the net effect of two clearly identifiable opposing tendencies: high fetal mitotic rates tend to increase susceptibility, while the relatively low fetal rates of metabolism of most foreign substances tend to reduce the consequences of exposure. When the latter factor predominates, an agent may be negligibly effective transplacentally, even though it may be very potent in adults. This occurs when the carcinogenicity of an agent depends on metabolic formation of very short-lived reactive intermediates that are produced inefficiently or not at all in fetal target tissues. On the other hand, when metabolism is not important, as with intrinsically reactive carcinogens such as the alkylating agents, fetal susceptibility to a given carcinogen may exceed that of adults by two or more decimal orders of magnitude. This potential for very high fetal risk is a major reason for emphasizing the importance of transplacental exposure in chemical carcinogenesis.

Further information on transplacental carcinogenesis can be found in a number of English, German, and Russian language reviews (36,59,73–75,103) and in several book-length monographs (in English) containing the proceedings of international conferences on this subject (76,82,101).

## IDENTIFICATION OF CHEMICAL CARCINOGENS

Chemical carcinogens are an exceedingly numerous and diverse group of substances, including such dissimilar materials as the gaseous vinyl chloride, the water-miscible liquid dimethylnitrosamine, the oil-soluble crystalline solid benzo[a]pyrene, the insoluble fibrous minerals comprising different forms of asbestos, and certain salts of several of the nonradioactive[1] heavy metals, including chromium, cadmium, and lead. Literally hundreds of the thousands of substances tested (106) have proved carcinogenic in one or more test systems. Although many of these are man-made synthetic organic chemicals, a significant number of natural products are also carcinogenic. These include metabolites of fungi and of other higher plants (aflatoxin, cycasin, safrole), naturally occurring products of combustion (benzo[a]pyrene), and substances that may form in the mammalian gastrointestinal tract from ingested precursors (nitrosamines from nitrite and secondary or tertiary amines). So many carcinogens have been identified that to maintain an accurate public sense of perspective, the U.S. National Cancer Institute has been obliged to publish a pamphlet documenting the fact that not everything causes cancer (61).

It is not possible accurately to predict that a substance is carcinogenic by inspection of its chemical structure. Moreover, many carcinogenic substances are complex mixtures that contain a minute quantity of one or more, often unknown, carcinogenic compounds. Benzo[a]pyrene, for example, was isolated originally as one of the active principles from 2 tons of carcinogenic coal tar pitch (13); aflatoxin $B_1$, the dominant carcinogen in toxic peanut meals contaminated by the fungus *Aspergillus flavus*, is found in such carcinogenic animal feeds at concentrations on the order of 1 to 10 ppm (111). Many carcinogens have other properties, such as mutagenicity, that serve provisionally to identify previously untested substances as suspected carcinogens, but proof of carcinogenicity can only come from accidental human exposures or from tests in animals. Although a wide variety of test species and modes of application of an agent have been used for this purpose (110), the method most generally employed involves lifetime feeding studies in mice and rats, beginning at or soon after weaning. The procedures for this have been well stand-

---

[1]Radionuclides are conventionally included with external sources of radiation as physical, rather than chemical, carcinogens.

ardized (86). Irrespective of the method used, a substance is generally considered carcinogenic if, in treated animals, to a statistically significant extent: (a) kinds of tumors not seen in controls appear; (b) a greater incidence or higher multiplicity of tumors develops than is seen in untreated animals; or (c) the latency for tumor development is shorter. These are purely phenomenological criteria for defining carcinogenicity, and although suitable for purposes of identifying possible risks to human health, they are not always adequate for research purposes. They do not, for example, allow a distinction to be made between agents capable of permanently converting normal cells to a neoplastic state and promoting agents that only enhance the development of overt tumors from preexisting latent, potentially neoplastic cells.

## METHODS FOR THE STUDY OF
## TRANSPLACENTAL CARCINOGENESIS

In addition to the basic principles of controlled experimentation that apply to conventional studies in carcinogenesis and the requirement for numbers of animals sufficient to attach statistically acceptable degrees of confidence to the results, adequate demonstration of transplacental[2] carcinogenesis in an experimental setting depends on adequate solutions to several technical problems unique to the transplacental route of exposure. Control of the timing of exposure is essential, since prenatal susceptibility to carcinogenesis is markedly dependent on stage of development. Measures must be devised to insure that transplacental exposure is the only exposure possible, so that an experiment in transplacental carcinogenesis does not inadvertently become one on combined pre- and postnatal effects. Finally, since it is the pregnant female that is directly subject to experimental manipulation rather than each conceptus individually, for statistical purposes it is all offspring in a litter combined, rather than each individual offspring, that represents a statistically independent unit. This can become extremely important when one is attempting to assess the significance of borderline carcinogenic effects.

Timing of exposure is best insured by timing the mating accurately, to within a tolerance of 1 day. This is most easily accomplished, with all commonly used laboratory species, by pairing proven breeders at the end of a day and separating them the following morning. The presence of copulation plugs in mice, and to a lesser extent rats, is useful confirmatory evidence of mating. The day after pairing, or the day a copulation plug is observed, is designated day 0 of gestation by some authors and day 1 by others and must be specified. It is generally not adequate simply to treat obviously pregnant animals and then to note the day of subsequent delivery and count backwards from the normal length of the gestation period. High doses of toxic agents given late in gestation may delay parturition by several days.

Transplacental carcinogenesis has been demonstrated in the offspring of animals exposed to chemicals by feeding or by stomach tube, by inhalation, by cutaneous

---

[2]The synonym diaplacental, used by those who prefer Greek to Latin prefixes, is encountered frequently in the European literature.

application, and, most commonly, by subcutaneous, intraperitoneal, or intravenous injection. Intraperitoneal injection, especially in oily vehicles, results in a slower rate of distribution of the agent throughout the mother's body, with lower but more prolonged blood levels than occur with intravenous injections. Although this may be useful, especially when testing agents with pharmacologic effects, the investigator should recall that even the most experienced investigators frequently miss the intended target when injecting intraperitoneally, injecting into the intestine, the gravid uterus, subcutaneously, or retroperitoneally rather than into the abdominal cavity (53,92). Accurate placement of intraperitoneal injections is easiest in anesthetized animals. Oral or intravenous administrations reduce the likelihood of wide fluctuations in tumor induction from litter to litter as a result of technical error and nonequivalent dosing; paravenous injection, which may occur when intravenous injection is attempted, is usually easily detected.

A more serious potential defect in transplacental carcinogenesis studies, however, is failure to control possible continued postnatal exposure of offspring via the treated mother's milk, fur, or excreta. It has been demonstrated that certain carcinogens given to lactating females may be transferred to suckling young in milk, and in quantities sufficient not only to induce tumor formation but to do so with such efficiency that transplacental effects of lower magnitude by the same agent may be completely obscured (62,63). To avoid false positive results of this sort, especially with chemically stable compounds with long biological half-lives, it is necessary to insure that the offspring of treated females, from the moment of birth, never nurse or come in contact with their natural mother. This is best accomplished by fostering[3] the young on untreated lactating females as has been done by a number of investigators in studies with the polynuclear aromatic hydrocarbons (10,77,104).

In contrast to the voluminous literature on identification of chemical carcinogens, relatively little is known of the transplacental effects of these substances. Those that have been satisfactorily tested and found active in one or more species as of December, 1979 are listed in Tables 1 to 4. In addition to these, diethylstilbestrol, the only known transplacental carcinogen for humans, is discussed separately. Besides man, transplacental carcinogenesis has been demonstrated in the mouse, rat, rabbit, two species of hamster, the pig, and the patas monkey.

## METABOLISM AND REACTIONS OF CHEMICAL CARCINOGENS

Chemical carcinogens that are small organic molecules, including all the known transplacental carcinogens with the possible exception of hormones, react rather indiscriminantly with the constituents of target cells. This occurs through a variety of metabolic and chemical processes that result in conversion of the agents (procarcinogens) to reactive derivatives (ultimate carcinogens), often via stable inter-

---

[3]This is readily accomplished by installing a treated, near-term pregnant female on a wire grid dividing a cage horizontally. A lactating female in the cage beneath the grid will usually gather up and care for the transplacentally exposed offspring that fall through the grid as they are delivered. Galvanized wire hardware cloth (4 mesh) is adequate for mice; poultry fencing is best for rats.

TABLE 1. *Direct-acting transplacental carcinogens*

| Compound | Species | Principal target organs | References |
|---|---|---|---|
| Sulfate and sulfonate esters | | | |
| Dimethyl sulfate | Rat | Nervous system | 21 |
| Diethyl sulfate | Rat | Nervous system | 21 |
| Methyl methanesulfonate | Rat | Nervous system | 41 |
| Propane sultone | Rat | Nervous system | 22 |
| Alkylnitrosoureas | | | |
| Methylnitrosourea | Rat | Nervous system | 2,40,100 |
| Ethylnitrosourea | Mouse | Lung, liver | 16,72,107 |
| | Mouse | Nervous system | 14 |
| | Rat | Nervous system | 2,19,24,37,38,40,43, 68,94,102 |
| | Syrian hamster | Nervous system | 37 |
| | Rabbit | Kidney | 25,32,91 |
| | Rabbit | Nervous system | 89,90 |
| | Patas monkey | Connective tissues | 78 |
| *n*-Propylnitrosourea | Rat | Nervous system | 39 |
| Other acylalkylnitrosamines | | | |
| Ethylnitrosobiuret | Rat | Nervous system | 23 |
| Methylnitrosourethane | Rat | Nervous system, kidney, liver | 97 |
| Miscellaneous | | | |
| Ethylurea + sodium nitrite | Rat | Nervous system | 67 |
| | Syrian hamster | Nervous system | 81 |
| | Rabbit | Kidney | 26 |
| Methylazoxymethanol | Rat | Nervous system, kidney, intestine | 45 |

mediate metabolites (proximate carcinogens). Ultimate carcinogens either are positively charged or have electron-deficient reactive centers. They are thus electrophilic and react (though at widely differing rates) with nucleophilic centers in both small molecules and in macromolecules to form covalently bound adducts. Recognition of this general phenomenon by James and Elizabeth Miller resulted in one of the most important and broadly valid unifying hypotheses in chemical carcinogenesis (52).

There are two major groups of such chemical carcinogens, direct-acting and metabolism-dependent. The former are not dependent on enzymes for conversion to chemically reactive intermediates. The best-understood direct-acting carcinogens are members of various classes of organic alkylating agents (46) and include the most potent of the known transplacental carcinogens. The alkylating agents react to varying extents with heteroatoms (N,S,O) in a wide variety of intracellular receptors including DNA; different agents have different product distributions (84). Reaction is by either unimolecular ($S_N1$) or bimolecular ($S_N2$) substitution. Compounds such as methyl methanesulfonate react directly with target molecules, e.g., glutathione (GSH) by $S_N2$:

$$CH_3SO_2\text{-}O\text{:}CH_3$$

$$H\text{-}\overset{\uparrow}{S}\text{-}G \longrightarrow CH_3SO_3^- + H\text{-}\underset{+}{\overset{CH_3}{\overset{|}{S}}}\text{-}G \xrightarrow{-H^+} G\text{-}S\text{-}CH_3$$

The alkylnitrosoureas decompose by unimolecular processes that generate highly reactive alkyldiazonium hydroxide intermediates that are too unstable to isolate. These react very rapidly by $S_N1$:

Both kinds of alkylating agents are included among the known transplacental carcinogens (Table 1).

TABLE 2. *Transplacental carcinogenesis by nitrosamines*

| Compound | Species | Principal target organs | References |
|---|---|---|---|
| Dialkylnitrosamines | | | |
| Dimethylnitrosamine | Rat | Kidney | 1 |
| | Syrian hamster | Digestive and urogenital systems | 6 |
| Diethylnitrosamine | Mouse | Lung, liver | 17,55 |
| | Mouse | Lung, liver, esophagus/ forestomach | 47 |
| | Rat | Kidney | 69,112 |
| | Syrian hamster | Trachea | 54,56,57,58 |
| Dipropylnitrosamine | Syrian hamster | Digestive and urogenital systems | 6 |
| Methylpropylnitrosamine | Syrian hamster | Liver, urinary tract | 4 |
| Dibutylnitrosamine | Syrian hamster | Upper respiratory tract | 5 |
| Stable metabolites of dialkylnitrosamines | | | |
| 2-Hydroxypropyl propylnitrosamine | Syrian hamster | Lung | 4 |
| 2-Oxopropyl propyl- nitrosamine | Syrian hamster | Liver | 4 |
| bis(2-Hydroxypropyl) nitrosamine | Syrian hamster | Nasal cavities, trachea, lung, liver | 4 |
| 4-Hydroxybutyl butyl- nitrosamine | Syrian hamster | Nasal cavities, trachea, lung, liver | 4 |
| Cyclic nitrosamines | | | |
| Nitrosohexamethyl- eneimine | Syrian hamster | Upper respiratory tract | 5 |
| Nitrosopiperidine | Syrian hamster | Digestive tract | 3 |

TABLE 3. *Hydrazines, triazenes, and aliphatic azo compounds with demonstrated transplacental carcinogenic activity*

| Compound | Species | Principal target organs | References |
|---|---|---|---|
| 1,2-Diethylhydrazine | Rat | Nervous system | 20 |
| 1-Methyl-2-benzyl-hydrazine | Rat | Nervous system, kidney | 18 |
| Azoxymethane | Rat | Nervous system, kidney | 18 |
| Azoxyethane | Rat | Nervous system | 20 |
| Azoethane | Rat | Nervous system | 20 |
| 1,1-Dimethyl-3-phenyltriazene | Rat | Nervous system, kidney | 18 |
| 1,1-Diethyl-3-phenyltriazene | Rat | Nervous system | 18 |
| 1,1-Diethyl-3-(3-pyridyl)triazene | Rat | Nervous system | 18 |
| N-(1-Methylethyl)-4-[(2-methylhydrazino)-methyl]benzamide (Procarbazine; Natulan) | Rat | Nervous system | 35 |

The vast majority of carcinogens are converted to analogous reactive electrophiles in one or more enzyme-mediated metabolic steps. Commonly, the first step is oxidative and is catalyzed by one of the cytochrome-containing monooxygenases or mixed-function oxidases (48). Diethylnitrosamine, for example, is hydroxylated at an $\alpha$-carbon atom, generating an ethyl-(1-hydroxyethyl) nitrosamine that is too unstable to isolate or prepare synthetically. It decomposes by a mechanism such as that illustrated above for methylnitrosourea, generating acetaldehyde and a molecule of nitrogen as by-products and an ethyldiazonium hydroxide intermediate that reacts by $S_N1$. Compounds containing a carbon–carbon double bond may be oxidized to epoxide derivatives which are potentially reactive by $S_N2$. Aromatic hydrocarbons are similarly metabolized to arene oxides which may be hydrolyzed to dihydrodiols by epoxide hydrase; these may then be oxidized to a second, sometimes more toxic, arene oxide. The most potent carcinogenic metabolite of benzo[a]pyrene arises from such a sequence through successive formation of the 7,8-oxide, 7,8-dihydrodiol, and 7,8-dihydrodiol-9,10-oxide (83). Aromatic amines can be oxidized to aminophenols via arene oxides or to hydroxylamines. The hydroxylamines are proximate carcinogens that are further metabolized to reactive electrophiles via sulfate conjugates (52), a metabolic path that also serves to activate certain of the heteroaromatic N-oxides such as 3-hydroxyxanthine to ultimate carcinogens (7). These react not only at heteroatoms but also with nucleophilic carbon atoms such as C-8 in guanine. Thus, both oxidative and conjugative pathways are important in production of ultimate carcinogenic metabolites of many compounds that are known to be transplacental carcinogens.

Both oxidative and conjugative enzymes are inducible by exposure to various substances, including substrates (48,49), and are generally present in uninduced

TABLE 4. *Metabolism-dependent transplacental carcinogens other than aliphatic nitrogen-containing compounds*

| Compound | Species | Principal target organs | References |
|---|---|---|---|
| Polynuclear aromatic hydrocarbons | | | |
| Benzo[a]pyrene | Mouse | Lung, skin[a] | 10,11[a] |
| Methylcholanthrene | Mouse | Lung | 95,104 |
| 7,12-Dimethylbenz[a]-anthracene | Mouse | Lung, skin[a], liver, ovary | 11[a], 28[a],29[a], 98,99 |
| | Rat | Nervous system, kidney | 60,70,77 |
| Heteroaromatic compounds and aromatic amines | | | |
| 3-Hydroxyxanthine | Rat | Liver, mammary glands | 7,8 |
| 2-(2-Furyl)-3-(5-nitro-2-furyl)acrylamide (Furylfuramide; AF-2) | Mouse | Lung | 64 |
| 4-Nitroquinoline-1-oxide | Mouse | Lung | 63 |
| o-Aminoazotoluene | Mouse | Liver | 27,30 |
| 4-Dimethylaminoazo-benzene | Mouse | Liver, lung | 30 |
| o-Toluidine | Mouse | Liver, lung | 30 |
| 3,3'-Dichlorobenzidine | Mouse | Liver, lung | 30 |
| Natural products of plant and fungal origin | | | |
| Aflatoxin | Rat | Liver | 31 |
| Methylazoxymethyl-β-D-glucopyranoside (Cycasin) | Rat | Nervous system, intestine | 88 |
| Safrole | Mouse | Kidney | 109 |
| Miscellaneous | | | |
| Ethyl carbamate | Mouse | Lung, skin[a], liver, ovary | 28[a],29[a],42, 44,62,65, 85,108 |
| Vinyl chloride | Rat | Blood vessels, kidney, Zymbal's gland | 50 |

[a]Skin tumorigenesis in mice occurred during postnatal topical application of croton oil or phorbol ester promoting agents.

fetal tissues at levels much lower than those found in adults (49). An exception is β-glucosidase, important in the metabolism of cycasin, which is present at highest levels in rat tissues during prenatal and early postnatal life (87).

## TRANSPLACENTAL EFFECTS

### Direct-Acting Carcinogens

Metabolism-independent, direct-acting alkylating agents are among the most potent of the known transplacental carcinogens, and their effects have been well characterized in rodent and, to a much lesser extent, in nonrodent species (Table

1). Ethylnitrosourea (ENU), the first such compound to be identified as a transplacental carcinogen (19), is also the most potent mutagen so far identified in mice (79). Ethylnitrosourea is one of the most thoroughly studied transplacental carcinogens and is representative of the direct-acting agents in its carcinogenic properties.

Offspring of rats given ENU during the final week of gestation are born apparently normal and without visible evidence of tumor. After growing to maturity, however, they selectively develop tumors of the cranial, spinal, and peripheral nerves, the spinal cord, and the brain (2,19,24,37,38,40,43,68,94,102; Fig. 1). Tumors of nonneural origin (kidney, breast) are found extremely infrequently. A single exposure is sufficient for carcinogenesis. The incidence of tumors among offspring of treated females and the multiplicity of induced tumors vary greatly with the stage of pregnancy at which ENU is given. Treatment on or before day 11 does not lead to tumor development during postnatal life, although it may be teratogenic if the dose is sufficiently large. However, beginning on day 12, the developing nervous system becomes increasingly susceptible to carcinogenesis, reaching a maximum shortly before birth and declining rapidly thereafter (37; Fig. 2). When different doses of ENU were given to pregnant rats on the 15th day of pregnancy, prior to the stage of maximum susceptibility, an increasing fraction of the pups developed tumors as the dose was increased (37). The multiplicity of tumors in a single tumor-bearing rat also increased with increasing dose. Comparable exposures resulted in much lower incidences of neurogenic tumors in adult rats; 15-day fetuses appeared at least 50-fold more susceptible than adults (37; Fig. 3). Transplacentally induced tumors of the nervous system developed more slowly at lower doses than at higher single doses (37; Fig. 4). Studies in other strains of rats revealed that although all were susceptible to carcinogenesis in the nervous system, some were much more susceptible than others (24).

Comparable studies with ENU in mice similarly showed that fetal susceptibility to carcinogenesis was negligible prior to the 12th day of gestation and that fetuses were more susceptible than adults to ENU (72,107). However, whereas tumors of the nervous system were occasionally seen in mice exposed transplacentally to ENU (14,16,107), the predominant carcinogenic effect was seen in the peripheral lung (Fig. 5) and in the liver (Fig. 6). Tumors are not seen in these organs in rats given ENU transplacentally. When ENU was given to pregnant rabbits relatively late in gestation, kidney tumors were the only neoplasms subsequently observed in the offspring (25,32,91). Only when the compound was given very early in pregnancy were tumors of the nervous system seen (89,90). Similarly, in one species of nonhuman primate, transplacental exposure to ENU led predominantly to tumors of blood vessels and other connective tissues in the offspring (78); tumors of the brain and its meninges have subsequently been observed, but infrequently (J. M. Rice, *unpublished data*).

Ethylnitrosourea, like other nitrosamides and nitrosamines, can be formed in the stomach and intestine from inorganic nitrite and a nitrosatable precursor. When pregnant rats, hamsters, or rabbits were fed ethylurea and sodium nitrite, tumors

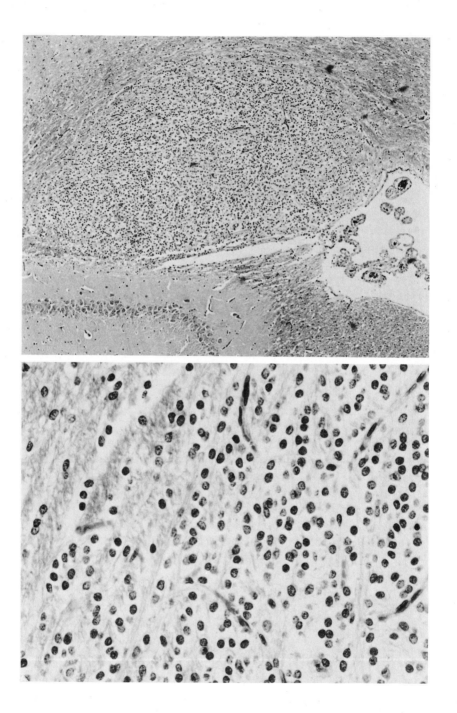

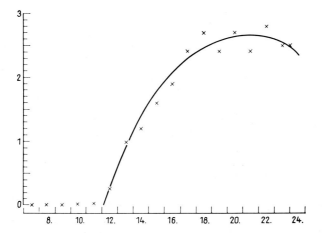

**FIG. 2.** Relation of neurogenic tumor development in the offspring to the day of gestation on which pregnant BD-IX rats were given a single intravenous injection of ethylnitrosourea [0.5 mmole (60 mg)/kg body weight]. The number of primary neurogenic tumors per rat is plotted against day of gestation. (From Ivankovic and Druckrey, ref. 37, with permission.)

like those resulting from transplacental exposure to ENU developed in the offspring (26,67,81).

Most other alkylating agents that have been tested for transplacental carcinogenic activity have been studied only in rats, in which they induce a spectrum of tumors very much like those seen in experiments with ENU. In the homologous series of alkylnitrosoureas, testing of the methyl, ethyl, *n*-propyl, *n*-butyl, *n*-pentyl, and benzyl compounds allowed an assessment of structure–activity relationships (37, 39,40). The methyl compound is a weaker transplacental carcinogen than its ethyl and *n*-propyl homologs, both of which are very potent. The *n*-butyl derivative is a weak transplacental carcinogen, and the *n*-pentyl and benzyl derivatives are inactive (39). Prediction of transplacental carcinogenicity from *a priori* considerations of chemical structure clearly is not a simple undertaking. In the case of the alkylnitrosoureas, transplacental carcinogenicity is approximately inversely correlated with chemical stability and oil/water partition coefficient except for the methyl compound. The spectrum of DNA adducts also changes with increasing alkyl chain

**FIG. 1.** Primary brain tumor in a male Lewis rat whose mother had received 0.2 mmole ethylnitrosourea/kg body weight intravenously on the 21st day of gestation. The rat developed paralysis 40 weeks after birth and at necropsy was found to have two large malignant schwannomas (in the intracranial portion of the left trigeminal nerve and in the cauda equina), an anaplastic oligodendroglioma of the lower cervical spinal cord, and two small gliomas in the brain. **Top:** Small primary glioma of the brain, characteristically located in the subcortical white matter and adjacent to the wall of a lateral ventricle, the choroid plexus of which is visible at right. Tumors of this size, less than 2 mm in diameter, are not visible on the surface of the brain and can be found only by careful dissection and examination after fixation. Grossly they appear in cut sections as well-defined translucent foci. Hematoxylin and eosin, ×55. **Bottom:** Higher magnification of the border of the tumor, a well-differentiated and highly vascular oligodendroglioma. ×330.

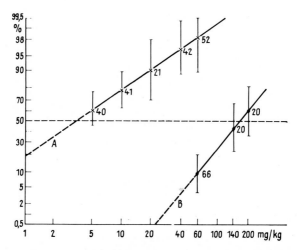

**FIG. 3.** Linear regression analysis of dose–response relationships for the induction of neurogenic tumors in BD-IX rats after a single intravenous injection of ethylnitrosourea. *A,* Prenatal exposure on day 15 of gestation; *B,* in adult rats. Confidence limits for $p = 0.05$ and numbers of rats contributing to each treatment group are indicated. (From Ivankovic and Druckrey, ref. 37, with permission.)

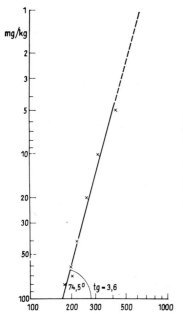

**FIG. 4.** Dependence of latency on dose for the development of neurogenic tumors in BD-IX rats in response to a single transplacental exposure to ethylnitrosourea on day 15 of gestation. The log–log plot of dose (*d*, mg/kg) versus time (*t*, days after birth) to appearance of signs of tumor reduces to the linear equation, $-\log d = 3.6 \log t + (constant)$. (From Ivankovic and Druckrey, ref. 37, with permission.)

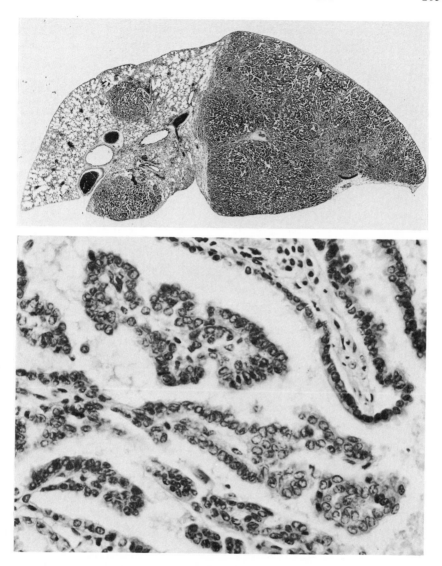

**FIG. 5.** Multiple pulmonary tumors in a female C3HfB/HeN mouse, 43 weeks after birth. The mouse had 16 lung tumors, 1 liver tumor, and a Schwannoma of the trigeminal nerve. Its mother had received a single intraperitoneal injection of ethylnitrosourea (0.5 mmole/kg) on day 15 of gestation. **Top:** Cross section of a lung lobe showing three independent lung tumors of different size. The small tumor at upper left is growing into a bronchiole. Hematoxylin and eosin, × 13.5. **Bottom:** Higher magnification of invasive portion of the tumor showing papillary pattern and cuboidal to low columnar epithelial tumor cells. Bronchiolar lining is at upper right. × 330.

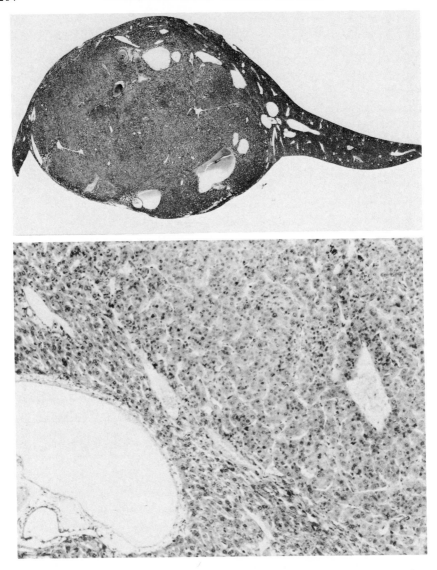

**FIG. 6.** Hepatocellular carcinoma in a male C3HfB/HeN mouse aged 50 weeks, transplacentally exposed to 0.5 mmole ethylnitrosourea/kg maternal body weight on day 14 of gestation. The mouse had 6 lung tumors, 9 liver tumors, and a trigeminal Schwannoma. **Top:** A single large tumor severely distorts the cross-sectional silhouette of the affected liver lobe. Hematoxylin and eosin, ×6.5. **Bottom:** Higher magnification illustrates the trabecular pattern of the tumor (upper right), the expansive growth of which compresses the bordering hepatic parenchyma. ×80.

length (84). Methylnitrosourea is both extremely reactive and extremely toxic; in fact, a lower incidence of neurogenic tumors is seen in the offspring of rats given both ENU and its methyl homolog successively than in rats given ENU alone (2). It appears that methylnitrosourea destroys a large fraction of the cells that would eventually have developed into tumors and that the maximum transplacental carcinogenicity associated with the ethyl and propyl compounds results at least in part from optimally rapid and selective chemical reactivity.

Methyl- and ethylnitrosoureas have been used by Tomatis and associates (100,102) to study the tumor incidence in the second ($F_2$) and third ($F_3$) generation descendants of animals directly exposed to the carcinogen while pregnant. In agreement with other investigators who have performed similar experiments with different carcinogens in both rats and mice (65,97,99), they found a low but significant excess incidence of tumors in the $F_2$ and/or $F_3$ generations. There is some evidence that this elusive effect is mediated through carcinogen-induced damage to the germ cells of $F_1$ females exposed while *in utero* (97). This potentially very important finding requires much further study.

## Metabolism-Dependent Carcinogens

Nitrosamines are metabolized by mixed-function oxidases to reactive alkylating metabolites with very short half-lives. Those that have been shown to possess transplacental carcinogenic activity are listed in Table 2.

The simplest member of the class, dimethylnitrosamine, induces renal tumors in adult rats when given as a single exposure or as a short series of treatments. When given to pregnant rats, similar tumors are induced in the offspring but at much lower rates than in the mothers and only if exposure occurs near the end of gestation (1). This is because conversion of this compound to its very reactive ultimate carcinogenic metabolites must occur in fetal target tissues where the necessary enzymes are present at very low levels (49). Most other nitrosamines are also less active transplacentally than in adults, but there are exceptions. Diethylnitrosamine, di-*n*-butyl-nitrosamine, and nitrosohexamethyleneimine are all transplacental carcinogens for the upper respiratory tract in the Syrian hamster; the last two are more active transplacentally than in adults (5), and diethylnitrosamine is slightly more carcinogenic transplacentally (58).

As with the direct-acting carcinogens, comparable exposure of different species to metabolism-dependent agents leads to different kinds of tumors in different target organs. When diethylnitrosamine is given to pregnant mice, tumors in the offspring are predominantly seen in the lung (17,55). In fact, tumors of the lung (Fig. 5) and liver parenchyma (Fig. 6) are the most commonly found neoplasms in the offspring of mice transplacentally exposed to most of the known transplacental carcinogens and are a common index of carcinogenicity in adults of this species (110). There are limits, however, to the generalization that similar types of tumors are induced in rodents by both direct and transplacental exposures. In the hamster, for example, although diethylnitrosamine affects the upper respiratory tract (not the lung) both prenatally and in adults, higher homologs with different organ specificities in adult hamsters do not affect the same organ systems in both fetus and adult. The 2-oxo and 2-hydroxy derivatives of di-*n*-propylnitrosamine, for example, affect the pancreas (along with the liver and other organs) in adult hamsters; pancreatic tumors are not seen in transplacentally treated offspring (4). Similarly, di-*n*-butylnitrosamine and its 4-hydroxy derivative are urinary bladder carcinogens in the adult rat but do not affect that organ when they are given transplacentally (4,5).

A wider range of tumor types and target organs is seen in offspring of rodents exposed to certain compounds with relatively stable proximate and ultimate carcinogenic metabolites. Rats that receive 7,12-dimethylbenz[*a*]anthracene transplacentally develop tumors in the nervous system, kidney, and blood vessels (60,-70,77), a wider range of organs than is affected by the direct-acting carcinogens. It is possible that this is caused in part by the transfer of ultimate carcinogenic metabolites of maternal origin to the fetus.

Whatever tumors are seen in the offspring of animals given carcinogens during pregnancy probably represent only a fraction of the potential tumor cells generated by such treatment. Skin tumors in mice transplacentally exposed to carcinogens can be demonstrated only when noncarcinogenic promoting agents are applied to the skin during postnatal life (11,28,29), and it is likely that latent tumor cells in other organs could also be revealed by similar treatment.

## Diethylstilbestrol

The synthetic, nonsteroid estrogen diethylstilbestrol (DES) was given to pregnant women to prevent miscarriage during the 1940s and 1950s. This prenatal exposure has since been associated with the development of vaginal adenosis and clear-cell adenocarcinoma of the vagina and cervix in female children of women given DES and related estrogens during pregnancy. The adenosis is a minor developmental anomaly that is very common in DES-exposed children; it is apparently not a precancerous lesion. Clear-cell adenocarcinoma of the lower female reproductive tract is a relatively rare disease, a fact that facilitated recognition of its relation to DES. It has been seen associated with a maternal history of DES treatment in children as young as 7 and in young women as old as 28 (34). At this time, DES remains the only agent known to have acted as a transplacental carcinogen in humans.

Experimentally, the transplacental effects of DES have been studied in the mouse (51,56), the Syrian hamster (80), and the Rhesus monkey (33). In none of these species has it produced both the carcinogenic and teratogenic effects characteristic of prenatal DES exposure in humans. In the monkey, transplacental DES exposure results in vaginal adenosis in female offspring, but, as yet, no adenocarcinomas have been observed (33). In the neonatal mouse, both DES and a wide variety of steroid hormones, including estrogens and nonestrogenic steroids, have been shown to induce a permanently altered state of differentiation in the squamous epithelium of the vagina (96). Squamous-cell carcinomas, very different from the human clear-cell carcinomas, can develop from this permanently altered epithelium. The endocrine effects of DES in relation to perinatal carcinogenesis have been extensively reviewed (76).

A major question still to be resolved concerns the mechanism of the carcinogenic effects of DES and whether this substance is metabolized to chemically reactive intermediates, which might classify it as a metabolism-dependent carcinogen. The primary effects of DES both in humans and experimental animals are on estrogen-responsive tissues, and it appears firmly established that the estrogenic activity of DES is at least partly responsible for its carcinogenic activity. Diethylstilbestrol given transplacentally to mice has been reported to increase slightly the incidence of lung tumors in offspring (66). This finding, if confirmed, would indicate that DES is also a metabolism-dependent chemical carcinogen. Much work is in progress on possible mutagenic and carcinogenic metabolites of DES (76).

## TRANSPLACENTAL EXPOSURE DURING BIOASSAYS FOR CARCINOGENICITY

Transplacental exposure is not routinely incorporated into bioassays of suspected carcinogens as conducted by the United States Government. Several agents, including DDT (105) and saccharin (9), have been tested for carcinogenicity by other organizations using test protocols that spanned two or more generations. In at least one case, animals were only marginally susceptible to carcinogenicity in conventional lifetime feeding studies, but they were clearly more susceptible when exposure was begun before conception and then continued throughout pre- and postnatal life (9).

A general approach to incorporation of prenatal exposure into conventional bioassays has been outlined (93). The rationale acknowledges greater technical problems associated with this approach to testing. However, these problems are outweighed by the possibility of significantly increasing the sensitivity of conventional bioassays by extending the period of exposure to the perinatal period. This proposal does not include procedures to identify transplacentally active carcinogens specifically. Such an extended approach may become more frequently adopted if regulatory agencies begin to require it in the course of safety assessment of new chemicals.

An alternative approach to screening new substances involves a combination of *in vivo/in vitro* techniques. Gravid test animals are exposed to suspected carcinogens. Then cultures are prepared from fetal tissues removed from these animals, and the cultures are evaluated for the appearance of potentially neoplastic cells (15,71). Such *in vivo/in vitro* approaches are presently undergoing development.

## REFERENCES

1. Alexandrov, V. A. (1968): Blastomogenic effect of dimethylnitrosamine on pregnant rats and their offspring. *Nature*, 218:280–281.
2. Alexandrov, V. A., and Napalkov, N. P. (1976): Experimental study of relationship between teratogenesis and carcinogenesis in the brain of the rat. *Cancer Lett.*, 1:345–350.
3. Althoff, J., Grandjean, C., Marsh, S., Pour, P., and Takahashi, M. (1977): Transplacental effects of nitrosamines in Syrian hamsters. II. Nitrosopiperidine. *Z. Krebsforsch.*, 90:71–77.

4. Althoff, J., Grandjean, C., and Pour, P. (1977): Transplacental effect of nitrosamines in Syrian hamsters. IV. Metabolites of dipropyl and dibutylnitrosamine. Z. Krebsforsch., 90:119–126.
5. Althoff, J., Pour, P., Grandjean, C., and Eagen, M. (1976): Transplacental effects of nitrosamine in Syrian hamsters. I. Dibutylnitrosamine and nitrosohexamethyleneimine. Z. Krebsforsch., 86:69–75.
6. Althoff, J., Pour, P., Grandjean, G. and Marsh, S. (1977): Transplacental effects of nitrosamines in Syrian hamsters. III. Dimethyl and dipropylnitrosamine. Z. Krebsforsch., 90:79–86.
7. Anderson, L. M., McDonald, J. M., Budinger, J. J., Mountain, I. M., and Brown, G. B. (1978): 3-Hydroxyxanthine: Transplacental effects and ontogeny of related sulfate metabolism in rats and mice. J. Natl. Cancer Inst., 61:1405–1410.
8. Anderson, L. M., Teller, M. N., Budinger, J. M., and Brown, G. B. (1978): Increased incidence of mammary tumors in rats after direct or transplacental exposure to 3-hydroxyxanthine. J. Natl. Cancer Inst., 61:1411–1414.
9. Arnold, D. L., Moodie, C. A., Grice, H. C., Charbonneau, S. M., Stavric, B., Collins, B. T., McGuire, P. F., Zawidzka, Z. Z., and Munro, I. C. (1980): Long-term toxicity of ortho-toluene sulfonamide and sodium saccharin in the rat. Toxicol. Appl. Pharmacol., 52:113–152.
10. Bulay, O. M., and Wattenberg, L. W. (1970): Carcinogenic effects of subcutaneous administration of benzo[a]pyrene during pregnancy on the progeny. Proc. Soc. Exp. Biol. Med., 135:84–86.
11. Bulay, O. M., and Wattenberg, L. W. (1971): Carcinogenic effects of polycyclic hydrocarbon carcinogen administration to mice during pregnancy on the progeny. J. Natl. Cancer Inst., 46:397–402.
12. Cayama, E., Tsuda, H., Sarma, D. S. R., and Farber, E. (1978): Initiation of chemical carcinogenesis requires cell proliferation. Nature, 275:60–62.
13. Cook, J. W., Hewett, C. L., and Hieger, I. (1933): The isolation of a cancer-producing hydrocarbon from coal tar. Parts I, II, and III. J. Chem. Soc., 395–405.
14. Denlinger, R. H., Koestner, A., and Wechsler, W. (1974): Induction of neurogenic tumors in C3HeB/FeJ mice by nitrosourea derivatives: Observations by light microscopy, tissue culture, and electron microscopy. Int. J. Cancer, 13:559–571.
15. DiPaolo, J. A., Nelson, R. L., Donovan, P. J., and Evans, C. H. (1973): Host mediated in vivo–in vitro assay for chemical carcinogenesis. Arch. Pathol., 95:380–388.
16. Diwan, B. A., and Meier, H. (1974): Strain- and age-dependent transplacental carcinogenesis by 1-ethyl-1-nitrosourea in inbred strains of mice. Cancer Res., 34:764–770.
17. Diwan, B. A., and Meier, H. (1976): Transplacental carcinogenic effects of diethylnitrosamine in mice. Naturwissenschaften, 63:487.
18. Druckrey, H. (1973): Chemical structure and action in transplacental carcinogenesis and teratogenesis. In: Transplacental Carcinogenesis, edited by L. Tomatis and U. Mohr, pp. 45–48. International Agency for Research on Cancer, Lyon.
19. Druckrey, H., Ivankovic, S., and Preussman, R. (1966): Teratogenic and carcinogenic effects in the offspring after single injection of ethylnitrosourea to pregnant rats. Nature, 210:1378–1379.
20. Druckrey, H., Ivankovic, S., Preussmann, R., Landschütz, C., Stekar, J., Brunner, U., and Schagen, B. (1968): Transplacental induction of neurogenic malignomas by 1,2-diethyl-hydrazine, azo- and azoxyethane in rats. Experientia, 24:561–562.
21. Druckrey, H., Kruse, H., Preussmann, R., Ivankovic, S., and Landschütz, C. (1970): Cancerogene alkylierende Substanzen. III. Alkyl-halogenide, -sulfate, -sulfonate, and ringspannte Heterocyclen. Z. Krebsforsch., 74:241–270.
22. Druckrey, H., Kruse, H., Preussmann, R., Ivankovic, S., Landschütz, C., and Gimmy, J. (1970): Cancerogene alkylierende Substanzen. IV. 1,3-Propansulton and 1,4-Butansulton. Z. Krebsforsch., 75:69–84.
23. Druckrey, H., and Landschütz, C. (1971): Transplacentare und neonatale Krebserzeugung durch Äthylnitrosobiuret (ÄNBU) an BD-IX Ratten. Z. Krebsforsch., 76:45–58.
24. Druckrey, H., Landschütz, C., and Ivankovic, S. (1970): Transplacentare Erzeugung maligner Tumoren des Nervensystems. II. Äthylnitrosoharnstoff an 10 genetisch definierten Rattenstämmen. Z. Krebsforsch., 73:371–386.
25. Fox, R. R., Diwan, B. A., and Meier, H. (1975): Transplacental induction of primary renal tumors in rabbits treated with 1-ethyl-1-nitrosourea. J. Natl. Cancer Inst., 54:1439–1448.
26. Fox, R. R., Diwan, B. A., and Meier, H. (1977): Transplacental carcinogenic effects of combined treatment of ethylurea and sodium nitrite in rabbits. J. Natl. Cancer Inst., 59:427–429.

27. Gel'shtein, V. I. (1961): [The incidence of tumors among offspring of mice exposed to orthoaminoazotoluene] (Rus.). *Vopr. Onkol.*, 7(10):58–64.
28. Goerttler, K., and Löhrke, H. (1976): Diaplacental carcinogenesis: Initiation with the carcinogens dimethylbenzanthracene (DMBA) and urethane during fetal life and postnatal promotion with the phorbol ester TPA in a modified 2-stage Berenblum/Mottram experiment. *Virchows Arch.* [*Pathol. Anat.*], 372:29–38.
29. Goerttler, K., and Löhrke, H. (1977): Diaplacental carcinogenesis: Tumor localization and tumor incidence in NMRI mice after diaplacental initiation with DMBA and urethane and postnatal promotion with the phorbol ester TPA in a modified 2-stage Berenblum/Mottram experiment. *Virchows Arch.* [*Pathol. Anat.*], 376:117–132.
30. Golub, N. I., Kolesnichenko, T. S., and Shabad, L. M. (1974): [Blastomogenic action of some nitrogen-containing compounds on the progeny of experimental mice] (Rus.). *Biull. Eksp. Biol. Med.*, 78:62–65.
31. Grice, H. C., Moodie, C. A., and Smith, C. D. (1973): The carcinogenic potential of aflatoxin or its metabolites in rats from dams fed aflatoxin pre- and postpartum. *Cancer Res.*, 33:262–268.
32. Guthert, H., Jackel, E. M., and Warzok, R. (1973): Zur karzinogenen Wirkung von *N*-Äthyl-*N*-nitrosoharnstoff (ÄNH) bei Kaninchen. *Zentralbl. Allg. Pathol.*, 117:461–471.
33. Hendrickx, A., Benirschke, K., Thompson, R. S., Ahern, J. K., Lucas, W. E., and Oi, R. H. (1979): The effects of prenatal diethylstilbestrol (DES) exposure on the genitalia of pubertal *Macaca mulatta*. I. Female offspring. *J. Reprod. Med.*, 22:233–240.
34. Herbst, A. L., Scully, R. E., and Robboy, S. J. (1979): Prenatal diethylstilbestrol exposure and human genital tract abnormalities. In: *Perinatal Carcinogenesis, NCI Monograph 51*, edited by J. M. Rice, pp. 25–34. United States Government Printing Office, Washington.
35. Ivankovic, S. (1972): Erzeugung von Malignomen bei Ratten nach transplacentarer Einwirkung von *N*-Isopropyl-α-2(methyl-hydrazino)-*p*-toluamid · HCl. *Arzneim. Forsch.*, 22:905–907.
36. Ivankovic, S. (1975): Praenatale Carcinogenese. In: *Handbuch der Allgemeinen Pathologie, Vol. 6, Part 7*, edited by H.-W. Altmann, F. Buchner, H. Cottier, E. Grundmann, G. Holle, E. Letterer, W. Masshoff, H. Meesen, F. Roulet, G. Seifert, and G. Siebert, pp. 941–1002. Springer-Verlag, Berlin, Heidelberg.
37. Ivankovic, S., and Druckrey, H. (1968): Transplacentare Erzeugung maligner Tumoren des Nervensystems. I. Äthylnitrosoharnstoff (ÄNH) an BD IX-Ratten. *Z. Krebsforsch.*, 71:320–360.
38. Ivankovic, S., Druckrey, H., and Preussmann, R. (1966): Erzeugung neurogener Tumoren bei den Nachkommen nach einmaliger Injektion von Äthylnitrosoharnstoff an Schwangere Ratten. *Naturwissenschaften*, 53:410–411.
39. Ivankovic, S., and Zeller, W. J. (1972): Transplacental blastomogen action of *n*-propyl-nitrosourea in BD rats. *Arch. Geschwulstforsch.*, 40:99–102.
40. Jänisch, W., Schreiber, D., Warzok, R., and Schneider, J. (1972): Die transplacentare Induktion von Geschwulsten des Nervensystems. Vergleichende Untersuchung der Wirksamheit von Methyl und Äthylnitrosoharnstoff. *Arch. Geschwulstforsch.*, 39:99–106.
41. Kleihues, P., Mende, C., and Reucher, W. (1972): Tumors of the peripheral and central nervous system induced in BD rats by prenatal application of methyl methane sulfonate. *Eur. J. Cancer*, 8:641–645.
42. Klein, M. (1952): The transplacental effect of urethan on lung tumorigenesis in mice. *J. Natl. Cancer Inst.*, 12:1003–1010.
43. Koestner, A., Swenberg, J. A., and Wechsler, W. (1971): Transplacental production with ethyl-nitrosourea of neoplasms of the nervous system in Sprague–Dawley rats. *Am. J. Pathol.*, 63:37–56.
44. Larsen, C. D. (1947): Pulmonary tumor induction by transplacental exposure to urethane. *J. Natl. Cancer Inst.*, 8:63–70.
45. Laqueur, G. L., and Spatz, M. (1978): Transplacental induction of tumours and malformations in rats with cycasin and methylazoxymethanol. In: *Transplacental Carcinogenesis*, edited by L. Tomatis and U. Mohr. pp. 59–64. International Agency for Research on Cancer, Lyon.
46. Lawley, P. D. (1976): Carcinogenesis by alkylating agents. In: *Chemical Carcinogens, ACS Monograph 173*, edited by C. E. Searle, pp. 83–244. American Chemical Society, Washington.
47. Likhachev, A. Y. (1971): [Transplacental blastomogenic action of *N*-nitrosodiethylamine in mice] (Rus.). *Vopr. Onkol.*, 17(1):45–50.
48. Lu, A. Y. H., and Levin, W. (1974): The resolution of the liver microsomal hydroxylation system. *Biochim. Biophys. Acta*, 344:205–240.

49. Lucier, G. W., Lui, E. M. K., and Lamartiniere, C. A. (1979): Metabolic activation/deactivation reactions during prenatal development. *Environ. Health Perspect.*, 29:7–16.
50. Maltoni, C. (1976): Predictive value of carcinogenesis bioassays. *Ann. N.Y. Acad. Sci.*, 271:431–443.
51. McLachlan, J. A. (1979): Transplacental effects of diethylstilbestrol in mice. In: *Perinatal Carcinogenesis, NCI Monograph 51*, edited by J. M. Rice, pp. 67–72. United States Government Printing Office, Washington.
52. Miller, E. C., and Miller, J. A. (1976): The metabolism of chemical carcinogens to reactive electrophiles and their possible mechanisms of action in carcinogenesis. In: *Chemical Carcinogens, ACS Monograph 173*, edited by C. E. Searle, pp. 737–762. American Chemical Society, Washington.
53. Miner, N. A., Koehler, J. and Greenaway, L. (1969): Intraperitoneal injection of mice. *Appl. Microbiol.*, 17:250–251.
54. Mohr, U., and Althoff, J. (1964): Mögliche diaplazentar carcinogene Wirkung von Diäthylnitrosamin beim Goldhamster. *Naturwissenchaften*, 51:515.
55. Mohr, U., and Althoff, J. (1965): Die diaplacentare Wirkung des Cancerogens Diäthylnitrosamin bei der Maus. *Z. Krebsforsch.*, 67:152–155.
56. Mohr, U., Althoff, J., and Authaler, A. (1966): Diaplacental effect of the carcinogen diethylnitrosamine in the golden hamster. *Cancer Res.*, 26:2349–2352.
57. Mohr, U., Althoff, J., Wrba, H. (1965): Diaplazentare Wirkung des Carcinogens Diäthylnitrosamin beim Goldhamster. *Z. Krebsforsch.*, 66:536–540.
58. Mohr, U., Reznik-Schuller, H., Reznik, G., and Hilfrich, J. (1975): Transplacental effects of diethylnitrosamine in Syrian hamsters as related to different days of administration during pregnancy. *J. Natl. Cancer Inst.*, 55:681–683.
59. Napalkov, N. P. (1971): [Experiments with transplacental carcinogenesis as a method of investigating the etiopathogenesis of tumors in children] (Rus.). *Vopr. Onkol.*, 17(8):3–15.
60. Napalkov, N. P., and Alexandrov, V. A. (1974): Neurotropic effects of 7,12-dimethylbenz[a]anthracene in transplacental carcinogenesis. *J. Natl. Cancer Inst.*, 52:1365–1366.
61. National Cancer Institute (1979): *Everything Doesn't Cause Cancer. NIH Publication No. 79-2039*. United States Government Printing Office, Washington.
62. Nomura, T. (1973): Carcinogenesis by urethan via mother's milk and its enhancement of transplacental carcinogenesis in mice. *Cancer Res.*, 33:1677–1683.
63. Nomura, T. (1974): Tumor induction in the progeny of mice receiving 4-nitroquinoline-1-oxide and *N*-methyl-*N*-nitrosourethan during pregnancy or lactation. *Cancer Res.*, 34:3373–3378.
64. Nomura, T. (1975): Carcinogenicity of the food additive furylfuramide in foetal and young mice. *Nature*, 258:610–611.
65. Nomura, T. (1975): Transmission of tumors and malformations to the next generation of mice subsequent to urethan treatment. *Cancer Res.*, 35:264–266.
66. Nomura, T., and Kanzaki, T. (1977): Induction of urogenital anomalies and some tumors in the progeny of mice receiving diethylstilbestrol during pregnancy. *Cancer Res.*, 37:1099–1104.
67. Osske, G., Warzok, R., and Schneider, J. (1972): Diaplazentare Tumorinduktion durch endogen gebildeten *N*-Äthyl-*N*-nitrosoharnstoff bei Ratten. *Arch. Geschwulstforsch.*, 40:244–247.
68. Pfaffenroth, M. J., and Das, G. D. (1979): *N*-Ethyl-*N*-nitrosourea-induced spinal tumors in an inbred strain of W albino rats. *J. Natl. Cancer Inst.*, 63:647–650.
69. Pielsticker, K., Wieser, O., Mohr, U., and Wrba, H. (1969): Diaplazentar induzierte Nierentumoren bei der Ratte. *Z. Krebsforsch.*, 69:345–350.
70. P'rvanova, L. G. (1978): [Carcinogenesis after two administrations of DMBA to rats in different life periods] (Rus.). *Vopr. Onkol.*, 24(11):96–99.
71. Quarles, J. M., Sega, M., Schenley, C. K., and Lijinsky, W. (1979): Transformation of hamster fetal cells by nitrosated pesticides in a transplacental assay. *Cancer Res.*, 39:4525–4533.
72. Rice, J. M. (1969): Transplacental carcinogenesis in mice by 1-ethyl-1-nitrosourea. *Ann. N.Y. Acad. Sci.*, 163:813–827.
73. Rice, J. M. (1973): An overview of transplacental chemical carcinogenesis. *Teratology*, 8:113–126.
74. Rice, J. M. (1976): Carcinogenesis: A late effect of irreversible toxic damage during development. *Environ. Health Perspect.*, 18:133–139.
75. Rice, J. M. (1979): Perinatal period and pregnancy: Intervals of high risk for chemical carcinogens. *Environ. Health Perspect.*, 29:23–27.

76. Rice, J. M. (1979): *Perinatal Carcinogenesis, NCI Monograph 51*. United States Government Printing Office, Washington.

77. Rice, J. M., Joshi, S. R., Shenefelt, R. E., and Wenk, M. (1978): Transplacental carcinogenic activity of 7,12-dimethylbenz[a]anthracene. In: *Carcinogenesis, Vol. 3, Polynuclear Aromatic Hydrocarbons*, edited by P. W. Jones and R. I. Freudenthal, pp. 413–422. Raven Press, New York.

78. Rice, J. M., Palmer, A. E., London, W. T., Sly, D. L., and Williams, G. M. (1978): Transplacental effects of ethylnitrosourea in the patas monkey. In: *Tumors of Early Life in Man and Animals*, edited by L. Severi, pp. 893–906. Perugia Quadrennial International Conferences on Cancer, Perugia.

79. Russell, W. L., Kelley, E. M., Hunsicker, P. R., Bangham, J. W., Maddux, S. C., and Phipps, E. L. (1979): Specific locus test shows ethylnitrosourea to be the most potent mutagen in the mouse. *Proc. Natl. Acad. Sci. U.S.A.*, 76:5818–5819.

80. Rustia, M. (1979): Role of hormone imbalance in transplacental carcinogenesis induced in Syrian golden hamsters by sex hormones. In: *Perinatal Carcinogenesis, NCI Monograph 51*, edited by J. M. Rice, pp. 77–87. United States Government Printing Office, Washington.

81. Rustia, M., and Shubik, P. (1974): Prenatal induction of neurogenic tumors in hamsters by precursors of ethylurea and sodium nitrite. *J. Natl. Cancer Inst.*, 52:605–608.

82. Severi, L. (1978): *Tumors of Early Life in Man and Animals*. Perugia Quadrennial International Conferences on Cancer, Perugia.

83. Sims, P., Grover, P. L., Swaisland, A., Pal, K., and Hewer, A. (1974): Metabolic activation of benzo[a]pyrene proceeds by a diol-epoxide. *Nature*, 252:326–328.

84. Singer, B. (1977): Sites in nucleic acids reacting with alkylating agents of differing carcinogenicity or mutagenicity. *J. Toxicol. Environ. Health*, 2:1279–1295.

85. Smith, W. E., and Rous, P. (1948): The neoplastic potentialities of mouse embryo tissues. IV. Lung adenomas in baby mice as a result of prenatal exposure to urethane. *J. Exp. Med.*, 88:529–554.

86. Sontag, J. M., Page, N. P., and Saffiotti, U. (1976): *Guidelines for Carcinogen Bioassay in Small Rodents, D.H.E.W. Publication No. (NIH) 76-801*. United States Government Printing Office, Washington.

87. Spatz, M. (1968): Hydrolysis of cycasin by β-glucosidase in skin of newborn rats. *Proc. Soc. Exp. Biol. Med.*, 128:1005–1008.

88. Spatz, M., and Laqueur, G. L. (1967): Transplacental induction of tumors in Sprague–Dawley rats with crude cycad material. *J. Natl. Cancer Inst.*, 38:233–245.

89. Stavrou, D., Dahme, E., and Schroder, B. (1977): Transplacentare neuroonkogene Wirkung von Äthylnitrosoharnstoff beim Kaninchen während der fruhen Graviditätsphase. *Z. Krebsforsch.*, 89:331–339.

90. Stavrou, D., Dahme, E., and Schroder, B. (1978): On the question of transplacental induction of neurogenic tumors in rabbits. In: *Tumors of Early Life in Man and Animals*, edited by L. Severi, pp. 445–452. Perugia Quadrennial International Conferences on Cancer, Perugia.

91. Stavrou, D., and Hanichen, T. (1975): Oncogene Wirkung von Äthylnitrosoharnstoff beim Kaninchen während der pranatalen Periode. *Z. Krebsforsch.*, 84:207–215.

92. Steward, J. P., Ornellas, E. P., Beernink, K. D., and Northway, W. H. (1968): Errors in the technique of intraperitoneal injection of mice. *Appl. Microbiol.*, 16:1418–1419.

93. Swenberg, J. A. (1979): Incorporation of transplacental exposure into routine carcinogenicity bioassays. In: *Perinatal Carcinogenesis, NCI Monograph 51*, edited by J. M. Rice, pp. 265–268, United States Government Printing Office, Washington.

94. Swenberg, J. A., Koestner, A., Wechsler, W., and Denlinger, R. H. (1972): Quantitative aspects of transplacental tumor induction with ethylnitrosourea in rats. *Cancer Res.*, 32:2656–2660.

95. Takahashi, G., and Yasuhira, K. (1973): Microautoradiographic and radiometric studies on the distribution of 3-methylcholanthrene in mice and their fetuses. *Cancer Res.*, 33:23–28.

96. Takasugi, N. (1979): Development of permanently proliferated and cornified vaginal epithelium in mice treated neonatally with steroid hormones and the implication in tumorigenesis. In: *Perinatal Carcinogenesis, NCI Monograph 51*, edited by J. M. Rice, pp. 57–66. United States Government Printing Office, Washington.

97. Tanaka, T. (1973): Transplacental induction of tumours and malformations in rats treated with some chemical carcinogens. In: *Transplacental Carcinogenesis*, edited by L. Tomatis and U. Mohr, pp. 100–111. International Agency for Research on Cancer, Lyon, France.

98. Tomatis, L. (1965): Increased incidence of tumors in $F_1$ and $F_2$ generations from pregnant mice injected with a polycyclic hydrocarbon. *Proc. Soc. Exp. Biol. Med.*, 119:743–747.
99. Tomatis, L., and Goodall, C. M. (1969): The occurrence of tumors in $F_1$, $F_2$, and $F_3$ descendants of pregnant mice injected with 7,12-dimethylbenz[*a*]anthracene. *Int. J. Cancer*, 4:219–225.
100. Tomatis, L., Hilfrich, J., and Turusov, V. (1975): The occurrence of tumours in $F_1$, $F_2$, and $F_3$ descendants of BD rats exposed to *N*-nitrosomethylurea during pregnancy. *Int. J. Cancer*, 15:385–390.
101. Tomatis, L., and Mohr, U. (1973): *Transplacental Carcinogenesis.* International Agency for Research on Cancer, Lyon, France.
102. Tomatis, L., Ponomarkov, U., and Turusov, U. (1977): Effects of ethylnitrosourea administration during pregnancy on three subsequent generations of BD VI rats. *Int. J. Cancer*, 19:240–248.
103. Tomatis, L., Turusov, V., and Guibbert, D. (1972): Prenatal exposure to chemical carcinogens. In: *Topics in Chemical Carcinogenesis*, edited by W. Nakahara, S. Takayama, T. Sugimura, and S. Odashima, pp. 445–459. University of Tokyo Press, Tokyo.
104. Tomatis, L., Turusov, V., Guibbert, D., Duperray, B., Malaveille, C., and Pacheco, H. (1971): Transplacental carcinogenic effect of 3-methylcholanthrene in mice and its quantitation in fetal tissues. *J. Natl. Cancer Inst.*, 47:645–651.
105. Turusov, V. S., Day, N. E., Tomatis, L., Gati, E., and Charles, R. T. (1973): Tumors in CF-1 mice exposed for six consecutive generations to DDT. *J. Natl. Cancer Inst.*, 51:983–997.
106. United States Public Health Service (1951,1957,1969, and succeeding volumes): *Survey of Compounds Which Have Been Tested for Carcinogenic Activity, USPHS Publication 149.* United States Government Printing Office, Washington.
107. Vesselinovitch, S. D., Koka, M., Rao, K. V. N., Mihailovich, N., and Rice, J. M. (1977): Prenatal carcinogenesis by ethylnitrosourea in mice. *Cancer Res.*, 37:1822–1828.
108. Vesselinovitch, S. D., Mihailovich, N., and Pietra, G. (1967): The prenatal exposure of mice to urethan and the consequent development of tumors in various tissues. *Cancer Res.*, 27:2333–2337.
109. Vesselinovitch, S. D., Rao, K. V. N., and Mihailovich, N. (1979): Transplacental and lactational carcinogenesis by safrole. *Cancer Res.*, 39:4378–4380.
110. Weisburger, J. H. (1976): Bioassays and tests for chemical carcinogens. In: *Chemical Carcinogens, ACS Monograph 173*, edited by C. E. Searle, pp. 1–23, American Chemical Society, Washington.
111. Wogan, G. N. (1966): Chemical nature and biological effects of the aflatoxins. *Bacteriol. Rev.*, 30:460–470.
112. Wrba, H., Pielsticker, K., and Mohr, U. (1967): Die diaplazentarcarcinogene Wirkung von Diäthylnitrosamin bei Ratten. *Naturwissenschaften*, 54:47.

*Developmental Toxicology*, edited by
C. A. Kimmel and J. Buelke-Sam. Raven Press,
New York © 1981.

# Transplacental Toxicology: Prenatal Factors Influencing Postnatal Fertility

J. A. McLachlan, R. R. Newbold, K. S. Korach, J. C. Lamb IV, and Y. Suzuki

*Transplacental Toxicology Group, Laboratory of Reproductive and Developmental Toxicology, National Institute of Environmental Health Sciences, Research Triangle Park, North Carolina 27709*

In recent years there has been a growing concern about the exposure of pregnant women to drugs or chemicals and the subsequent overt effects on their offspring. Transplacental toxicology includes defects (morphological, biochemical, or behavioral) induced at any stage of gestation and detected or expressed later in life. Thus, functional abnormalities of the immune system, neurological defects, or appearance of tumors that are noticed in adult life may be linked to exposure to toxic agents in the prenatal period. Certain developing organ systems may be at particular risk for these long-term consequences or latent expression of toxic effects induced during the prenatal period.

For example, the development of the genital tract and subsequent attainment of fertility is a process that is susceptible to disruption by environmental agents. In most eutherian mammals, including mice and humans, the female fetus is extremely vulnerable to germ cell toxicants, since the development of the oocyte occurs prenatally with no new germ cells formed after birth (9,132). Therefore, any change induced in the fetal oocyte by chemicals during the prenatal period may result in a decreased reproductive capacity of the offspring that will not be evident until much later in the animal's life when sexual maturity is reached. Reduced fertility in the offspring may be the most obvious consequence of prenatal exposure to toxic environmental chemicals. It could also include the possibility of long-term genetic damage to the developing germ cell and/or transplacental carcinogenic changes in fetal organs. A dramatic and well-known example of long-term transplacental toxicological effects is that of diethylstilbestrol (DES). Exposure to this compound during human pregnancies has been associated with a low incidence of vaginal

---

Dr. Lamb's present address is National Toxicology Program, Research Triangle Park, North Carolina 27709.
Dr. Suzuki's present address is Asia University, Tokyo 180, Japan.

clear-cell adenocarcinoma in the female offspring (53). More recently, compromised reproductive capacity in both male (47) and female (7,52,108,115) offspring has been suggested.

To help understand the role of *in utero* environmental influences on the establishment of normal reproductive function, this chapter will discuss some prenatal factors that affect subsequent postnatal fertility. Development of the central nervous system (CNS), the hypothalamic–pituitary–gonadal axis, and the liver, or other target organ metabolic patterns will be considered, as well as development of the germ cell and genital tract. Emphasis will be given to studies in experimental animals in the hope that toxicologic and biologic principles pertinent to all species may be established.

Figure 1 summarizes the important events in the attainment of sexual maturity and some of the consequences of alterations in this complex process. The mature reproductive tract is susceptible to chemical insults that can decrease fertility in either a temporary or permanent manner. These should be considered for comparison to effects induced by chemicals during development. The gonads, reproductive tract, and neuroendocrine system are all vulnerable to chemical toxicity by different

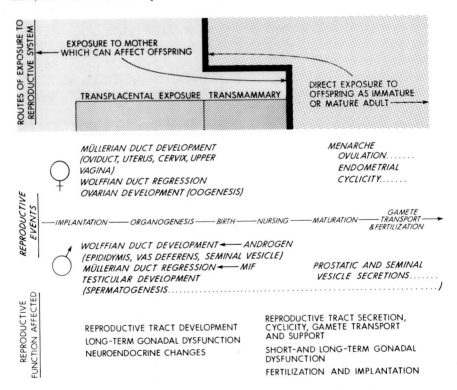

**FIG. 1.** Sensitive factors for the induction of reproductive toxicity.

mechanisms. Differences in susceptibility between males and females can also be described in their respective reproductive organ systems. The ability to predict chemical toxicity in mature animals also may be confounded by the presence of cyclic changes that can alter either the response of the target organ or, as in the case of spermatogenic maturation, the response of the specific cells in a certain stage of development or growth. Initially, testing for normal fertility after chemical exposures can best be verified by the outcome of mating. A more complete understanding of fertility can be gained only after criteria are met that insure that the studies test for all possible effects. This would include, for example, the verification that the germ cell line has not been decreased or otherwise compromised. Therefore, in the male, the complete sperm cycle must be evaluated to ensure that no specific stage of sperm development has been disrupted. Normal ovulation and oviductal transport, fertilization, and blastocyst implantation are all important endpoints in evaluating female fertility.

Altered reproductive function not associated with acute chemical exposures still leaves the possibility of prior exposures, since early chemical insults can, of course, induce either genetic or ontogenic anomalies that may only be expressed in later life. Sexual maturation, as it relates to toxicity, should not only be considered to include the neonatal to pubertal periods, but also the prenatal development of the reproductive system. Human reproductive tract development begins in the first trimester of pregnancy. During this period, the male and female components of the developing genital tract are expressed, and the reproductive tract attains features characteristic of the genotype. However, since both male (Wolffian) and female (Müllerian) reproductive duct systems are present in all embryonic mammals, the developing reproductive tract possesses a unique susceptibility to chemical insults during the time preceding the regression of one or the other of the duct systems. Furthermore, the sexual differentiation of an asexual gonad during this period of development may also be susceptible to chemical insult. The inhibition of ovarian germ cell mitosis by a chemical may lead to irreversible sterility or decreased fertility in the female, since as indicated, the total complement of oogonia is present at birth. Spermatogonia, in contrast to oogonia, are capable of mitotic divisions after birth and will increase in number at puberty. However, in the male, inhibition or delay of testicular descent of one or both testes can lead to sterility or decreased fertility.

Considering the developmental changes associated with reproductive tract organogenesis, it is apparent that embryonic chemical exposure is a special toxicological problem. The once popular misconception that the placenta is a universal shield against all exogenous chemical insults must be discarded to consider the toxic potential of chemicals as they relate to pregnant women and to the reproductive development of their offspring. Since the developing reproductive system exposed to chemicals *in utero* presents complex problems, we will discuss, first, impaired fertility after postnatal exposure to chemicals; this may provide insights into chemical or drug effects before birth.

## REPRODUCTIVE ALTERATIONS ASSOCIATED WITH
## CHEMICAL EXPOSURES

### Postnatal Exposure

Problems with reproduction can result from a variety of different mechanisms. One obviously would be an effect of a chemical on the differentiated reproductive tract itself. Another involves an indirect action on reproduction by interaction with other extragonadal tissues such as the pituitary, hypothalamus, or brain. Normally, neuroendocrine target organs function to synthesize and secrete trophic hormones and related releasing factors (107). In addition, these organs are the response sites of feedback inhibition (79). The exact mechanisms by which chemicals can alter neuroendocrine function are not clearly understood.

From the compounds listed in Table 1, there are two possible neuroendocrine effects that may result in impaired reproduction. The first effect is produced by examples in the general class of "tranquilizer" type compounds, including reserpine, chlorpromazine, and perphenazine. Reserpine has been reported to block ovulation in rats (22). This effect is presumably caused by the compound's action on endogenous catecholamines which, secondarily, influences the ability of the sympathetic nervous system to stimulate gonadotropin release (22,23). Chlorpromazine and perphenazine, both phenothiazine derivatives, have a pronounced effect on the hypothalamus (56). Their reported inhibition of ovulation involves a complete hypothalamic suppression (103) which would bring about a decrease in gonadotropin levels by suppressing gonadotropin-releasing factor synthesis and/or release.

The second possible way in which chemicals might alter reproduction does not involve CNS depression but involves, rather, a more direct action of a chemical at neuroendocrine centers. In one case, the chemicals seem to possess intrinsic gonadal steroid hormonal activity; in the other, they do not possess steroid hormone-like activity. The role of steroid hormones in the development of normal sexual behavior has been well established (48).

Pesticides, for example, chlordecone (Kepone®) and $o,p'$-DDT, are foreign compounds that possess significant estrogenic activity (91) (Table 1). The induction of persistent vaginal estrus (PVE) in rats (48) has been taken as an indication of the effect of chlordecone on gonadotropin secretion (43). Further studies will be required to determine if the effects of pesticides on gonadotropins are actually a result of the steroid-like activity of the compounds. In one report, neonatal administration of $o,p'$-DDT was shown to partially block the increase in serum levels of luteinizing hormone (LH) that follows ovariectomy (45). Thus, alteration in the hypothalamic–ovarian axis may play a role in anovulation observed in these rats.

Other organochlorine pesticides (e.g., dieldrin, aldrin, and mirex) have been reported to alter reproduction, but these compounds failed to demonstrate any estrogenic activity in rats exposed neonatally (43). Dieldrin (10) and aldrin (25) have been reported to have significant effects on reproduction. The dieldrin study

TABLE 1. *Some compounds reported to alter fertility after postnatal exposure*

| Compound | Alteration in | Sex | Species |
|---|---|---|---|
| **Herbicides** | | | |
| Diquat | Spermatogenesis (98) | Male | Mouse |
| Paraquat | Spermatogenesis (98) | Male | Mouse |
| Polychlorinated biphenyls (PCB) | Neuroendocrine function (42) | Female | Rat |
| Polychlorinated biphenyls (PCB) | Reproductive capacity (57,93) | Female | Rat, mouse |
| Polychlorinated biphenyls (PCB) | Reproductive tract (106) | Male | Mouse |
| Yalane | Spermatogenesis (123) | Male | Rat |
| **Fungicides** | | | |
| Maneb | Spermatogenesis and reproductive tract (95,113) | Male | Rat |
| Cineb | Spermatogenesis and reproductive tract (95,113) | Male | Rat |
| Captan | Spermatogenesis and reproductive tract (19,20) | Male | Mouse |
| **Pesticides** | | | |
| Mirex | Neuroendocrine function (41,43) | Female | Rat |
| Aldrin | Reproductive capacity (25) | Male | Dog |
| Aldrin | Neuroendocrine (43) | Female | Rat |
| DDT | Reproductive capacity (25) | Male | Dog |
| DDT | Endocrine and reproductive organs (94) | Male | Mouse |
| DDT | Neurological system (44,45) | Female | Rat |
| DDT | Reproductive organs (44,51) | Female | Rat |
| Chlordecone (Kepone®) | Neurological system (16,43) | Female | Rat |
| Chlordecone (Kepone®) | Reproductive tract function (35,84) | Female | Rat |
| Chlordane | Reproductive tract (128) | Female | Mouse |
| Chlordane | Reproductive tract (70) | Male | Rat |
| Dichlorvos (DDVP) | Spermatogenesis (61) | Male | Rat |
| Carbaryl | Neuroendocrine (113,114) | Both | Rat |
| Methyl parathione + DDT | Spermatogenesis (30) | Male | Rat |
| Lindane | Spermatogenesis (29) | Male | Rat |
| Polychloropinene | Testes, reproductive tract (80) | Male | Mouse, rat |
| Dieldrin | Neuroendocrine (43) | Female | Rat |
| Dieldrin | Neurological (25) | Male | Dog |
| 1,2-Dibromo-3-chloropropane (DBCP) | Testes (81) | Male | Human |
| Ethylene dibromide | Gonads (2) | Male | Bull |

*(contd.)*

TABLE 1. *(Continued)*

| Compound | Alteration in | Sex | Species |
|---|---|---|---|
| Metals, organometals, and other inorganic elements | | | |
| Mercury (Hg) | Gonads (67) | Male | Mouse, rat |
| Methylmercury | Testes (34,105) | Male | Mouse, rat |
| | Reproductive capacity (60) | Male | Rat |
| Lead (Pb) | Reproductive capacity (54) | Both | Rat |
| | Testes and reproductive tract (36) | Male | Rat |
| Selenium (Se) | Ovary (33) | Female | Pig |
| Cadmium (Cd) | Testes, reproductive tract (26,31) | Male | Rat |
| Aluminum | Testes (59) | Male | Rat |
| Boron | Gonad (68,126) | Male | Rat |
| Food additives, components, or contaminants | | | |
| Metanil yellow | Testes (117) | Male | Rat |
| Dimethylnitrosamine | Reproductive tract (3) | Both | Mouse, rat |
| Monosodium glutamate | Reproductive organs (64) | Both | Hamster |
| Experimental and therapeutic drugs | | | |
| Quinacrine-HCl | Reproductive tract (18,58) | Female | Rat |
| Chlorambucil | Testes (49) | Male | Human |
| Caffeine | Testes (40) | Male | Rat |
| Triethylenemelamine (TEM) | Testes (20) | Male | Mouse |
| Cyclophosphamide | Testes (13,37) | Male | Human, rat |
| Sodium nitrite | Reproductive tract (3) | Female | Mouse |
| Imipramine-HCl | Reproductive tract (3) | Female | Mouse |
| Halothane | Reproductive tract (130) | Female | Mouse |
| Nitrous oxide | Testes (62) | Male | Rat |
| Theobromine | Testes (40) | Male | Rat |
| Idenopyridine | Testes (55) | Male | Dog |
| 5-Bromodeoxyuridine | Testes (6) | Male | Rat |
| Busulfan | Testes (1) | Male | Rat |
| Epinephrine | Suppressed ovulation (23) | Female | Rabbit |
| Norepinephrine | Suppressed ovulation (23) | Female | Rabbit |
| Amphetamine | Suppressed ovulation (23) | Female | Rabbit |
| Serotonin | Suppressed ovulation (23) | Female | Rabbit |
| BCNU | Reproductive capacity (120) | Male | Rat, rabbit |
| Phenacetin | Testes (14) | Male | Rat |
| Reserpine | Ovulation blocked (22,103) | Female | Mouse, rat |
| Chlorpromazine | Ovulation blocked (103) | Female | Mouse |
| Perphenazine | Ovulation blocked (103) | Female | Mouse |
| Promazine | Ovulation blocked (103) | Female | Mouse |
| Other chemicals | | | |
| Ethanol | Testes, reproductive tract (122) | Male | Rat |

*(contd.)*

TABLE 1. *(Continued)*

| Compound | Alteration in | Sex | Species |
|---|---|---|---|
| Δ⁹-Tetrahydrocannabinol | Reproductive tract (11) | Female | Rat |
| Tris(2,3-dibrompropyl) phosphate | Testes (96) | Male | Rabbit |
| Diethyl adipate | Testes (116) | Male | Mouse |
| Dibutylphthalate (DBP) | Testes (17) | Male | Rat |
| Ethylene oxide cyclic tetramer | Testes (69) | Male | Rat |
| Dimethylbenzanthracene (DMBA) | Testes (1) | Male | Rat |
| Hexachlorophene | Reproductive capacity (46) | Male | Rat |

[a]This list is not comprehensive but is representative of compounds that have been categorized by use.

(10) involved the treatment of male rats with low levels of the compound. The resulting serum LH levels were found to be appreciably decreased as a result of the treatment. Beagle dogs were used in the aldrin study (25). Mating, birth rate, and mammary development were significantly decreased. Mirex was suggested by Fuller and Draper (41) to block induced ovulation by decreasing LH release. The mechanism by which these types of compounds decrease reproductive function and exert an effect on gonadotropin secretion awaits further experimentation, since it appears these compounds may be affecting neuroendocrine target organs directly (e.g., pituitary/hypothalamus) and not peripheral endocrine organs (e.g., uterus).

Chlordane, like DDT and dieldrin, is a central nervous system stimulant. It also has been reported to induce hepatic metabolism of testosterone after treatment of adult rats (127). This apparently results in lack of androgen-induced growth in the seminal vesicle (70). There are few other reports of chlordane exposure to the male reproductive tract.

Another compound that has been studied, although there are only a few reports, is benzene hexachloride. Lindane is the most active isomer of this chemical. Dikshith and Datta (30) studied changes after intratesticular injections of lindane and found degenerative changes, necrosis, and cellular proliferation in the intertubular and intratubular regions.

An additional factor that is often overlooked in considering reproductive toxicology is the part of the integrative function of the reproductive system involving steroid synthesis and secretion. Steroid synthesis from either the adrenal glands or gonadal tissue (i.e., ovary and testis) is of unquestionable importance in reproductive physiology (121). Any alteration in steroidogenic processes occurring in these organs can have major effects on the reproductive function of the organism. For example, in the pregnant female, delays in implantation of the blastocyst (15) or parturition (131) may result in subfertility. Therefore, it is apparent that steroid hormone balance needs to be controlled. During the normal reproductive cycle in the female, and particularly during pregnancy, the organism utilizes metabolism and plasma protein binding as a means of controlling the circulating levels of free active hormones (90,129). Although few studies have addressed the question of the influence of environmental chemicals on steroid synthesis, there have been a limited number of reports suggesting an alteration of steroid hormone balance by an effect on metabolizing enzymes. In addition, certain pesticides possess estrogenic steroid hormone activity (42–44), and these chemicals appear to act through the steroid receptor mechanism (91). An exposure to chemicals possessing steroid activity could alter the steroid balance in the whole animal and thereby alter reproductive function.

In addition to the factors discussed above, the effect of environmental chemicals on the liver (97) may indirectly affect reproduction. In 1970, Lincer and Peakall (71) demonstrated that exposure of birds to Arochlor® 1254 or 1262 [trade names for polychlorinated biphenyl (PCB) containing 54% chlorine and 62% chlorine, respectively] increased hepatic estrogen metabolism. Recently, additional studies (28) have described specific effects of PCBs on steriod-metabolizing enzymes (e.g., 5α-reductase and 16β-hydroxylase activities) and have suggested use of these enzyme activities as biochemical markers. Studies by Wassermann and Wassermann (124) have indicated that PCB increased glucocorticoid levels. This effect was induced by the stress characteristic of the PCB on the body in general and not specifically on the adrenal gland (125). Further studies will be required to ascertain the exact site and mechanism of chemical effects on steroidogenesis and reproduction.

It has been postulated that DDT, aldrin, dieldrin, chlordane, parathion, and other organochlorine and organophosphorus compounds, because of their effect on microsomal enzyme activity may, through alterations of normal body metabolism, influence hormone-dependent factors involved in reproduction (21,63,99,127).

The process by which a chemical exerts its effects, whether through direct action, through altered steroid synthesis, through changes in the activity of steroid-metabolizing enzymes, or through interference with receptor interactions, is ultimately important for extrapolation to other chemicals or species.

## Prenatal Exposure

Although it has been known for some three decades that the mammalian conceptus can be damaged by exposure to chemicals during early development (110,111,119), there are relatively few studies concerning prenatal exposure to foreign chemicals and the subsequent postnatal fertility of the offspring.

### Effects on the Female

In most mammals, the female fetus is especially vulnerable to agents that damage the germ cell, since the formation of all of the oocytes occurs during fetal life (132). Cytological and biochemical evidence shows that the mitotic activity and DNA synthesis of oocytes cease by birth in both the mouse (101) and human (4,5) and resume again only at the time of ovulation and fertilization of the mature egg.

Therefore, chemicals that affect the female germ cell during oogenesis may be expected to have a lasting effect on the fertility of the female.

As seen in Fig. 2, when mouse fetuses were exposed to procarbazine, a common antineoplastic agent reported to interfere with DNA synthesis (66), either before (day 10), during (day 12), or after (day 17) peak oocyte DNA synthetic periods, the subsequent fertility of the female offspring was decreased (87). These results

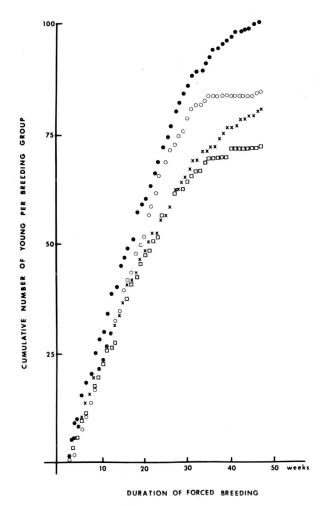

**FIG. 2.** Total reproductive capacity of female mice exposed prenatally to procarbazine. Timed pregnant CD-1 mice were treated subcutaneously with procarbazine (160 mg/kg) on days 10 (×), 12 (□), or 17 (○) of gestation and compared to mice treated with saline (●) on day 12. Reproductive capacity of female offspring was determined by repetitive forced breeding in which females were housed continuously with untreated fertile males, removed when noticeably pregnant, allowed to deliver their young, and immediately returned to the male. Total reproductive capacity was expressed as the cumulative number of live young born per female during the period of observation (J. A. McLachlan and R. L. Dixon, *unpublished observations*).

suggest the likelihood of a particular period of sensitivity during oogenesis to long-term toxicologic effects on fertility. The most pronounced effect occurred in females exposed during the peak of oocyte DNA synthesis, corresponding to days 12 and 13 in the mouse (12). Severe alterations in gonadal morphology were apparent in these animals (Fig. 3, bottom).

Further examination of Fig. 2 demonstrates the advantage of repeated forced breeding throughout the animal's reproductive life to determine effects on fertility; effects that are obvious late in the breeding regimen are not apparent during the first few matings. Thus, agents that alter DNA synthesis, such as alkylating agents [e.g., busulfan, (Table 2)], can be expected to interfere with germ cell replication and development. Diamond et al. (27) reported marked ovarian hypoplasia in a small-for-gestational-age infant from a mother treated with busulfan for leukemia. Administration of busulfan to pregnant rats can also alter the gonadal morphology of the offspring (39). This is a good example of biological principles, which, although established in animals, seem to cross species lines and may be applicable to humans. Ionizing radiation produces some of the same toxicities seen following exposure to radiomimetic alkylating agents. Peters (100) has described the effects of prenatal radiation exposure on ovarian morphology and reproductive capacity of female offspring.

Fetal ovaries may also be a target site for the action of some environmental pollutants, particularly polycyclic aromatic hydrocarbons (PAH); PAH are known to deplete primordial germ cells in adult rodents and primates (32,38). In fact, exposure of mice *in utero* to dimethylbenzanthracene results in depletion of both male and female germ cells at birth and infertility after maturation (76,78). Similar results have been obtained with benzo(*a*)pyrene (75,77).

Fetal germ cells are not the only target for prenatal exposure to chemicals that may lead to subfertility. In 1971, Herbst and his colleagues reported the association between maternal treatment with the synthetic estrogen DES and vaginal adenocarcinoma in female offspring (53). In order to evaluate the transplacental toxicity of DES and other hormonally active environmental chemicals, pregnant mice were treated in our laboratory with the compound on days 9 through 16 of gestation. Again, repetitive forced breeding of the female offspring revealed a dose-related decrease in reproductive capacity (85). Impaired ovarian function did contribute to subfertility, but the major cause seemed to be related to lesions in the genital tract (89). Thus, the mouse as a model system indicates that DES-induced subfertility may be an important concern. Earlier clinical studies by Pomerance (102) suggested that anovulatory bleeding and infertility may be a problem in DES-exposed human female offspring. In fact, recent clinical reports describe alterations in reproductive tract function, such as menstrual irregularities and subfertility, in prenatally DES-exposed females (7,8,52,108,115).

### Effects on the Male

Unlike the mammalian female, the male continues to produce germ cells throughout postnatal life. Although many compounds are recognized as toxicants that affect

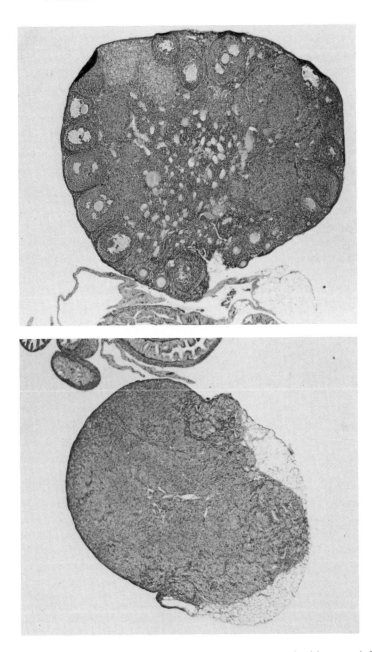

**FIG. 3. Top:** Photomicrograph of an ovary from a 6-week-old control female. **Bottom:** Photomicrograph of an ovary from a 6-week-old female mouse exposed prenatally to procarbazine (160 mg/kg) on day 12 of gestation. Note absence of follicles and germ cells.

TABLE 2. *Some compounds reported to alter fertility after prenatal exposure*[a]

| Compound given to mother | Major effects in offspring | Species |
|---|---|---|
| Methoxychlor | Reduced fertility in males and females (50) | Rat |
| Dimethylbenzanthracene (DMBA) | Gonadal dysplasia and reduced fertility in males and females (24,77,78) | Mouse |
| Benzo(a)pyrene | Gonadal dysplasia and reduced fertility in males and females (75,76) | Mouse |
| Diethylstilbestrol (DES) | Genital tract abnormalities and reduced fertility in females (85) | Mouse |
| Diethylstilbestrol (DES) | Genital tract abnormalities and reduced fertility in females (7,8,52,108,115) | Human |
| Diethylstilbestrol (DES) | Genital tract abnormalities and reduced fertility in males (85,88) | Mouse |
| Diethylstilbestrol (DES) | Genital tract abnormalities including sperm (47) | Human |
| Methyl methanesulfonate | Sterility in males (65) | Rat |
| Procarbazine | Reduced fertility in females (87) | Mouse |
| Cyclophosphamide | Reduced fertility in males and females (118) | Mouse |
| Clomid | Reproductive tract (83) | Rat |
| Busulfan | Gonadal dysplasia in males and females (39) | Rat |
| Cyanoketone | Altered estrous cycles (109) | Rat |

[a]This list is not comprehensive but represents some examples of chemical compounds reported to alter fertility after prenatal exposure. Three-generation studies of reproductive capacity were excluded since postnatal and prenatal contributions cannot be separated.

germ cells in adult males, there is little known about the effects of transplacental toxicants on the germ cells in male fetuses (Table 2). Abundant toxicological studies investigating spermatogenesis in adult animals have indicated that the effects of various toxicants on spermatogenesis may involve several sites of action. Certain compounds may act directly on the germ cells, probably at the level of DNA, RNA, and protein synthesis. The germ cell-damaging effects of prenatal exposure to procarbazine (87) and DMBA (78) on spermatogenesis have been described. These seem to be mediated by a toxic effect directly on the immature germ cell but are manifested by reduced fertility in the mature male.

Other compounds may act by interfering with the normal hormonal function regulating spermatogenesis. However, the detailed mechanism of the transplacental toxicological action of these compounds on fetal spermatogonia has not yet been elucidated. For example, studies on the male offspring of women treated with DES during pregnancy report that average values for sperm density and total motile spermatozoa per ejaculate were less than half those of controls. Furthermore, the number of abnormal sperm in the DES-exposed group was significantly greater than in the control group (47). With the mouse as a model, again our studies seem to be particularly relevant, since 60% of male offspring were sterile (88). Gonadal abnormalities in the mouse included cryptorchid testes and reduction in number of spermatogonia in approximately 63% of the males 9 to 10 months of age.

In addition to germ cell alterations in the male, the developing reproductive tract is especially vulnerable to toxicants. As shown in Fig. 1, both male and female fetuses, at sexually undifferentiated stages, have two pairs of genital ducts, Wolffian and Müllerian. During crucial periods of sexual differentiation, fetal testes produce two major kinds of hormones; the androgens induce development and differentiation of the Wolffian ducts to form male reproductive accessory organs, whereas Müllerian inhibiting factor (MIF) causes regression of Müllerian ducts in male fetuses. Therefore, there is a possibility that prenatal treatment with compounds that antagonize the effects of these hormones from the fetal testes may induce a failure of organogenesis in the male accessory reproductive organs. In fact, certain compounds given prenatally cause morphological abnormalities in the male reproductive tract in later life, as shown in Table 2. Studies on male mice exposed prenatally to DES show some anatomical abnormalities in the urogenital tracts; for example, 42% of male offspring treated prenatally with DES have epididymal cysts, and 63% of these animals have nodular enlargement of seminal vesicles or coagulating glands. A similar observation of epididymal cysts and prostatic inflammation is also recognized in DES-exposed human males; affected males of both species have undescended testes. In addition to these abnormalities, the male reproductive accessory glands in DES-treated male mice have homologous structures (derived from Müllerian ducts) to those of females, such as oviducts, a uterus, and an upper vagina. Furthermore, histological studies have demonstrated that most of the epididymal cysts are formed by Müllerian duct remnants (Y. Suzuki and J. A. McLachlan, *unpublished observations*).

### Other Transplacental Effects on Extragenital Reproductive Function

Unlike the biological factors involved in mutagenesis and teratogenesis, reproduction is a highly integrated function that involves a behavioral component. Thus, even in the absence of direct toxic effects on the endocrine system or the genital tract, compounds that alter behavior may result in essentially infertile animals. It is well known, for example, that exposure to androgenic or estrogenic hormones in the perinatal period can result in irreversible abnormalities in sexual behavior and subsequent infertility (48). Less well known are experiments that demonstrate that common environmental chemicals including $o,p'$-DDT (92) and chlordecone (43) produce similar long-lasting effects. As described previously (104), these effects may be related to the weak estrogenic properties of this class of chemicals. Therefore, the central nervous system in the developing male or female is, to some extent, more vulnerable to damage resulting in impaired fertility than that previously described in mature individuals. Thus, development of the integrative behavior so necessary to reproduction may be susceptible to disruption by psychotropic agents as well as hormonally active xenobiotics.

An additional comparison between developing and mature organisms can be made for reproductive toxicity effects mediated by the liver. As described earlier, compounds that alter hepatic metabolism of gonadal hormones can alter the reproductive characteristics of the affected individual. During neonatal development of the rat, compounds such as TCDD (74) and PCB (72,73) have been demonstrated to exert a long-lasting effect on hepatic function. Whether this imprinting of hepatic enzymes by perinatal chemical experience is a general biological phenomenon remains to be established; however, these data suggest that *in utero* exposure to environmental agents may result in compromised fertility later in life by altered function not only in the genital tract but also in extragenital systems as well. Moreover, functional abnormalities induced *in utero* often are long-lasting, whereas those that follow adult treatment are more frequently of short duration. Obvious exceptions to this generalization include irreversible germ cell depletion in both mature and immature females treated with alkylating agents or polycyclic aromatic hydrocarbons.

Of concern in the evaluation of a chemical's transplacental toxicity is whether the effect observed in a mature animal is associated with factors induced *in utero* or from the persistence of the compound into the later period of observation. Methoxychlor, a methoxy analog of DDT, was fed to pregnant rats, and the offspring were later studied for reproductive tract function. It was determined that both females and males showed decreased reproductive capacities at maturity (50). Unlike DDT, methoxychlor is not stored in adipose tissue and is not found to persist in tissues, suggesting that a chemical does not have to remain in the target tissue to induce a latent effect at that site.

Finally, when one evaluates chemicals for reproductive toxicity, the specificity of effect is an important consideration. Reports of chemically induced reproductive failure occasionally ignore the health status of the animal after chemical exposure. In evaluating chemicals for effects on reproduction, it is critical to determine the place of observed reproductive effects within the general toxicity profile of the compound. For example, in a report on ethylene dibromide (112), reproductive effects were observed only at exposure levels associated with mortality and morbidity. Likewise, in the evaluation of transplacental toxicity studies, effects on reproductive performance in offspring are most meaningful in the absence of acute toxicities to the mother and gross malformations in the young.

## SUMMARY

The attainment of sexual maturity, including normal fertility, is a remarkably complex process requiring many sequential environmental cues. Blocked or abnormal cues are associated with a disruption in this sensitive process and may lead to compromised reproductive capacity.

The unique sensitivity of the developing reproductive system, as demonstrated by long-term infertility related to prenatal exposure to DES in mice and humans, suggests special vulnerability during this period. Thus, even though exposure to chemicals during *in utero* life may not always be associated with abnormalities readily apparent at birth, the subsequent capacity of an organism to reproduce itself may be altered; the significance of this capacity to the survival of a species needs no further elaboration. The differential sensitivity of the fetal and adult reproductive systems is exemplified by the ovarian response in mice to DMBA. The dose of DMBA and the time to ovarian atrophy were both significantly less following prenatal exposure than following postnatal exposure (78).

The relationship of these observations in experimental animals to humans is not yet established. Comparable results obtained in mice and humans exposed *in utero* to DES suggest that the fetal period may be an especially vulnerable time for induction of reproductive abnormalities. Thus, inclusion of the study of the transplacental toxicity of environmental chemicals that may result in impaired reproduction in offspring is necessary in the safety evaluation of any compound. Of more general concern may be the observation that many common environmental chemicals possess weak estrogenic activity that compromises reproductive processes in immature animals exposed to them (86). The recent hypothesis (82) that depletion of female germ cells in mice by polycyclic aromatic hydrocarbons may be a good model for human female exposures to smoking and industrial pollution compels us to consider this possibility.

## REFERENCES

1. Ahlquist, K. A. (1966): Enzyme changes in rat testis produced by the administration of busulfan and 7,12-dimethylbenz-*a*-anthracene. *J. Reprod. Fertil.*, 12:377.
2. Amir, D. (1973): The sites of the spermicidal action of ethylene dibromide in bulls. *J. Reprod. Fertil.*, 35:519–525.
3. Anderson, J. M., Giner-Sorolla, A., and Ebeling, D. (1978): Effects of imipramine, nitrite, and dimethylnitrosamine on reproduction in mice. *Res. Commun. Chem. Pathol. Pharmacol.*, 19(2): 311–327.
4. Baker, T. G. (1963): A quantitative and cytological study of germ cells in human ovaries. *Proc. R. Soc. Lond. [Biol.]*, 158:417–433.
5. Baker, T. G. (1971): Radiosensitivity of mammalian oocytes with particular reference to the human female. *Am. J. Obstet. Gynecol.*, 110:746–761.
6. Barasch, J. M., and Bressler, R. S. (1977): The effect of 5-bromodeoxyuridine on the postnatal development of the rat testis. *J. Exp. Zool.*, 200:1–8.
7. Barnes, A. (1979): Menstrual history of young women exposed *in utero* to diethylstilbestrol. *Fertil. Steril.*, 32(2):148–153.
8. Berger, M. J., and Goldstein, D. P. (1980): Impaired reproductive performance in DES-exposed women. *Obstet. Gynecol.*, 55(1):25–27.
9. Biggers, J. D., and Schuetz, A. W. (1972): *Oogenesis*. University Park Press, Baltimore.
10. Blend, M. J., and Lehnert, B. E. (1973): Luteinizing hormone (LH) serum levels and body weight/ organ weight ratios in male rats fed low levels of dieldrin. In: *Pesticides and the Environment: A Continuing Controversy*, edited by W. B. Diechmann, p. 189. Medical Book Corp, New York.
11. Borgen, L. A., Davis, W. M., and Pace, H. B. (1971): Effects of snythetic $\Delta^9$-tetrahydrocannabinol on pregnancy and offspring in the rat. *Toxicol. Appl. Pharmacol.*, 20:480–486.
12. Borum, K. (1961): Oogenesis in the mouse. *Exp. Cell Res.*, 24:495.
13. Botta, J. A., Jr., Hawkins, H. C., and Weikel, J. H., Jr. (1974): Effects of cyclophosphamide on fertility and general reproductive performance of rats. *Toxicol. Appl. Pharmacol.*, 27:602–611.
14. Boyd, E. M. (1971): Sterility from phenacetin. *Clin. Pharmacol.*, (March–April):96–102.
15. Briggs, M. H., and Brotherton, J. (1970): *Steroid Biochemistry and Pharmacology*. Academic Press, New York.
16. Cannon, S. B., and Kimbrough, R. D. (1979): Short-term chlordecone toxicity in rats including effects on reproduction, pathological organ changes, and their reversibility. *Toxicol. Appl. Pharmacol.*, 47:469–476.

17. Cater, B. R., Cook, M. W., Gangolli, S. D., and Grasso, P. (1977): Studies on dibutyl phthalate-induced testicular atrophy in the rat: Effect on zinc metabolism. *Toxicol. Appl. Pharmacol.*, 41:609–618.
18. Ciaccio, L. A., Hill, J. L., and Kincl, F. A. (1978): Observation on toxic effects of quinacrine hydrocholoride (in rodents). *Contraception*, 17:231–236.
19. Collins, T. F. X. (1972): Dominant lethal assay. I. Captan. *Food Cosmet. Toxicol.*, 10:353.
20. Collins, T. F. X. (1972): Effect of captan and triethylenemelamine (TEM) on reproductive fitness of DBA/2J mice. *Toxicol. Appl. Pharmacol.*, 23:277–287.
21. Conney, A. H., Welch, R. M., Kuntzman, R., and Burnes, J. J. (1967): Effects of pesticides on drug and steroid metabolism. *Clin. Pharmacol. Ther.*, 8:2.
22. Coppola, J. A., Leonardi, R. G., and Lippmann, W. (1966): Ovulatory failure in rats after treatment with brain norepinephrine depletors. *Endocrinology*, 78:225–228.
23. Currie, G. N., Black, D. L., Armstrong, D. T., and Greep, R. O. (1969): Blockade of ovulation in the rabbit with catecholamines and sympathomimetics. *Proc. Soc. Biol. Med.*, 130:598–602.
24. Davis, G. J., McLachlan, J. A., and Lucier, G. W., (1978): The effect of 7,12-dimethylbenz-*a*-anthracene (DMBA) on the prenatal development of gonads in mice. *Teratology*, 17:33A.
25. Deichmann, W. B., MacDonald, W. E., Beasley, A. G., and Cubit, D. (1971): Subnormal reproduction in beagle dogs induced by DDT and aldrin. *Indust. Med. Surg.*, 40(2):10–20.
26. Der, R., Fahim, A., Yousef, M., and Fahim, M. (1976): Environmental interaction of lead and cadmium on reproduction and metabolism of male rats. *Research Commun. Chem. Pathol. Pharmacol.*, 14(4):689–714.
27. Diamond, I., Anderson, M. M., and McCreache, S. R. (1960): Transplacental transmission of busulfan (Myleran®) in a mother with leukemia. *Pediatrics*, 25:85–90.
28. Dieringer, C. S., Lamartiniere, C. A., Schiller, C. M., and Lucier, G. W. (1979): Altered ontogeny of hepatic steroid-metabolizing enzymes by pure polychlorinated biphenyl congeners. *Biochem. Pharmacol.*, 28:2511–2514.
29. Dikshith, T. S., and Datta, K.K. (1972): Effect of intratesticular injection on lindane and endrin on the testes of rats. *Acta Pharmacol. Toxicol. (Kbh.)*, 31:1–10.
30. Dikshith, T. S., and Datta, K. K. (1972): Pathologic changes induced by pesticides in the testes and liver of rats. *Exp. Pathol. (Jena)*, 7:309–316.
31. Dixon, R. L., and Lee, I. P. (1976): Methods to assess reproductive effects of environmental chemicals: Studies of cadmium and boron administration orally. *Environ. Health Perspect.*, 13:49.
32. Dobson, R. L., Koehler, C. G., Felton, J. S., Kwan, T. C., Weubbles, B. J., and Jones, D. C. L. (1978): Vulnerability of female germ cells in developing mice and monkeys to tritium, gamma rays, and polycyclic aromatic hydrocarbons. In: *Developmental Toxicology of Energy-Related Pollutants*, edited by D. D. Mahlum, M. R. Sikov, P. L. Hackett, and F. D. Andrew, pp. 1–14. Technical Information Center, United States Department of Energy, Washington.
33. Edwards, M. J., Hartley, W. J., and Hansen, E. A. (1977): Selenium and lowered reproductive efficiency in pigs. *Aust. Vet. J.*, 53(11):553–554.
34. Epstein, S. S., and Shafner, H. (1968): Chemical mutagens in the human environment. *Nature*, 219:385–387.
35. Eroschenko, V. P., and Wilson, W. O. (1974): Photoperiods and age as factors modifying the effects of Kepone in Japanese quail. *Toxicol. Appl. Pharmacol.*, 29:329.
36. Fahim, M. S., Webb, M., Hilderbrand, D. C., and Russel, R. L.(1972): Effect of lead acetate on male reproduction. *Fed. Proc.*, 31:272.
37. Fairley, K. F., Barrie, J. U., and Johnson, W. (1972): Sterility and testicular atrophy related to cyclophosphamide therapy. *Lancet*, 1:568–569.
38. Felton, J. S., Kwan, C., Wuebbles, B. J., and Dobson, R. L. (1978): Genetic differences in polycyclic-aromatic-hydrocarbon metabolism and their effects on oocyte killing in developing mice. In: *Developmental Toxicology of Energy-Related Pollutants*, edited by D. D. Mahlum, M. R. Sikov, P. L. Hackett, and F. D. Andrew, pp. 15–26. Technical Information Center, United States Department of Energy, Washington.
39. Forsberg, J. G., and Olivecrona, H. (1966): The effect of prenatally administrated busulfan on rat gonads. *Biol. Neonate*, 10:180–192.
40. Friedman, L., Weinberger, M. A., Farber, T. M., Moreland, F. M., Peters, E. L., Gilmore, C. E., and Khan, M. A. (1979): Testicular atrophy and impaired spermatogenesis in rats fed high levels of the methylxanthines caffeine, theobromine, or theophylline. *J. Environ. Pathol. Toxicol.*, 2:687–706.

41. Fuller, G. B., and Draper, S. W. (1975): Effect of Mirex on induced ovulation in immature rats. *Proc. Soc. Exp. Biol. Med.*, 148:414–417.
42. Gellert, R. J. (1978): Uterotrophic activity of polychlorinated biphenyls (PCB) and induction of precocious reproductive aging in neonatally treated female rats. *Environ. Res.*, 16:123–130.
43. Gellert, R. J. (1978): Kepone, mirex, dieldrin, and aldrin: Estrogenic activity and the induction of persistent vaginal estrus and anovulation in rats following neonatal treatment. *Environ. Res.*, 16:131–138.
44. Gellert, R. J., Heinrichs, W. L., and Swerdloff, R. S. (1972): DDT homologue estrogen-like effects on the vagina, uterus, and pituitary of the rat. *Endocrinology*, 91:4.
45. Gellert, R. J., Heinrichs, W. L., and Swerdloff, R. S. (1974): Effects of neonatally-administered DDT homologs on reproductive function in male and female rats. *Neuroendocrinology*, 16:84–94.
46. Gellert, R. J., Wallace, C. A., Wiesmeier, E. M., and Shuman, R. M. (1978): Topical exposure of neonates to hexachlorophene: Longstanding effects on mating behavior and prostatic development in rats. *Toxicol. Appl. Pharmacol.*, 43:339–349.
47. Gill, W. B., Schumacher, G. F. B., Bibbo, M., Straus, F. H. II, and Schoenberg, H. W. (1979): Association of diethylstilbestrol exposure *in utero* with cryptorchidism, testicular hypoplasia and semen abnormalities. *J. Urol.*, 122:36–39.
48. Gorski, R. A. (1971): Gonadal hormones and the perinatal development of neuroendocrine function. In: *Frontiers in Neuroendocrinology*, edited by L. Martini and W. F. Ganong, pp. 237–282. Oxford University Press, New York.
49. Guesry, P., Lenoir, G., and Broyer, M. (1978): Gonadal effects of chlorambucil given to prepubertal and pubertal boys for nephrotic syndrome. *J. Pediatr.*, 92(2):299–303.
50. Harris, S. J., Cecil, H. C., and Bitman, J. (1974): Effect of several dietary levels of technical methoxychlor on reproduction in rats. *J. Agric. Food Chem.*, 22(6):969–973.
51. Heinrichs, W. L., Gellert, R. J., Bakke, J. L., and Lawrence, N. L. (1971): DDT administered to neonatal rats induces persistent estrus syndrome. *Science*, 173:642–643.
52. Herbst, A. L., Hubby, M. M., Blough, R. R., and Azizi, F. (1980): A comparison of pregnancy experience in DES-exposed and DES-unexposed daughters. *J. Reprod. Med.*, 24(2):62–69.
53. Herbst, A. L., Ulfelder, H., and Poskanzer, D. C. (1971): Adenocarcinoma of the vagina: Association of maternal stilbestrol therapy with tumor appearance in young women. *N. Engl. J. Med.*, 284:878.
54. Hilderbrand, D. C., Der, R., Griffin, W. T., and Fahim, M. S. (1973): Effect of lead acetate on reproduction. *Am. J. Obstet. Gynecol.*, 115:1058–1065.
55. Hodel, C., and Suter, K. (1978): Reversible inhibition of spermatogenesis with an indenopyridine (20–438). *Arch. Toxicol. [Suppl.]*, 1:323–326.
56. Jarvik, M. E. (1965): Drugs used in the treatment of psychiatric disorders. In: *The Pharmacological Basis of Therapeutics*, edited by L. S. Goodman and A. Gilman, pp. 159–180. Macmillan, New York.
57. Jonsson, H. T., Jr., Keil, J. E., Gaddy, R. G., Loadholt, C. B., Hennigar, G. R., and Walker, E. M., Jr. (1975/1976): Prolonged ingestion of commercial DDT and PCB; effects on progesterone levels and reproduction in the mature female rat. *Arch. Environ. Contam. Toxicol.*, 3:479–490.
58. Joseph, A. A., and Kinncl, F. A. (1974): Toxic and antifertility effects of quinacrine hydrochloride in rats. *Am. J. Obstet. Gynecol.*, 119:978–981.
59. Kamboj, V. P., and Kar, A. B. (1964): Antitesticular effects of metallic salt and rare earth salts. *J. Reprod. Fertil.*, 7:21–28.
60. Khera, K. S. (1973): Reproductive capability of male rats and mice treated with methyl mercury. *Toxicol. Appl. Pharmacol.*, 24:167–177.
61. Krause, W., and Homola, S. (1974): Alterations of the seminiferous epithelium and the Leydig cells of the rat testis after the application of dichlorvos (DDVP). *Bull. Environ. Contam. Toxicol.*, 11(5):429–433.
62. Kripke, B. J., Kelman, A. D., Shah, N. K., Balogh, K., and Handler, A. H. (1976): Testicular reaction to prolonged exposure to nitrous oxide. *Anesthesiology*, 14(2):104–113.
63. Kupfer, D. (1969): Influence of chlorinated hydrocarbons and organophosphate pesticides on metabolism of steroids. *Ann. N. Y. Acad. Sci.*, 160:244–253.
64. Lamperti, A. (1976): The effects of neonatally-administered monosodium glutamate on the reproductive system of adult hamsters. *Biol. Reprod.*, 14(3):362–369.
65. Lang, R. (1977): Heritable translocation test and dominant-lethal assay in male mice with methyl methanesulfonate. *Mutat. Res.*, 48:75–88.

66. Lee, I. P., and Dixon, R. L. (1972):Effects of procarbazine on spermatogenesis determined by velocity sedimentation cell separation technique and serial mating. *J. Pharmacol. Exp. Ther.*, 181:219–226.
67. Lee, I. P., and Dixon, R. L. (1975): Effects of mercury on spermatogenesis studied by velocity sedimentation cell separation and serial mating. *J. Pharmacol. Exp. Ther.*, 194:171–181.
68. Lee, I. P., Sherins, R. J., and Dixon, R. L. (1968): Evidence for induction of germinal aplasia in male rats by environmental exposure to boron. *Toxicol. Appl. Pharmacol.*, 45:557–590.
69. Leong, B. K. J., Ts'o, T. O. T., and Chenoweth, M. B. (1974): Testicular atrophy from inhalation of ethylene oxide cyclic tetramer. *Toxicol. Appl. Pharmacol.*, 27:342–354.
70. Levin, W., Welch, R. M., and Conney, A. H. (1969): Inhibitory effect of phenobarbital or chlordane pretreatment on the androgen-induced increase in seminal vesicle weight in the rat. *Steroids*, 13:155–161.
71. Lincer, J. L., and Peakall, D. B. (1970): Metabolic effects of polychlorinated biphenyls in the American kestrel. *Nature*, 228:783–784.
72. Lucier, G. W., and McDaniel, O. S. (1979): Developmental toxicology of the halogenated aromatics: Effects on enzyme development. *Ann. N.Y. Acad. Sci.*, 77:449–457.
73. Lucier, G. W., McLachlan, J. A., and Davis, G. J. (1978): Transplacental toxicology of the polychlorinated and polybrominated biphenyls. In: *Developmental Toxicology of Energy-Related Pollutants*, edited by D. D. Mahlum, M. R. Sikov, P. C. Hackett, F. D. Andrew, pp. 188–203. Technical Information Center, United States Department of Energy, Washington.
74. Lucier, G. W., Sonawane, B. R., McDaniel, O. S., and Hook, G. E. R. (1975): Postnatal stimulation of hepatic microsomal enzymes following administration of TCDD to pregnant rats. *Chem. Biol. Interact.*, 11:15–26.
75. MacKenzie, K. M. (1981): Infertility in mice exposed *in utero* to benzo(*a*)pyrene. *Biol. Reprod.* (*submitted*).
76. MacKenzie, K. M., Lucier, G. W., and McLachlan, J. A. (1979): Infertility in mice exposed prenatally to benzo-*a*-pyrene (BP). *Teratology*, 19:38A.
77. MacKenzie, K. M., Lucier, G. W., and McLachlan, J. A. (1979): Infertility in mice following prenatal exposure to 9,10-dimethyl-1,2-benzanthracene (DMBA). In: *Proceedings of the 12th Annual Meeting of the Society for the Study of Reproduction*, p. 30A., Quebec.
78. MacKenzie, K. M., Lucier, G. W., and McLachlan, J. A. (1980): Reproductive failure in mice exposed prenatally to 9,10-dimethyl-1,2-benzanthracene. *J. Reprod. Fertil.* (*submitted*).
79. Mahesh, V. B., Muldoon, T. G., Eldridge, J. C., and Korach, K. S. (1972): Studies in the regulation of FSH and LH secretion by gonadal steroids. In: *Gonadotropins*, edited by B. B. Saxena, C. G. Beling, and H. M. Gandy, pp. 730–742. John Wiley and Sons, New York.
80. Makovskaya, E. I., Shamrai, P. F., and Grigor, E. N. N. (1972): Structural and histochemical changes of internal secretion glands during polychlorpinene poisoning. *Vrach. Delo.*, 2:128–131.
81. Marshall, S., Whorton, D., Krauss, R. M., and Palmer, W. S. (1978): Effect of pesticides on testicular function. *Urology*, XI(3):257.
82. Mattison, R., and Thorgeirsson, S. S. (1978): Smoking and industrial pollution, and their effects on menopause and ovarian cancer. *Lancet*, 1:187.
83. McCormack, S. A., and Clark, J. H. (1979): Clomid administration to the pregnant rat causes abnormalities of the reproductive tract in offspring and mothers. *Science*, 204:629–631.
84. McFarland, L. Z., and Lacy, P. B. (1969): Physiologic and endocrinologic effects of the insecticide Kepone in the Japanese quail. *Toxicol. Appl. Pharmacol.*, 15:441–450.
85. McLachlan, J. A. (1977): Prenatal exposure to diethylstilbestrol in mice: Toxicological studies. *J. Toxicol. Environ. Health*, 2:527–537.
86. McLachlan, J. A. (1980): *Estrogens in the Environment.* Elsevier/North-Holland, New York.
87. McLachlan, J. A., and Dixon, R. L. (1973): Reduced fertility in female mice exposed prenatally to procarbazine. *Fed. Proc.*, 32:745.
88. McLachlan, J. A., Newbold, R. R., and Bullock, B. (1975): Reproductive tract lesions in male mice exposed prenatally to diethylstilbestrol. *Science*, 190:991–992.
89. McLachlan, J. A., Newbold, R. R., and Bullock, B. C. (1980): Long-term effects on the female mouse genital tract associated with prenatal exposure to diethylstilbestrol. *Cancer Res.*, 40:3988–3999.
90. Migeon, C. J., Bertrand, J., and Wall, P. E. (1957): Physiological disposition of 4-$^{14}$C cortisol during late pregnancy. *J. Clin. Invest.*, 36:1350–1362.

91. Nelson, J. A. (1974): Effects of dichlorodiphenyltrichloroethane (DDT) analogs and polychlorinated biphenyl (PCB) mixture of 17β-³H estradiol binding to rat uterine receptor. *Biochem. Pharmacol.*, 23:447–451.
92. Nelson, J. A., Struck, R. F., and James, R. (1978): Estrogenic activities of chlorinated hydrocarbons. *J. Toxicol. Environ. Health*, 4:325–340.
93. Orberg, J. (1978): Effects of pure chlorbiphenyls (2,4′,5-trichlorobiphenyl and 2,2′,4,4′,5,5′-hexachlorobiphenyl) on the reproductive capacity in female mice. *Acta Pharmacol. Toxicol. (Kbh.)*, 42:323–327.
94. Orberg, J., and Lundberg, C. (1974): Some effects of DDT and PCB on the hormonal system in the male mouse. *Environ. Physiol. Biochem.*, 4:116–120.
95. Orlova, N. V., Khovayeva, L. A., and Akineheva, M. Y. (1971): Specific features of the action produced by pesticides of different chemical structure on warm-blooded animals. *Vopr. Pitan.*, 30:32.
96. Osterberg, R. E., Bierbower, G. W., and Hehir, R. M. (1977): Renal and testicular damage following dermal application of the flame retardant Tris(2,3-dibromopropyl) phosphate. *J. Toxicol. Environ. Health*, 3:979–987.
97. Parke, D. V. (1968): *The Biochemistry of Foreign Compounds*. Pergamon Press, London.
98. Pasi, A., Embree, J. W., Jr., and Eisenlord, G. H. (1974): Assessment of the mutagenic properties of diquat and paraquat in the murine dominant lethal test. *Mutat. Res.*, 26:171–175.
99. Peakall, D. B. (1967): Pesticide-induced enzyme breakdown of steroids in birds. *Nature*, 216:505.
100. Peters, H. (1969): The effect of radiation in early life on the morphology and reproductive function of the mouse ovary. In: *Advances in Reproductive Physiology*, edited by A. McLaren, pp. 149–185. Logos Press, London.
101. Peters, H., and Crone, M. (1967): DNA synthesis in oocytes of mammals. *Arch. Anat. Microsc. Morphol. Exp.*, 56(Suppl. 3–4):160–170.
102. Pomerance, W. (1973): Post-stilbestrol secondary syndrome. *Obstet. Gynecol.*, 42:12–18.
103. Purshottam, N., Mason, M., and Pincus, G. (1961): Induced ovulation in the mouse and the measurement of its inhibition. *Fertil. Steril.*, 12:346–352.
104. Rall, D. P., and McLachlan, J. A. (1980): Potential for exposure to estrogens in the environment. In: *Estrogens in the Environment*, edited by J. A. McLachlan, pp. 199–202. Elsevier/North-Holland, New York.
105. Rohrborn, G. (1968): Mutagenicity tests in mice. *Humangenetik*, 6:345–361.
106. Sanders, O. (1975): Effects of a polychlorinated biphenyl (PCB) on sleeping times, plasma corticosteroids, and testicular activity of white-footed mice. *Environ. Physiol. Biochem.*, 5:308–313.
107. Schally, A. V., Redding, T. W., and Arimura, A. (1973): Effect of sex steroids on pituitary responses to LH and FSH-releasing hormone *in vitro*. *Endocrinology*, 93:893–902.
108. Schmidt, G., Fowler, W. C., Talbert, L. M., and Edelman, D. A. (1980): Reproductive history of women exposed to diethylstilbestrol *in utero*. *Fertil. Steril.*, 33(1):21–24.
109. Shapiro, B., Goldman, A. S., and Root, A. W. (1974): Prenatal interference with the onset of puberty, vaginal cyclicity and subsequent pregnancy in the female rat. *Proc. Soc. Exp. Biol. Med.*, 145:334–339.
110. Shepard, T. H. (1973): *Catalog of Teratogenic Agents*. Johns Hopkins University Press, Baltimore.
111. Shepard, T. H., Nelson, T., Oakley, G. P., and Lemire, R. J. (1971): Collection of human embryos and fetuses. In: *Monitoring, Birth Defects and Environment: The Problem of Surveillance*, edited by E. B. Hook, D. T. Janerich, and I. H. Porter, pp. 29–43, Academic Press, New York.
112. Short, R. D., Winston, J. M., Hong, C. B., Minor, J. L., Lee, C. C., and Seifter, J. (1979): Effects of ethylene dibromide on reproduction in male and female rats. *Toxicol. Appl. Pharmacol.*, 49:97–105.
113. Shtenberg, A. I., Orlova, N. V., and Torchinskill, A. M. (1973): Action of pesticides of different chemical structures on the gonads and embryogenesis of experimental animals. *Gig. Sanit.*, 38:16–20.
114. Shtenberg, A. I., and Rybakova, M. N. (1968): Effects of carbaryl on the neuroendocrine system of rats. *Food Cosmet. Toxicol.*, 6:461–467.
115. Siegler, A. M., Wang, C. F., and Friberg, J. (1979): Fertility of the diethylstilbestrol exposed offspring. *Fertil. Steril.*, 31(6):601–607.

116. Singh, A. R., Lawrence, W. H., and Autian, J. (1975): Dominant lethal mutations and antifertility effects of di-2-ethylhexyl adipate and diethyl adipate in male mice. *Toxicol. Appl. Pharmacol.*, 32:566–576.
117. Singh, G. B., and Khanna, S. K. (1972): Effect of intratesticular administration of metanil yellow in rats. *Exp. Pathol. (Jena)*, 7:172–175.
118. Sotomayer, R. E., and Cumming, R. B. (1975): Induction of translocations by cyclophosphamide in different germ cell stages in male mice: Cytological characterization and transmission. *Mutat. Res.*, 27(3):375–388.
119. Strobino, B. R., Kline, J., and Stein, Z. (1978): Chemical and physical exposures of parents: Effects on human reproduction and offspring. In: *Early Human Development*, edited by S. J. Hutt and C. Hutt, pp. 371–399. Elsevier/North-Holland Biomedical Press, New York.
120. Thompson, D. J., Molello, J. A., Strebing, R. J., Dyke, I. L., and Robinson, V. B. (1974): Reproduction and teratology studies with oncolytic agents in the rat and rabbit. I. 1,3-bis(2-Chloroethyl)-1-nitrosourea (BCNU). *Toxicol. Appl. Pharmacol.*, 30:422–439.
121. Turner, C. D. (1966): *General Endocrinology, Fourth Edition*, W. B. Saunders, Philadelphia.
122. Van Thiel, D. H., Gavaler, J., and Lester, R. (1975): Alcohol is a direct testicular toxin. *Clin. Res.*, 23:941–942.
123. Voytenko, G. A., and Medved, I. L. (1973): The effect of certain thiocarbamates on the generative function. *Gig. Sanit.*, 38:111–114.
124. Wassermann, D., and Wassermann, M. (1972): Ultrastructure of adrenal zona fasiculata in rats receiving polychlorinated biphenyls (PCB's). *17th International Congress of Occupational Health*.
125. Wassermann, D., Wassermann, M., Cucos, S., and Djavaherian, M. (1973): Function of adrenal gland–zona fasiculata in rats receiving polychlorinated biphenyls. *Environ. Res.*, 6:334–338.
126. Weir, R. J., Jr., and Fisher, R. S. (1972): Toxicologic studies on borax and boric acid. *Toxicol. Appl. Pharmacol.*, 23:351–364.
127. Welch, R. M., Levin, W., and Conney, A. M. (1967): Insecticide inhibition and stimulation of steroid hydroxylases in rat liver. *J. Pharmacol. Exp. Ther.*, 155:167–173.
128. Welch, R. M., Levin, W., Kuntzman, R., Jacobson, M., and Conney, A. H. (1971): Effect of halogenated hydrocarbon insecticides on the metabolism and uterotropic action of estrogens in rats and mice. *Toxicol. Appl. Pharmacol.*, 19:234–246.
129. Westphal, U. (1971): *Steroid–Protein Interactions*. Springer-Verlag, New York.
130. Wharton, R. S., Mazze, R. I., Baden, J. M., Hitt, B. A., and Dooley, J. R. (1978): Fertility, reproduction and postnatal survival in mice chronically exposed to halothane. *Anesthesiology*, 48:167–174.
131. Zarrow, M. X., Yochim, J. M., and McCarthy, J. L. (1964): *Experimental Endocrinology. A Sourcebook of Basic Techniques*. Academic Press, New York.
132. Zuckerman, S. S. (1962): *The Ovary,Vols. I and II*. Academic Press, New York.

*Developmental Toxicology*, edited by
C. A. Kimmel and J. Buelke-Sam. Raven Press,
New York © 1981.

# Behavioral Assessment of the Postnatal Animal: Testing and Methods Development

Jane Adams and Judy Buelke-Sam

*Perinatal and Postnatal Evaluation Branch, Division of Teratogenesis Research, National Center for Toxicological Research, Food and Drug Administration, Jefferson, Arkansas 72079*

The central nervous system (CNS) appears to be especially susceptible to toxic insult during its extended development, and evidence is rapidly accumulating to suggest that functional alterations can result from perinatal exposure levels lower than those producing overtly toxic signs (3,16,23,36,42,57,87,91,111,124,125,128, 133,139,149,154,159,160). This prolonged susceptibility of the nervous system has led both neurotoxicologists and teratologists to search for more sensitive indicators of toxicity via the assessment of CNS functional integrity following prenatal and/or neonatal exposures. Physiological, biochemical, and behavioral investigations are all necessary complementary approaches to evaluating CNS function. However, this chapter will be limited only to special considerations of and progress being made in the development of behavioral screening systems.

## BASIC CONSIDERATIONS IN TEST SYSTEM DEVELOPMENT

No single approach or behavioral test battery has been identified as the most reliable, sensitive, and economic means of detecting behavioral dysfunction following developmental insult. There are two major factors that contribute to this state of affairs. First, our understanding of "normal" behavior and its underlying mechanisms is far from complete. Much research is still required within the many disciplines that contribute to this basic knowledge. Second, only recently have scientists begun to direct their efforts toward evaluating general approaches and specific methodologies of these disciplines for direct application to prospective screening of new drugs and chemicals. The identification of the ultimate test system must wait; however, the development of a currently defined, effective test strategy cannot. The legal mandates and moral obligation to detect potential behavioral teratogens require it.

Several different strategies (49,107,132,152,153) and behavioral test batteries (25,63,149) for behavioral teratology have been proposed. All represent attempts to evaluate at different ages behaviors that rely on various CNS subsystem functions and to do this in some orderly and progressive fashion. In addition, there have been several recent reviews of the basic research area and important considerations in test system development (19,22,35,36,47,111). Together, these reports offer a good introduction to the current status of behavioral teratology, and the interested reader is referred to these for a more complete review of the subject.

## Detection Versus Delineation of Toxicity

The goal of a behavioral teratology screening system is to prevent, or at least reduce, human developmental exposures that cause behavioral dysfunctions. The effective achievement of this goal hinges on both the detection of neurotoxic actions and the subsequent delineation of the type(s), degree(s), and mechanism(s) of neurotoxicity. With the growing number of new substances to be tested, the greatest need is for a rapid, reliable, yet accurate prediction of neurotoxic potential. Once neurotoxic properties are detected, they need to be more fully delineated to allow more precise estimation across species of the actual human risk involved. Behavioral evaluations will play an important role in both levels of testing, although the general approach to system development may be rather different for the two. In both cases, however, it is assumed that the animals "appear" physically normal; test results from subjects already showing overt toxic signs are not very informative toxicologically (110).

In primary-level screening designed to detect toxicity, the major concern is that a behavioral teratogen not be missed. Therefore, a broad range of CNS functions needs to be evaluated. Although behavioral teratology testing may include evaluation of CNS functions that have been shown to be affected following adult exposures, it should not be limited to such evaluations. Embryo/fetotoxic effects are the result of changes produced during the exposure period and of the developmental events occurring at that time (110,148,155). Therefore, developmental treatment effects may be expressed upon functions other than those affected in the mature CNS (107,110,111). Apical test methods, by definition, are not highly specific measures but instead measure effective integration of sensory, motor, motivational, learning, and/or memory processes (22). The use of a few such methods would provide overlap in the evaluation of contributing neurological systems and might provide the best chance of identifying a behavioral teratogen as well as the greatest assurance that such a compound would not go undetected.

The prolonged period of CNS development would suggest that a broad exposure period also be used in primary screening. Initial acute and subchronic pharmacological/toxicological evaluations carried out in mature organisms may provide information on appropriate dose ranges for such behavioral teratology testing. And just as the developmental exposure period may dictate the toxic response, the toxic response may dictate the most appropriate period for evaluating behavior (19,47). Thus, when little is known about the behavioral teratogenic potential of a compound, a system to detect such toxicity should include a broad exposure period and a developmental series of tests that sample a broad range of CNS functions. This approach should also be used in studies of new agents that belong to the same pharmacological class as known behavioral teratogens. We simply do not know enough about structure–activity relationships to limit CNS functional evaluations at the outset (37,79).

There are at least two advantages to be gained when such a system is applied early in the overall screening hierarchy. First, either the same animals or animals from the same litters may be used in evaluations of one or more other postnatal functions as described in preceding chapters. Although the possibility of multiple test interactions exists, coincident assessment of other endpoints, e.g., reproductive capabilities, immune competence, etc., provides the opportunity both to evaluate relative system sensitivities and better describe the overall toxicologic profile of the agent under study. Second, the integrative nature of behavior makes it possible to detect a variety of adverse effects that may be secondarily expressed as alterations in behavior, e.g., altered thermoregulatory capacity, respiratory inadequacy, metabolic disturbances, etc. Such "secondary" effects are of utmost concern to the basic researcher, and a good deal of effort is often spent controlling for such confounding influences (36,47,132). In primary screening, however, the goal is to detect toxicity, and at this stage it is more important to know that something is wrong than to know what is wrong.

Depending on the results of primary screening and the economic and/or therapeutic value of the agent, secondary behavioral testing may be warranted. Once "target functions" have been suggested by primary testing, subsequent evaluations may include more sophisticated and selective behavioral techniques, perhaps in other species, chosen specifically to help delineate the type(s) and degree(s) of toxicity produced. For example, primary screening in albino rats may suggest that visual function is impaired. Characterization of visual dysfunction using simple procedures is very difficult in nonpigmented animals. Therefore, one or more psychophysical techniques may be deemed appropriate in pigmented rats and/or in another species. Also necessary at this stage are more selective exposure regimens and testing schedules as well as many procedural controls to isolate a direct neurotoxic effect from other indirect actions (19,47). For example, cross-fostering procedures may be employed to control for continued neonatal exposure via the milk and also altered maternal behavior and/or inadequate lactation during early postnatal life. Such procedures may be warranted at this stage, although they would be too costly and time consuming at the primary screening level (20).

At this point, pharmacological or chemical class, as well as primary test results, may suggest target functions for evaluation. For example, it is very likely that a new sedative–hypnotic drug might require different functional assessments, exposure, and testing schedules than would an organochlorine pesticide. The potential use of such agents dictates the probability of exposure and the populations at greatest risk; obviously, these differ. Also different are the spectra of "intended" effects and commonly associated adverse side effects of these two classes of agents. Thus, secondary behavioral evaluations should be flexibly designed with agent specificity in mind. However, the selection of agent-specific procedures should not preclude evaluation of any new compound at the primary screening level.

## Procedural Considerations

There are several procedural aspects that should be considered prior to or in conjunction with the establishment of a behavioral teratology test system. These include selection of the test subject, the use of a variety of positive and negative controls to define system reliability and sensitivity, test validation, and standardization of selected methods and procedures. Consideration of these aspects in the early stages of test system development may directly contribute to the selection or elimination of individual behavioral methods. These considerations are important at all levels of behavioral teratology testing. However, they are particularly important in primary screening where the major concern is that a toxic effect be detected. The following points apply to such detection.

1. Buelke-Sam and Kimmel (19), Rodier (110), and Coyle et al. (36) have discussed a variety of considerations in subject selection, and the reader is referred to these sources for more complete discussion. However, for economic and historical reasons, rodents appear the most likely subjects for primary behavioral teratology screening. The use of other species to investigate specific behavioral deficits is often appropriate, but usually at secondary test levels.

2. Establishing the "normal" behavioral profile of the subject population is a critical element of any primary screening battery. Such efforts coincidently provide valuable historical information about subject behavior and the utility of the methods being used to monitor that behavior. Once an adequate historical control population has been tested using a given behavioral method, the inherent variability of that method can be assessed. We are applying an approach to evaluate behavioral teratologic methods that was proposed by Nelson and Holson (86) for more conventional teratologic endpoints, e.g., fetotoxicity and weight reduction. First, the magnitude of treatment-effect the procedure should detect is determined, e.g., a 25% change in response. Using historical variance data, one can then determine the minimum number of subjects needed to demonstrate such an effect at a given confidence level using the statistical method of Winne (156).

In our laboratory, we have evaluated the ontogeny of two neuromotor responses in rats using this method: the surface righting reflex and negative geotaxic response (93). When coefficients of variation ($CV = 100 \times SD/\bar{X} \times 100$) were calculated for each measure, righting reflex response times were more variable (larger CVs) than were negative geotaxic turning times both within and across pups. Such variability inherently contributes to increased or decreased methods sensitivity in uncovering toxic effects. For example, given the variability we have found in righting times on the first of three trials at postnatal day 2, a sample size of 80 litters per treatment group would be needed to detect a 25% change in righting times at the $p = 0.05$ level. The variability of repeated measures would require 66 litters per group to demonstrate a comparable change. However, the lower CVs obtained for negative geotaxis suggest that this measure may be potentially useful for early detection of neuromotor dysfunction. Given the variability observed in our control population on the first of three trials on postnatal day 8, a sample size of 13 litters per group would be required to demonstrate a 25% change in turning times; variability for repeated measures on this day would require that 17 litters per group be used.

Butcher et al. (24) have suggested another potential methodological use for historical control performance data. Once the normal range of behavior is defined for a particular method by repeated use, and the sensitivity of the method established using several positive control agents, then new compounds could be tested without reference to a concurrent positive control group. Appropriate test administration would be assured by demonstrating that the mean and variance of the negative controls fell within the established range of historical data. Under such circumstances, a test group not differing from controls could more confidently be evaluated as not showing a toxic effect. Such an approach would be of economic benefit to a primary screening program, as the time and number of animals required to include concurrent positive controls in such testing are very great. However, the initial use of known behavioral teratogens to define sensitivity and validity of behavioral methods is indeed essential (19,24).

3. In the primary screening context, a valid test is one that detects postnatal behavioral dysfunction following prenatal insult. The key issue is whether the observed behavioral change is a result of exposure to the agent under study. Tilson et al. (145) have proposed a systematic approach to validating behavioral toxicologic methods that appears to be applicable to screening. This approach compares compounds known to produce specific neurotoxic actions through the use of a battery of tests selected to detect a range of possible effects and to overlap in terms of functions evaluated. Test validation is achieved by showing that methods presumed to measure similar functions detect similar behavioral changes. Those techniques assumed to assess different processes are used to distinguish neurotoxic profiles. This approach assumes the use of well-defined, consistent procedures, adequate historical control information, and positive control agents with defined neurotoxic actions. Such efforts are needed in the development of behavioral teratology test systems. Availability of data resulting from tests that have been validated in this fashion is essential to risk estimation. The utilization of nonvalidated test procedures is of little value within a primary screening system.

4. There is considerable polarization in the scientific community concerning regimentation imposed by standardized procedures, even for primary detection screens (19,20,105,107,108,153). Opponents of standardized testing suggest that it may threaten the potential for development of new, more sensitive indicators of behavioral dysfunction and that strict adherence to an established battery may lead to "false" negative results because a particularly relevant test may not have been included in the battery. However, uniformity of behavioral methods and procedures is necessary to assure both comparability of results within and across laboratories (150) and the value of such data in risk estimation. The inconsistencies and seeming contradictions reported in the animal literature for several identified behavioral teratogens (e.g., lead and alcohol) as well as behavioral test methods (e.g., open field activity measures) clearly support this view.

Although the lack of comparability across laboratories precludes the integration of information essential for making decisions related to compound safety, there is no reason why researchers should be limited to only standardized tests. Indeed, the selection of such tests can only result from the information that is currently available on particular methods. The incorporation of new and better tests can only result from the development and subsequent standardization of other techniques. Therefore, the coincident evaluation of other methods would offer the potential for comparison of the reliability and sensitivity of the standard and new behavioral methods. If such a comparative approach were used and a particular behavioral method were shown to be less sensitive to known behavioral teratogens or to be a correlate of a simpler, less expensive, or more reliable method, such data would warrant the appropriate removal and substitution of techniques into the standard test battery. Any test battery could then be updated in light of new information concerning its sensitivity. This approach would provide the best opportunity for both state-of-the-art safety evaluation and innovative progress in the expanding field of behavioral teratology.

## CURRENT PRACTICES AND NEW DIRECTIONS IN BEHAVIORAL EVALUATION

In order to assess the behavioral teratogenic effects of any chemical, a test battery must sample from multiple behavioral endpoints. Ideally, six component subsystems should be evaluated: (a) physical growth and maturation, (b) reflex and motor development, (c) sensory function, (d) activity and reactivity levels, (e) learning and memory abilities, and (f) functioning in neurotransmitter systems. Ideally, these component systems should be evaluated throughout the lifespan of the animal, since behavioral deficits might be expressed in three major ways (49,131). First of all, a retardation in the rate of development of certain functions could occur. Second, alterations in the adult levels of function could be manifest. Third, an impairment in responding because of the premature onset of aging could occur. In order to comprehensively evaluate the behavioral teratogenic potential of any agent, a multiplicative, longitudinal approach is necessary.

An evaluation of the literature and survey information collected by Buelke-Sam and Kimmel (19) reveals the following information on currently used behavioral screening techniques: (a) behavioral evaluations are primarily based on the assessment of reflex and motor development, locomotor activity, and "sensory functioning"; (b) "sensory" evaluations are typically carried out in conjunction with other measures such as startle reflex testing or discrimination learning procedures; (c) behavioral studies also typically involve the evaluation of biological endpoints such as physical growth and maturation; and (d) most behavioral testing is done on adolescent or young adult animals, with the exception of reflex and motor development tests.

This information indicates that state-of-the-art testing in any given laboratory rarely involves sampling from all of the subsystems of behavior or a longitudinal approach to the detection of behavioral dysfunction. The incorporation of these two critical elements would be a positive step toward the creation of a test battery capable of providing answers to questions concerning compound safety. The significance and logistics of implementing a screening program utilizing a life-span approach will be considered first, followed by a discussion of the methods that are available for the evaluation of functioning in the six component systems outlined above. In the latter segment, techniques in current use and methods with promise for application in the screening framework will be discussed.

## Longitudinal Testing

A life-span approach could provide information on the rates of maturation and decline of function in experimental animals. By 6 weeks of age, the central nervous system of the rat in many ways approximates that of the adult (71,115). It may be conjectured that this time frame is comparable to the first 12 to 15 years of human life. In children, acceleration or retardation in development during that extensive maturational period has been shown to have significant impact on later function (14,15,26,39,76,78,100,120). Surprisingly, however, within a screening context, the ontogeny of function has generally not been evaluated except within the motor system (19). Information on alterations in rate of development in other systems must be obtained because of its importance not only as an endpoint in detecting toxicity but also to provide insight into the mechanisms underlying behavioral dysfunction. It may well be easiest to see the relationship between structure and function during the time period when the parallels unfold so rapidly.

The lack of life-span approaches in evaluation of behavioral teratogens may not simply reflect a lack of awareness of their importance. Methods have not been available that permit the evaluation of abilities in preweanling animals, i.e., tests that are compatible with the response capabilities of young animals (5,27,53,115). Also, a life-span approach would require holding animals to old age for further testing, and this would be costly. Strongly needed are methods suitable for testing very young animals and methods that may be diagnostic of adult function or of the onset of behavioral changes related to premature aging. In the discussions that follow on methods appropriate for the assessment of different behavioral functions, early testing will be addressed. The need for methods that are predictive of later dysfunction may be much more difficult to meet. At present, one may only advocate that at least a small sample of animals involved in behavioral teratology studies be maintained for testing at older ages and that the correlation between early and late behavioral manifestations be investigated.

## Categories of Behavioral Function

### Physical Growth and Maturation

An evaluation of an animal's general physical characteristics is important not only as an endpoint in the detection of toxicity but also as an aid in the interpretation of behavioral data. The presence of body weight differences in animals from different treatment groups may confound the results of several behavioral tests. For example, measurements of motor activity accomplished by mechanical devices such as jiggle cages or stabilimeters are influenced by animal weight (108). Interpretation of the results of such tests is limited when control or correction for such differences has not been accomplished. From a screening standpoint, differences in body weight alone provide significant information on the developmental toxicity of the chemical under evaluation.

Recording body weight and physical landmarks such as time of eye opening and incisor eruption is currently a matter of routine and has been proposed in most specific test batteries (49,63,132,147). The functional relevance of differences in the attainment of certain physical landmarks is not clear. Although the day of eye opening has been interpreted as an indicator of development in the CNS (68,158), this assumption does not appear to be valid. Schapiro et al. (119) compared biochemical, neurophysiological, and behavioral indices of CNS development in rats treated with thyroxine or cortisol with those of control animals. Although both hormonally treated groups showed an earlier age of eye opening than did controls, the thyroxine-treated group showed an acceleration in CNS development, whereas the cortisol group demonstrated retardation. Thus, although age of eye opening may be a correlate of serious alterations, it does not appear to be a reliable predictor of the type of altered neural development produced by insult. In addition, it may be more appropriate to compare physical landmark data in treated animals with historical control information, since variability may be too high for adequate statistical power to be reached when small numbers of litters are used. One must consider historical information so that the biological significance of a statistically significant difference may be evaluated.

## Reflex and Motor Development

Buelke-Sam and Kimmel (19) reported that reflex and motor development are the most widespread of all behavioral endpoints assessed in developmental toxicity studies. In developmental psychobiology, the neuromuscular system has been more thoroughly studied than any other in the developing animal. Methods used to assess neuromotor development in the rat were first introduced by Tilney and Kubie (143), further investigated by Bolles and Woods (17), and extended somewhat by Fox (43). The responses most frequently evaluated are the righting reflex, negative geotaxic response, auditory startle reflex, pivoting, grasping, and placing reflexes. These methodologies have remained virtually unchanged since their introduction in 1931. Other methods in current use have derived from studies by Altman et al. (5,6) and include evaluations of rotorod balancing, traversing rods, grasping and hanging duration, and locomotion. Measurement of the ontogeny of swimming behavior (119) is also a common technique for the evaluation of neuromotor development.

As previously mentioned, the neuromotor system is the only system commonly evaluated according to the ontogeny of function. The two most common behaviors evaluated are surface righting and auditory startle (19). Table 1 presents a sampling of studies in which alterations in these two reflexes have been investigated following prenatal exposures. In the majority of cases, treatment differences have not been detected by these tests, although other measures have often shown differences. When these tests have shown treatment effects, the effects usually have been accompanied by physical differences in the animals. These results question the utility of monitoring development of these two reflexes. The reader is referred particularly to our earlier discussion on the variability of the righting reflex measure. Other evaluations of motor development may be more useful, particularly those that have already been standardized by Tilson, Mitchell, and Cabe (145). Evaluations of motor development must be considered as apical endpoints in detecting toxicity, since the performance of certain responses is known to be influenced by testing conditions used and motivational state of the animals (45).

## Sensory Function

The direct evaluation of sensory function requires the use of extensive psychophysical testing (64,157). Unfortunately, psychophysical testing is too labor intensive and time consuming to be feasible within a primary screening context. The reader should consult Stebbins (135) or Geschieder (46) for excellent catalogs of psychophysical techniques if such measures are of interest.

The majority of researchers surveyed by Buelke-Sam and Kimmel (19) evaluated sensory systems only in conjunction with other measures such as auditory startle reflex testing or discrimination learning tests. This type of evaluation bears only "face validity" as a measure of the integrity of sensory function. Whereas an auditory startle test or a visual discrimination task may purport to evaluate a given sensory system, the information provided on actual sensory abilities is mainly of a dichotomous nature, i.e., the animal hears or does not hear, does or does not discriminate light from dark, etc.

One behavioral response that appears to be sensitive to a variety of sensory stimulus conditions is ultrasonic vocalization of neonatal rodents (13). Changes in vocalization rate have been reported to occur as a function of olfactory (4,90), thermal (51,88), and tactile (89) stimulus conditions. Different stimuli show different patterns of eliciting vocalization as a function of the age of the animal and corresponding maturational changes in the organism. Few neonatal responses show such systematic changes that are easily quantified and are related to easily quantifiable stimuli. The measurement of ultrasounds could potentially offer an assessment of the rate of development of sensitivity to various stimuli. Only a few studies have investigated the influence of prenatal treatment on the vocalization rates of rodent pups (1,2,56), but the results appear quite promising. Further work is needed to determine the utility of measuring ultrasounds as an indicant of responsiveness to sensory stimuli within a screening framework.

Measurements of responsiveness to sensory stimulation are by necessity indirect and apical. Since responsiveness to stimuli can only be measured through the

TABLE 1. Summary of studies in which the development of surface righting and/or auditory startle has been evaluated

| Agent | Species | Physical differences | Differences Righting | Differences Startle | Other behavioral differences | Source |
|---|---|---|---|---|---|---|
| Baygon | Albino CD | Yes | —[a] | Yes | Yes | 113 |
| Cannabis smoke | Wistar rats | Yes | No | — | Yes | 44 |
| Carbon monoxide | Long–Evans rats | Yes | No | — | Yes | 40 |
| Chlorazepate dipotassium | Long–Evans rats | Yes | No | No | Yes | 58 |
| Cyclophosphamide | Swiss–Webster mice | Yes | Yes | — | Yes | 99 |
| Diazepam | Sprague–Dawley rats | Yes | No | No | Yes | 25 |
| Ethanol | Sprague–Dawley rats | Yes | No | — | Yes | 72 |
| Fenfluramine | Sprague–Dawley rats | Yes | No | — | Yes | 25 |
| 5-Azacytidine | Mice | Yes | Yes | — | Yes | 112 |
| Hydroxyurea | Sprague–Dawley rats | Yes | No | No | No | 18 |
| Lead | Long–Evans rats | Yes | — | No | Yes | 91 |
| MAMA | Long–Evans rats | Yes | Yes | — | Yes | 65 |
| Maneb | CD rats | Yes | — | No | No | 62 |
| Phencyclidine | Cox Swiss albino mice | No | No | — | Yes | 48 |
| Phencyclidine | Sprague–Dawley rats | Yes | No | — | Yes | 61 |
| Prochlorperazine edisylate | Sprague–Dawley rats | Yes | No | — | Yes | 25 |
| Propoxyphene | Sprague–Dawley rats | Yes | No | — | Yes | 25 |
| Protein malnutrition | Wistar rats | Yes | Yes | Yes | Yes | 138 |
| Restraint stress | Porton–Wistar/ola rats | Yes | — | Yes | Yes | 11 |
| Undernutrition | Hooded Lister rats | Yes | No | Yes | Yes | 127 |
| Vitamin A | Sprague–Dawley rats | Yes | Yes | — | Yes | 25 |

[a]Dashes indicate that the test was not conducted.

animal's performance, factors such as behavioral state, motivation, and perceptual and neuromotor capacity intervene in any stimulus–response chain. Therefore, when interpreting the results of a behavioral test that purports to evaluate sensory function, the possible confounding of results by these intervening variables must be considered (34). Apical tests provide useful information for the detection of toxicity but can only provide direction for further investigations aimed at the delineation of dysfunction. In answering the treatment effect question at a primary screening level, such apicality is acceptable and, in fact, may be desirable. In order to elucidate the action(s) of a behavioral teratogen, further specific sensory testing that involves extensive procedural controls to investigate the influence of such intervening variables must be undertaken.

### Activity and Reactivity Levels

An animal's "activity level" is used here to refer to the incidence of spontaneous locomotor behavior that occurs within the context of a particular physical testing environment. The most common devices now used to monitor activity levels are the open field and the activity wheel (19). These two measures have been evaluated in several critical reviews (108,109,140,151), and the reader should consult these sources for an analysis of these and numerous other ways of measuring activity level. In brief, neither of the two devices elicits reliable behavioral response patterns principally because of the influence of variable environmental conditions during testing. Procedural variables are rarely controlled to the extent necessary to permit a meaningful comparison of data obtained in different laboratories (109,151). Reiter and MacPhail (108) evaluated several activity measurement techniques specifically in regard to their potential use in toxicity testing and concluded that information was insufficient to permit the selection of any one "most appropriate" technique. The selection of the apparatus should be based on the components of activity that the experimenter wishes to measure (i.e., gross motor behavior, ambulation, stereotypical responses) and on whether a quantitative or qualitative type of measurement is desired (108). Furthermore, to maximize the probability of detection of behavioral teratogenic effects on activity, a testing environment that yields low levels of spontaneous activity could be selected if hyperactivity is hypothesized, or one that yields a high activity level could be utilized when hypoactivity is predicted (109).

Activity measurement has been conducted most frequently in adolescent and young adult animals in behavioral teratology studies (19). However, the assessment of developmental activity patterns may also be of value within a screening context. Several studies in the rat have shown that a peak in activity level occurs between 14 and 16 days of age in normally developing animals (29,31,74,101). The development of brainstem catecholaminergic systems has been implicated as a mediator for the rise in activity seen during this period (30). A decline in activity to adult levels is seen in the third and fourth postnatal weeks. Data presented by Erinoff et al. (38) suggest that the maturation of neuronal systems that utilize dopamine as a neurotransmitter is necessary for this suppression in activity to occur. This contention is further supported by other studies of experimental dopamine depletion (121,122). An evaluation of developmental activity patterns could also provide an indirect means of assessing the maturation of certain neurochemical systems.

An animal's reactivity level is defined as its responsiveness to an external stimulus. Evaluations of reactivity primarily involve the measurement of startle responses. Within the screening context, the auditory startle response has usually been interpreted as an index of development of auditory function and has usually been scored dichotomously as present or absent. In a few studies, the amplitude of air puff or auditory startle responses has been quantitatively measured electronically (18,25,144). The incorporation of precise measurement of the magnitude of startle responses increases the informational value and sensitivity of startle response data at little additional cost or change in labor intensity for the experimenter. Thus, measurement of reactivity in conjunction with the measurement of habituation of startle responses should be considered important tools in the screening of behavioral teratogenic compounds. Data supporting this will be presented in the discussion on learning measures that follows.

### *Learning and Memory Abilities*

In the assessment of learning and memory function, the most common methods in use are active and passive avoidance, simple operant tasks, and instrumental behavior in water, T or Y mazes (19). These tests are typically conducted in young adult animals and not in preweaning or aged animals. This approach may provide data that show treated and control animals to be functionally similar or dissimilar as adults, but no information is obtained regarding the rate of development of such responses or the rate of decline in function with age. Since an alteration in the information-processing ability of an animal is perhaps least obvious when only subtle changes are involved (22), rigorous tests must be utilized to uncover such deficits in function. As pointed out by Butcher (22), behavioral teratogenic agents that may produce deficits in learning or memory abilities must be identified in the laboratory because this sort of cause–effect relationship has such a low probability for clinical detection. Learning measures for use in adult animals are numerous; for excellent procedural reviews, the reader should consult Kling and Riggs (64), Burt (21), or Hulse et al. (55).

The remainder of this discussion is devoted to methods that afford an assessment of learning and memory skills in neonatal as well as adult animals. Criteria for inclusion in this discussion are that the methods be appropriate to the restricted response capabilities of neonatal animals and that testing require only a limited amount of time per animal. In addition, an effort has been made to include methods representative of different forms of learning. It must be recognized that different tests measure different types of function: learning is not a unitary process (141). Two broad classes of learning exist: habituation, which implies decreases in already existing responses to particular stimuli, and "associative" learning, which involves the acquisition of a response to a previously neutral stimulus as a result of temporal association or reinforcement contingencies (141). Two major subclasses of associative learning are classical and instrumental conditioning. Table 2 presents the techniques that appear to be most promising for use within a primary screening framework. In the discussion that follows, only the one task for which the most extensive ontogenetic data are available is discussed for each major category of learning.

Campbell and Stehouwer (32) have presented an excellent series of studies on the ontogeny of habituation and sensitization in the rat. In brief, habituation is the process that occurs when an organism ceases to respond to a stimulus that is repeatedly presented (50,141). The detailed operational definition of habituation involves nine criteria as put forth by Thompson and Spencer (142). Only response systems that show all or most of these criteria can technically be considered as models of the habituation phenomenon. One response system that does so and can be used in a developmental approach is the shock-induced limb withdrawal response (32). The type of response elicited by electric shock varies with developmental age, although threshold sensitivity does not (136). Three- and 6-day old animals respond by diffuse squirming, whereas 10- and 15-day-olds show discrete withdrawal responses. This qualitative change in the response appears to be related to the maturation of inhibitory mechanisms that modulate diffuse neuronal activity. The change from diffuse to discrete responding occurs at about day 8 or day 9 for the forelimb withdrawal response (32,137) and for head turning elicited by an air puff (41).

Among the quantitative endpoints of interest in the habituation paradigm are the amplitude and latency of the elicited responses. Response latency decreases with development such that 15-day-olds show response latencies two to three times shorter than 3-day-olds (32). This is correlated with increased myelination of axons in the neural response pathway (60). Response amplitudes increase with age to an asymptotic level reached about day 15. Optimal procedural variables such as shock intensity and length of the interstimulus interval also vary as a function of age (32). Retention of habituation learning is not shown by 3- and 6-day-olds but is present in both 10- and 15-day-old animals.

Overall, it thus appears that ontogenetic changes in habituation learning and retention could be assessed by testing at 6, 10, and 15 days of age. Given an 8-sec interstimulus interval, this measure would require approximately 20 min testing time per animal. It is therefore an ideal measure of simple learning phenomena which might yield important information on the rate of neural development. The same paradigm can be used on neonatal and adult animals, providing the potential for a longitudinal approach to treatment influences on simple learning abilities.

Shock avoidance responding has been chosen as a representative of instrumental learning because it occurs rapidly, can be demonstrated in a short test period, and because shock has been shown to induce equivalent levels of motivation across a wide range of ages (27,32). Nagy (80) reviewed the literature on shock avoidance learning with primary emphasis on whether or not learning and memory capabilities

TABLE 2. *Tests suitable for an ontogenetic analysis of learning in rodents*

| Test | Earliest age at which acquisition has been shown | Earliest age at which 24-hr retention shown | Variables with developmental significance | Possible critical testing ages | Testing time estimated/animal(s) | References |
|---|---|---|---|---|---|---|
| **Habituation** | | | | | | |
| Habituation of forelimb withdrawal | 3 days | 10 days | Response latency Response amplitude Retention Shock intensity Interstimulus interval length | 6–15 days | 20 min/animal | 32 136 |
| Habituation of air puff startle | 1 day | — | Rate of habituation | 6–12 days | 40–60 min/ animal | 41 |
| Prepulse inhibition and habituation of the acoustic startle response | 12 days | — | Prepulse modification Response amplitude Interstimulus interval | 12–16 days | 40 min/animal | 92 |
| **Instrumental learning** | | | | | | |
| Straight alley shock escape | 5 days | 9 days | Number of competing responses | 5–9 days | 60–80 min/ animal | 81 |
| Discriminated escape in T-maze | 9 days | 11 days | Number of correct choice-point turns Number of competing responses | 7–13 days | 60–80 min/ animal | 83 85 |
| Step-down passive avoidance | 7 days | 19 days | Number of trials to criterion | 7–19 days | 15–25 min/ animal | 102 |
| Appetitive learning in straight-alley runway | 10 days | 12 days | Partial reinforcement extinction effects | 10–15 days | 30–40 min/ animal | 7–9 33 |
| **Classical conditioning** | | | | | | |
| Odor aversion learning | 2 days | 6–8 days under certain conditions (see text) | CS–UCS interval Stimulus-preexposure effect | 4–8 days | 35 min/litter | 115 |

for instrumental responding developed within the limited age range of 5 to 20 days. Many early investigators concluded that instrumental learning could not take place until a certain level of postnatal maturation had occurred, approximately 15 to 20 days (28). Unfortunately, however, this suggestion was based on studies that utilized dependent measures that might have been beyond the limited sensory and response capabilities of neonatal animals (80).

Nagy and co-workers conducted a series of studies on the development of learning and memory in mice in the straight escape runway, a T maze, and a passive avoidance paradigm using procedures and performance requirements appropriate to the abilities of young animals. For the straight escape task, learning was shown at 5 days of age, and 24-hr retention was first shown at 9 days of age (81,82,102). The T-maze task was somewhat more complicated in that it required the correct choice of a turn in order for the animal to avoid shock. In this task, acquisition was not shown prior to day 9 (83), and 24-hr retention was not exhibited until 11 days of age, although enhanced performance was shown in 10-day-olds trained on day 9 as compared to naive 10-day-old animals. Passive avoidance studies on mice 7, 11, 15, 19, and 100 days of age conducted by Ray and Nagy (102) showed an inverted-U-shaped function for the acquisition and retention of this task. The 15-day-old animals required more acquisition trials than other age groups. The differences shown by 15-day-olds may not represent a lack of inhibitory control but, a by-product of the increased spontaneous activity levels known to occur in animals of this age (28,29,80,102). Collectively, these data have been interpreted as supporting the contention that young mice are capable of associative learning.

In a screening context, it appears that retention may be more sensitive to developmental insult than is acquisition. The effects of hypothyroidism and under-nutrition on T-maze learning have been investigated (77,84). Early exposure to excess thyroid hormone has been reported to advance early stages of CNS maturation (10,117,118). Murphy and Nagy (77) found no differences in acquisition of the T-maze task in thyroxine-treated animals, although a 2-day acceleration in the appearance of 24-hr memory was shown. When CNS maturation was experimentally retarded through postnatal undernutrition, mice also showed no difference in acquisition of the T-maze task but showed a 2-day delay in the emergence of 24-hr retention for the learned avoidance response. Incorporation of discriminated avoidance learning utilizing the T maze and testing on days 7, 9, 11, and 13 might provide important information on the ontogeny of retention of associative learning.

The acquisition and retention of classical conditioning in the newborn rat has received little attention, although it has been investigated in other species (73, 134,146), perhaps most thoroughly in the human infant (69,70,123).

The ontogeny of odor aversion learning, a form of classical conditioning, has been systematically investigated in rats by Rudy and Cheatle (114,115). The testing paradigm involves placing an animal in scented bedding [the conditioned stimulus (CS)], then, after some interval, injecting it with lithium chloride (LiCl), an illness-inducing agent [the unconditioned stimulus (UCS)]. The animal is then returned to the scented bedding for a duration of 30 min or to its home cage. The acquisition of the learned aversion is tested in conjunction with its retention several days following the CS–UCS pairing. The dependent measure of interest is the proportion of time (within 150 sec) that the animal spends over the CS-scented shavings versus over bedding with a novel odor.

An excellent review of this work may be found in Rudy and Cheatle (115). In brief, even 2-day-old animals acquire behavioral aversions to the scent paired with LiCl-induced illness and show retention of this learning when tested 6 days later. Under conditions in which injection is given immediately following exposure to the CS scent, 2-day-olds learn and retain as well as 14-day-olds or even adult animals. However, manipulation of the length of the interval between exposure and injection and the animal's previous exposure to the olfactory CS have revealed important age-related differences. When a 15-min delay exists between exposure and injection, 2- and 4-day-old animals cannot learn the CS–UCS association, although 6- and 8-day-olds can acquire the aversion. Preexposure to the conditioned stimulus 4 hr prior to a CS–UCS pairing interferes with acquisition of the task in 8-day-olds but not in 2-day-olds. It thus appears that for both of these procedural variables, the memory mechanisms influenced by olfactory stimulation are more fully developed in 8- than in 2-day-old rat pups. Investigation of the delayed learning and the stimulus preexposure effects in 2-, 4-, 6-, and 8-day-old animals could provide significant information on the rate of maturation of these memory processes in studies of developmental toxicity.

The habituation, instrumental learning, and classical conditioning data presented above all indicate the 8- to 11-day age period to be of particular importance in the development of memory abilities. It is therefore recommended that this time period be investigated in behavioral teratology protocols so that possible differences in the development of retention abilities can be assessed.

### Functioning in Neurotransmitter Systems

Investigation of major behavioral processes that involve a particular neurotransmitter system provides information on the functional integrity of a given system. Such investigations usually employ specific drugs known to affect a transmitter system and the measurement of changes in behavioral responses that result following administration of the drugs (29,59,95,129). Alterations in the threshold level or qualitative aspects of response in treated versus control animals could suggest differences in underlying neurochemical systems. Many compounds are known to produce changes in postnatal neurochemical systems when exposures occur during the pre- or perinatal period (125). However, identifying changes in actual CNS levels of particular neurochemical substances alone cannot answer questions regarding the functional significance of these changes. Therefore, investigations of the functional development of responsiveness to psychotropic agents and of behavioral systems thought to depend on specific neurotransmitter systems are warranted (129). The current state of knowledge on the correlation between discrete behaviors of an organism and underlying physiological processes is limited (125).

The following discussion will address the ontogenetic appearance of a few behavioral responses thought to result from function in certain neurotransmitter systems and behavioral patterns shown in developmental administration of psychoactive drugs.

As mentioned previously, the developmental activity peak appears to be related to functioning in the catecholaminergic system (30,38,121,122). Therefore, an early ontogenic assessment of spontaneous activity levels might provide some indication of maturation in central catecholaminergic function, particularly the dopaminergic system.

Some information suggests that the ontogeny of swimming behavior also may reflect catecholaminergic development (67,116,119). Perinatal thyroxine and corticosterone treatments, which influence the rate of CNS development, have been shown to influence the maturation of swimming behavior (119). Compared to controls, this development is accelerated by perinatal thyroxine and delayed by perinatal cortisol treatment. Lengvari et al. (67) have shown that neonatal thyroxine and corticosterone treatment significantly affect the developmental pattern of hypothalamic and mesencephalic catecholamines in directions consistent with accelerated or delayed CNS development.

Porsolt et al. (95) have shown in rats that the duration of immobility induced by forced swimming is influenced primarily by agents that modify central catecholamine activity. Immobilization is exhibited by untreated rats and mice when they are placed in the water within a restricted space from which escape is not permitted (94,96–98). This immobilization is characterized by floating in a slightly hunched but upright posture, and only those movements necessary to keep the head above water are observed. Agents that modify central catecholamines appear to alter inversely the duration of immobility; i.e., agents that increase catecholamine activity decrease the duration of the response, and agents that reduce catecholamine activity act to increase the duration (95). The immobilization response appears to be most prevalent in normally developing rats between days 32 and 36 (J. Adams, *personal observations*). Investigation of spontaneous levels of immobilization at 29, 35, and 41 days of age might be particularly informative in comparing maturational rates in treated and control animals.

Interestingly, decreased behavioral responsiveness to drugs that act on the catecholamine system has been noted during this period (12,66,103,104). Lanier and Isaacson (66) reported that rats 18 to 22 days or 45 to 49 days of age responded to amphetamine through increased open field activity, whereas 34- to 38-day-old rats did not show increased activity levels at any dose tested. In the "hole poke" apparatus, animals of this age have been shown to respond to amphetamine but to a lesser extent than younger or older animals (130). A decreased behavioral responsiveness to clonidine, an $\alpha$-adrenergic receptor-stimulating agent, and to apomorphine, a dopaminergic receptor-stimulating agent, has also been shown around 35 days of age in rats (103,104). Additionally, this age group shows an increased sensitivity to haloperidol-induced catalepsy as compared to younger and older animals (130). Haloperidol is a catecholaminergic receptor-blocking agent. Overall, it appears that the period around day 35 may be of particular interest in examining drug responsiveness. The changes in responsiveness during this period relative to earlier and later developmental ages suggest that significant developmental changes are occurring around this time. Therefore, investigations of responsiveness to catecholaminergic agents in 25-, 35-, and 45-day-old animals may be used to uncover differences in maturational rate in treated and contol animals.

Drugs that either increase synaptic serotonin or directly stimulate postsynaptic serotonin receptors produce a cluster of behaviors in rats (52,59,75,126). This behavioral syndrome is characterized by resting tremor, rigidity, reciprocal forepaw treading, Straub tail, hindlimb abduction, and lateral head weaving. The behavioral patterns produced by the serotonin precursor, 5-hydroxytryptophan, and the agonists, 5-methoxy-$N$,$N$-dimethyltryptamine and $p$-chloroamphetamine represent a valuable tool for estimating functional activity in central serotonergic systems. Jacobs (59) has studied the ontogeny of this behavioral syndrome in neonatal rats and found that it is not present prior to day 14 but is evident at 17 days of age.

Thus, assessment of ontogenetic behavioral effects of psychopharmacological agents may provide a means of investigating functional maturation in the nervous system. An excellent review of this approach may be found in Spear (129). Often drug responsiveness either does not appear until a certain age is reached or does not follow a monotonic pattern of emergence. Such information may suggest particularly sensitive ages for testing. The utilization of pharmacological manipulations in adult animals who have been developmentally exposed to a toxin might also be useful in providing information on differences in dosage thresholds for the expression of defined behavioral changes (59) or for "challenging" the integrity of a given response system (54,106,144).

In adult animals, pharmacological challenges have been successful at "uncovering" treatment effects not revealed under nonstimulated conditions. Hughes and Sparber (54) investigated operant learning in animals prenatally treated with methylmercury and found no differences until an amphetamine "challenge" was given. The administration of such psychoactive agents to treated animals may help to unmask treatment effects that can be compensated for under normal task demands (54).

Administering psychoactive agents to developmentally exposed adult animals can also be used to provide information on drug sensitivity. Behavioral teratogens, by altering underlying neurochemical systems, may alter the threshold for a given drug-induced response. Reiter et al. (106) demonstrated a reduced sensitivity to amphetamine-induced activity effects in animals perinatally exposed to lead. An increased sensitivity to amphetamine-induced activity changes has recently been reported in the female offspring of animals who received prenatal amphetamine exposure on days 12 to 15 of gestation (3). In combination, these data suggest that pharmacological challenges may be a valuable tool for both early detection of ontogenetic expressions of neurotoxicity and uncovering functional deficits in apparently normal adults.

## SUMMARY

The current inability to specify a single approach or specific behavioral test battery does not outweigh the necessity for behavioral teratology screening. Any test system should include a hierarchy of behavioral evaluation. Initial, primary screening to detect toxicity should include a broad developmental series that measures multiple CNS subsystem functioning. Secondary testing may include more sophisticated and specific techniques chosen to help delineate the types and degrees of toxicity produced. Several examples have been presented of currently available behavioral methods that show promise for early detection of behavioral dysfunction. However, the utility of these techniques can only be determined through efforts involving standardization and validation of the methods themselves.

Anatomical, biochemical, and behavioral evaluations are complementary means of assessing CNS function, and such combined approaches to behavioral teratology may help to delineate toxic actions involved in the production of behavioral deficits. Such information contributes not only to data interpretation but also to extrapolation. A rodent does not possess the complex nervous system or behavioral repertoire of man. Thus, there seems little reason to assume that a rodent will display the same overt manifestations as man following developmental neurotoxic insult. However, if particular neural structures and/or biochemical pathways are discerned to be the susceptible targets of insult, then a better estimate can be made of potential risk to the developing human. The first step toward achieving this goal is the use of the best available methods to evaluate potential behavioral teratogens, while continued efforts are made in the development and validation of more sensitive indicators of toxicity.

## ACKNOWLEDGMENTS

The authors wish to express their appreciation to Rose Huber and Cindy Hartwick for their precision, patience, and good nature throughout the preparation of this manuscript.

## REFERENCES

1. Adams, J. (1979): Behavioral assessment of the teratogenic effects of prenatal exposure to ethanol in the rat. *Teratology*, 19(2):17A.
2. Adams, J. (1980): Neonatal vocalizations following prenatal hypervitaminosis A in the rat. *Teratology*, 21(2):25A.
3. Adams, J., Buelke-Sam, J., and Kimmel, C. A. (1980): Postnatal behavioral alterations in rats exposed prenatally to low doses of *d*-amphetamine. In: *Proceedings of International Society for Developmental Psychobiology*. Cincinnati, p.29.
4. Adams, J., and Holcomb, P. (1980): Odor condition as a determinant of vocalization rate and signal duration in neonatal rat pups. In: *Proceedings of International Society for Developmental Psychobiology*. Cincinnati, p. 44.
5. Altman, J., Brunner, R. L., Bulert, F. G., and Sudershan, K. (1974): The development of behavior in normal and brain-damaged infant rats, studied with homing as motivation. In: *Drugs and the Developing Brain*, edited by A. Vernadakis and N. Weiner, pp. 321–350. Plenum Press, New York.

6. Altman, J., and Sudershan, K. (1975): Postnatal development of locomotion in the laboratory rat. *Anim. Behav.*, 23:896–920.
7. Amsel, A. (1979): The ontogeny of appetitive learning and persistence in the rat. In: *Ontogeny of Learning and Memory*, edited by N. A. Spear and B. A. Campbell, pp. 189–224. Lawrence Erlbaum Associates, Hillsdale, New Jersey.
8. Amsel, A., Burdette, D. R., and Letz, P. (1976): Appetitive learning, patterned alternation, and extinction in 10-day-old rats with nonlactating suckling as the reward. *Nature*, 262:816–818.
9. Amsel, A., Letz, R., and Burdette, D. R. (1977): Appetitive learning and extinction in 11-day-old rat pups: Effects of various reinforcement conditions. *J. Comp. Physiol. Psychol.*, 91:1156–1167.
10. Balazs, R., and Richter, D. (1973): Effects of hormones on the biochemical maturation of the brain. In: *Biochemistry of the Developing Brain, Vol. 1*, edited by W. Himwich, pp. 38–69. Marcel Dekker, New York.
11. Barlow, S. M., Knight, A. F., and Sullivan, F. M. (1978): Delay in postnatal growth and development of offspring produced by maternal restraint stress during pregnancy in the rat. *Teratology*, 18(2):211–240.
12. Bauer, R. H., and Duncan, D. L. (1975): Differential effects of *d*-amphetamine in mature and immature rats. *Physiol. Behav.*, 3:312–316.
13. Bell, R. W. (1974): Ultrasounds in small rodents: Arousal-produced and arousal-producing. *Dev. Psychobiol.*, 7(1):39–42.
14. Berges, M., Lezine, E., Harrison, A., and Boisselier, F. (1972): The "syndrome of the post-premature child": A study of its significance, Part 1. *Early Child Dev. Care*, 1:239–284.
15. Berges, M., Lezine, E., Harrison, A., and Boisselier, F. (1973): The "syndrome of the post-premature child": A study of its significance, Part II. *Early Child Dev. Care*, 2:61–94.
16. Bignami, G. (1976): Behavioral pharmacology and toxicology. *Annu. Rev. Pharmacol.*, 16:329–366.
17. Bolles, R. C., and Woods, P. S. (1964): The ontogeny of behavior in the albino rat. *Anim. Behav.*, 12:427–441.
18. Brunner, R. L., McLean, M., Vorhees, C. V., and Butcher, R. E. (1978): A comparison of behavioral and anatomical measures of hydroxyurea-induced abnormalities. *Teratology*, 18(3):379–384.
19. Buelke-Sam, J., and Kimmel, C. A. (1979): Development and standardization of screening methods for behavioral teratology. *Teratology*, 20:17–29.
20. Burkhalter, J. E., and Balster, R. L. (1979): Behavioral teratology evaluation of trichloromethane in mice. *Neurobehav. Toxicol.*, 1:199–205.
21. Burt, G. S. (1975): Use of behavioral techniques in the assessment of environmental contaminants. In: *Behavioral Toxicology*, edited by B. Weiss and V. G. Laties, pp. 241–264. Plenum Press, New York.
22. Butcher, R. E. (1976): Behavioral testing as a method for assessing risk. *Environ. Health Perspect.*, 18:75–81.
23. Butcher, R. E., Hawver, K., Burbacher, J., and Scott, W. (1975): Behavioral effects from antenatal exposure to teratogens. In: *Aberrant Development in Infancy: Human and Animal Studies*, edited by N. R. Ellis, pp. 161–167. Lawrence Erlbaum Associates, Hillsdale, New Jersey.
24. Butcher, R. E., Hoar, R. M., Nolan, G. A., and Vorhees, C. V. (1979): Inter-laboratory comparison of behavioral testing. *J. Assoc. Off. Anal. Chem.*, 62:840–843.
25. Butcher, R. E., and Vorhees, C. V. (1979): A preliminary test battery for the investigation of the behavioral teratology of selected psychotropic drugs. *Neurobehav. Toxicol. [Suppl.]*, 1:207–212.
26. Cameron, J., Livson, N., and Bayley, N. (1967): Infant vocalizations and their relationship to mature intelligence. *Science*, 157:331–333.
27. Campbell, B. A. (1967): Developmental studies of learning and motivation in infra-primate mammals. In: *Early Behavior: Comparative and Developmental Approaches*, edited by H. W. Stevenson, E. H. Hess, and H. L. Rheingold, pp. 43–72. John Wiley and Sons, New York.
28. Campbell, B. A., and Coulter, X. (1976): Neural and psychological processes underlying the development of learning and memory. In: *Habituation: Perspectives from Child Development, Animal Behavior, and Neurophysiology*, edited by T. J. Tighe and R. N. Leaton, pp.129–157. Lawrence Erlbaum Associates, Hillsdale, New Jersey.
29. Campbell, B. A., Lytle, L. D., and Fibiger, H. C. (1969): Ontogeny of adrenergic arousal and cholinergic inhibitory mechanisms in the rat. *Science*, 166:637–638.
30. Campbell, B. A., and Mabry, P. D. (1973): The role of catecholamines in behavioral arousal during ontogenesis. *Psychopharmacology*, 31:253–264.

31. Campbell, B. A., and Raskin, L. A. (1978): Ontogeny of habituation and sensitization in the rat. In: *Ontogeny of Learning and Memory*, edited by N. A. Spear and B. A. Campbell, pp. 67–100. Lawrence Erlbaum Associates, Hillsdale, New Jersey.
32. Campbell, B. A., and Stehouwer, D. J. (1979): Ontogeny of habituation and sensitization in the rat. In: *Ontogeny of Learning and Memory*, edited by N. A. Spear and B. A. Campbell, pp. 67–100. Lawrence Erlbaum Associates, Hillsdale, New Jersey.
33. Chen, J. S., and Amsel, A. (1980): Learned persistence at 11–12 days but not at 10–11 days in infant rats. *Dev. Psychobiol.*, 13(5):481–491.
34. Clifton, R. K., and Nelson, M. N. (1976): Developmental study of habituation in infants: The importance of paradigm, response system, and state. In: *Habituation: Perspectives from Child Development, Animal Behavior, and Neurophysiology*, edited by T. J. Tighe and R. N. Leaton, pp. 159–205. Lawrence Erlbaum Associates, Hillsdale, New Jersey.
35. Coyle, I., Wayner, M. J., and Singer, G. (1976): Behavioral teratogenesis: A critical evaluation. *Pharmacol. Biochem. Behav.*, 4:191–200.
36. Coyle, I., Wayner, M. J., and Singer, G. (1980): Behavioral teratogenesis: A critical evaluation. In: *Advances in the Study of Birth Defects, Vol. 4, Neural and Behavioral Teratology*, edited by T. V. N. Persuad, pp. 111–133. University Park Press, Baltimore.
37. Davis, W. M., Bedford, J. A., Buelke-Sam, J. L., Guinn, M. M., Hatoum, H. T., Waters, I. W., Wilson, M. C., and Braude, M. C. (1978): Acute toxicity and gross behavioral effects of amphetamine, four methoxyamphetamines, and mescaline in rodents, dogs and monkeys. *Toxicol. Appl. Pharmacol.*, 45:49–62.
38. Erinoff, L., MacPhail, R. C., Heller, A., and Seiden, L. S. (1979): Age-dependent effects of 6-hydroxydopamine on locomotor activity in the rat. *Brain Res.*, 64:195–205.
39. Faust, M. S. (1960): Developmental maturity as a determinant in prestige of adolescent girls. *Child Dev.*, 31:173–184.
40. Fechter, L. D., and Annau, Z. (1980): Prenatal carbon monoxide exposure alters behavioral development. *Neurobehav. Toxicol.*, 2(1):7–11.
41. File, S. T., and Scott, E. M. (1976): Acquisition and retention of habituation in the preweanling rat. *Dev. Psychobiol.*, 9:97–107.
42. Fox, D. A., Overmann, S. R., and Woolley, D. E. (1979): Neurobehavioral ontogeny of neonatally lead-exposed rats. II. Maximal electroshock seizures in developing and adult rats. *Neurotoxicology*, 1:149–170.
43. Fox, M. W. (1965): Reflex ontogeny and behavioral development of the mouse. *Anim. Behav.*, 13:234–241.
44. Fried, P. A. (1976): Short and long-term effects of prenatal cannabis inhalation upon rat offspring. *Psychopharmacology*, 50:285–291.
45. Gard, C., Hard, E., Larsson, K., and Petersson, V. (1967): The relationship between sensory stimulation and gross motor behavior during the postnatal development in the rat. *Anim. Behav.*, 15:563–567.
46. Gescheider, G. A. (1976): *Psychophysics: Methods and Theory*. Lawrence Erlbaum Associates, Hillsdale, New York.
47. Golub, M. S. (1980): Behavioral teratogenesis. In: *Advances in Perinatal Medicine*, edited by A. Milunsky, E. Friedman, and L. Gluck, pp. 231–293. Plenum Press, New York.
48. Goodwin, P. J., Perez, V. J., Eatwell, J. C., Palet, J. L., and Jaworski, M. T. (1980): Phencyclidine: Effects of chronic administration in the female mouse on gestation, maternal behavior, and the neonates. *Psychopharmacology.*, 69(1):63–67.
49. Grant, L. D. (1976): Research strategies for behavioral teratology studies. *Environ. Health Perspect.*, 18:85–94.
50. Groves, P. M., and Thompson, R. F. (1970): Habituation: A dual process theory. *Psychol. Rev.*, 77(5):419–450.
51. Hart, F. H., and King, J. A. (1966): Distress vocalizations of young in two subspecies of *Peromyscus maniculatus*. *J. Mammal.*, 47:287–293.
52. Holman, R. B., Elliot, G., Kramer, A., Seagraves, E., and Barchas, J. (1977): Stereotypy and hyperactivity in rats receiving ethanol and a monoamine oxidase inhibitor. *Psychopharmacology*, 54:237–239.
53. Horowitz, F. D. (1975): Visual attention, auditory stimulation, and language discrimination in young infants. *Monogr. Res. Child Dev.*, 39:5–6.

54. Hughes, J. A., and Sparber, S. B. (1978): *d*-Amphetamine unmasks postnatal consequences of exposure to methylmercury in utero: Methods for studying behavioral teratogenesis. *Pharmacol. Biochem. Behav.*, 8:365–375.
55. Hulse, S. H., Fowler, H., and Honig, W. K., editors (1978): *Cognitive Processes in Animal Behavior*. Lawrence Erlbaum Associates, Hillsdale, New Jersey.
56. Hunt, L., Smotherman, W., Wiener, S., and Levine, S. (1976): Nutritional variables and their effect on the development of ultrasonic vocalizations in rat pups. *Physiol. Behav.*, 17(6):1037–1039.
57. Iwata, S., Ichimura, M., Matsuzawa, Y., Takasaki, Y., and Sasaoka, M. (1979): Behavioral studies in rats treated with monosodium L-glutamate during the early stages of life. *Toxicol. Lett.*, 4:345–357.
58. Jackson, V., DeMyer, W., and Hingtgen, J. (1980): Delayed maze-learning in rats after prenatal exposure to clorazepate. *Arch. Neurol.*, 37(6):350–351.
59. Jacobs, B. L. (1976): An animal model for studying central serotonergic synapses. *Life Sci.*, 19:777–786.
60. Jacobson, M. (1970): *Developmental Neurobiology*. Holt, Rinehart and Winston, New York.
61. Jordan, R. L., Young, T. R., Dinwiddie, S. H., and Harry, G. J. (1979): Phencyclidine-induced morphological and behavioral alterations in the neonatal rat. *Pharmacol. Biochem. Behav.*, 11:39–45.
62. Kavlock, R., and Chernoff, N. (1978): Postnatal toxicity of maneb, EBIS, and ETU in rats. *Toxicol. Appl. Pharmacol.*, 45(1):358.
63. Kimmel, C. A. (Chairperson) (1977): Final report of the Committee on Postnatal Evaluation of Animals Subjected to Insult During Development. Manuscript available from chairperson, National Center for Toxicological Research, Jefferson, Arkansas.
64. Kling, J. A., and Riggs, L. A., editors (1971): *Woodworth and Schlosberg's Experimental Psychology*. Holt, Rinehart and Winston, New York.
65. Lai, H., Quock, R. M., Makous, W., Horita, A., and Jen, L. S. (1978): Methylazoxymethanol acetate: Effect of postnatal injection on brain amines and behavior. *Pharmacol. Biochem. Behav.*, 8(3):251–257.
66. Lanier, L. P., and Isaacson, R. L. (1977): Early developmental changes in the locomotor response to amphetamine and their relation to hippocampal function. *Brain Res.*, 126:567–575.
67. Lengvari, I., Branch, B. J., and Taylor, A. N. (1980): Effects of perinatal thyroxine and/or corticosterone treatment on the ontogenesis of hypothalamic and mesencephalic norepinephrine and dopamine content. *Dev. Neurosci.*, 3:59–65.
68. Levine, S. (1960): Stimulation in infancy. *Sci. Am.*, 202(6):80–86.
69. Lipsitt, L. P. (1967): Learning in the human infant. In: *Early Behavior: Comparative and Developmental Approaches*, edited by H. W. Stevenson, E. H. Hess, and H. L. Rheingold, pp. 225–247. John Wiley and Sons, New York.
70. Lipsitt, L. P., and Kaye, H. (1964): Conditioned sucking in the human newborn. *Psychon. Sci.*, 1:29–30.
71. Mabry, P. D., and Campbell, B. A. (1977): Developmental psychopharmacology. In: *Handbook of Psychopharmacology, Vol. 7*, edited by L. L. Iverson, S. D. Iverson, and S. H. Snyder, pp. 393–444. Plenum Press, New York.
72. Martin, J. C., Martin, D. C., Sigman, G., and Radow, B. (1977): Offspring survival, development, and operant performance following maternal ethanol consumption. *Dev. Psychobiol.*, 10(5):435–446.
73. Mason, W. A., and Harlow, H. F. (1958): Formation of conditioned responses in infant monkeys. *J. Comp. Physiol. Psychol.*, 51:68–70.
74. Melberg, P. E., Ahlenius, S., Engel, J., and Lundborg, P. (1976): Ontogenetic development of locomotor activity and rate of tyrosine hydroxylation. *Psychopharmacologia*, 49:119–123.
75. Metys, J., and Dlabac, A. (1980): Action of psychotropic drugs on behavioral syndrome induced by 5-hydroxytryptophan in rats. *Act. Nerv. Super. (Praha)*, 22(2):94–96.
76. Moore, T. (1967): Language and intelligence: A longitudinal study of the first eight years. *Hum. Dev.*, 10:881–906.
77. Murphy, J. M., and Nagy, Z. M. (1976): Neonatal thyroxine stimulation accelerates the maturation of both locomotor and memory processes in mice. *J. Comp. Physiol. Psychol.*, 90:1082–1091.
78. Mussen, P. H., and Jones, M. C. (1957): Self conceptions, motivations, and interpersonal attitudes of late and early maturing boys. *Child Dev.*, 28:243–256.
79. Myers, R. D. (1974): *Handbook of Drug and Chemical Stimulation of the Brain: Behavioral, Pharmacological and Physiological Aspects*. Van Nostrand Reinhold Co., New York.

80. Nagy, Z. M. (1979): Development of learning and memory processes in infant mice. In: *Ontogeny of Learning and Memory*, edited by N. A. Spear and B. A. Campbell, pp. 101–133. Lawrence Erlbaum Associates, Hillsdale, New Jersey.

81. Nagy, Z. M., Misanin, J. R., Newman, J. A., Olsen, P. L., and Hinderliter, C. F. (1972): Ontogeny of memory in the neonatal mouse. *J. Comp. Physiol. Psychol.*, 81:380–393.

82. Nagy, Z. M., and Mueller, P. W. (1973): Effect of amount of original training upon onset of a 24-hour memory capacity in neonatal mice. *J. Comp. Physiol. Psychol.*, 85:151–159.

83. Nagy, Z. M., and Murphy, J. M. (1974): Learning and retention of a discriminated escape response in infant mice. *Dev. Psychobiol.*, 7:185–192.

84. Nagy, Z. M., Porada, K. J., and Anderson, J. A. (1977): Undernutrition by rearing in large litters delays the development of reflexive, locomotor, and memory processes in mice. *J. Comp. Physiol. Psychol.*, 91:682–696.

85. Nagy, Z. M., and Sandman, M. (1973): Development of learning and memory of T-maze training in neonatal mice. *J. Comp. Physiol. Psychol.*, 83:19–26.

86. Nelson, C. J., and Holson, J. F. (1978): Statistical analysis of teratologic data: Problems and advancements. *J. Environ. Pathol. Toxicol.*, 2:187–199.

87. O'Callaghan, J. P., and Holtzman, S. G. (1977): Prenatal administration of levorphanol or dextrophan to the rat: Analgesic effect of morphine in the offspring. *J. Pharmacol. Exp. Ther.*, 200:255–262.

88. Okon, E. (1970): The effect of environmental temperature on the production of ultrasounds by isolated non-handled albino mouse pups. *J. Zool.*, 162:71–83.

89. Okon, E. (1970): The ultrasonic responses of albino mouse pups to tactile stimuli. *J. Zool.*, 162:485–492.

90. Oswalt, G. L., and Meier, G. W. (1975): Olfactory, thermal, and tactual influences on infantile ultrasonic vocalization in rats. *Dev. Psychobiol.*, 8(2):129–135.

91. Overmann, S. R., Fox, D. A., and Woolley, D. E. (1979): Neurobehavioral ontogeny of neonatally lead-exposed rats. I. Reflex development and somatic indices. *Neurotoxicology*, 1:125–147.

92. Parisi, T., and Ison, J. R. (1979): Development of the acoustic startle response in the rat: Ontogenetic changes in the magnitude of inhibition by prepulse stimulation. *Dev. Psychobiol.*, 12(3):219–230.

93. Phillips, M., Adams, J., and Buelke-Sam, J. (1980): Righting vs. negative geotaxis: A methodological evaluation. *Teratology*, 21:60A–61A.

94. Porsolt, R. D., Anton, G., Blavet, N., and Jalfre, M. (1978): Behavioral despair in rats: A new model sensitive to antidepressant treatments. *Eur. J. Pharmacol.*, 47:379–391.

95. Porsolt, R. D., Bertin, A., Blavet, N., Daniel, M., and Jalfre, M. (1979): Immobility induced by forced swimming in rats: Effects of agents which modify central catecholamine and serotonin activity. *Eur. J. Pharmacol.*, 57:201–210.

96. Porsolt, R. D., Bertin, A., and Jalfre, M. (1977): Behavioral despair in mice: A primary screening test for anti-depressants. *Arch. Int. Pharmacodyn. Ther.*, 229:327–331.

97. Porsolt, R. D., Bertin, A., and Jalfre, M. (1978): Behavioral despair in rats and mice: Strain differences and the effects of imipramine. *Eur. J. Pharmacol.*, 51:291–294.

98. Porsolt, R. D., LaPichon, M., and Jalfre, M. (1977): Depression: A new animal model sensitive to antidepressant treatments. *Nature*, 266:730–732.

99. Preache, M. M., and Gibson, J. E. (1976): Effects of cyclophosphamide treatment in newborn mice on the development of swimming and reflex behavior and on adult behavioral performance. *Dev. Psychobiol.*, 9(6):555–567.

100. Ramey, C. T., Starr, R. H., Pallas, J., Whitten, C. F., and Reed, V. (1975): Nutrition, response-contingent stimulation, and the maternal deprivation syndrome: Results of an early intervention program. *Merrill-Palmer*, 2:44–53.

101. Randall, P. K., and Campbell, B. A. (1976): Ontogeny of behavioral arousal in rats: Effect of maternal and sibling presence. *J. Comp. Physiol. Psychol.*, 90:453–459.

102. Ray, D., and Nagy, Z. M. (1978): Emerging cholinergic mechanisms and the ontogeny of response inhibition in the mouse. *J. Comp. Physiol. Psychol.*, 92:335–349.

103. Reinstein, D. K., and Isaacson, R. L. (1977): Clonidine sensitivity in the developing rat. *Brain Res.*, 135:378–382.

104. Reinstein, D. K., McClearn, D., and Isaacson, R. L. (1978): The development of responsiveness to dopaminergic agents. *Brain Res.*, 150:216–223.

105. Reiter, L. W. (1980): Neurotoxicology: Meet the real world. *Neurobehav. Toxicol.*, 2:73–74.

106. Reiter, L., Anderson, G., Lackey, J., and Cahill, D. (1975): Developmental and behavioral changes in the rat during chronic exposure to lead. *Environ. Health Perspect.*, 12:119–123.
107. Reiter, L., Heavner, G., Ruppert, P., and Kidd, K. (1980): Short-term vs. long-term neurotoxicity: The comparative behavioral toxicity of triethyltin in newborn and adult rats. In: *Effects of Foods and Drugs on the Development and Function of the Nervous System: Methods for Predicting Toxicity*, edited by R. Gryder and V. Frankos, pp. 144–154. United States Government Printing Office, Washington.
108. Reiter, L. W., and MacPhail, R. C. (1979): Motor activity: A survey of methods with potential use in toxicity testing. *Neurobehav. Toxicol. [Suppl.]*, 1:53–66.
109. Robbins, T. W. (1977): A critique of the methods available for the measurement of spontaneous motor activity. In: *Handbook of Psychopharmacology, Vol. 7*, edited by L. L. Iversen, S. D. Iversen, and S. H. Snyder, pp. 37–82. Plenum Press, New York.
110. Rodier, P. (1976): Critical periods for behavioral anomalies in mice. *Environ. Health Perspect.*, 18:79–83.
111. Rodier, P. (1978): Postnatal functional evaluations. In: *Handbook of Teratology, Vol. 4*, edited by J. G. Wilson and F. C. Fraser, pp. 397–428. Plenum Press, New York.
112. Rodier, P. M., Reynolds, S. S., and Roberts, W. N. (1979): Behavioral consequences of interference with CNS development in the early fetal period. *Teratology*, 19(3):327–336.
113. Rosenstein, L., and Chernoff, N. (1978): Spontaneous and evoked EEG changes in perinatal rats following *in utero* exposure to Baygon: A preliminary investigation. *Bull. Environ. Contam. Toxicol.*, 20(5):624–632.
114. Rudy, J. W., and Cheatle, M. D. (1977): Odor-aversion learning in neonatal rats. *Science*, 198:845–846.
115. Rudy, J. W., and Cheatle, M. D. (1979): Ontogeny of associative learning: Acquisition of odor aversions by neonatal rats. In: *Ontogeny of Learning and Memory*, edited by N. A. Spear and B. A. Campbell, pp. 157–188. Lawrence Erlbaum Associates, Hillsdale, New Jersey.
116. Schapiro, S. (1968): Some physiological, biochemical, and behavioral consequences of neonatal hormone administration: Cortisol and thyroxine. *Gen. Comp. Endocrinol.*, 10:214–228.
117. Schapiro, S. (1971): Hormonal and environmental influences on rat brain development and behavior. In: *Brain Development and Behavior*, pp. 307–334, edited by M. B. Sterman, D. J. McGinty, and A. M. Adinolfi. Academic Press, New York.
118. Schapiro, S., and Norman, R. J. (1967): Thyroxine: Effects of neonatal administration on maturation, development, and behavior. *Science*, 155:1279–1281.
119. Schapiro, S., Salas, M., and Vukovich, K. (1970): Hormonal effects on ontogeny of swimming ability in the rat: Assessment of central nervous system development. *Science*, 193:146–151.
120. Sell, Elsa J. (1980): *Follow-up of the High Risk Newborn—A Practical Approach*. Charles C. Thomas, Springfield, Illinois.
121. Shaywitz, B. A., Klopper, J. H., Yager, R. D., and Gordon, J. W. (1976): Paradoxical response to amphetamine in developing rats treated with 6-hydroxydopamine. *Nature*, 261:153–155.
122. Shaywitz, B. A., Yager, R. D., and Klopper, J. H. (1976): Selective brain dopamine depletion in developing rats: An experimental model of minimal brain dysfunction. *Science*, 191:305–308.
123. Siqueland, E. R., and Lipsitt, L. P. (1966): Conditioned head turning in the human newborn. *J. Exp. Child Psychol.*, 3:356–376.
124. Sjoden, P.-O., and Soderberg, U. (1978): Phenoxyacetic acid: Sublethal effects. *Ecol. Bull. (Stockh.)*, 27:149–164.
125. Slotkin, T. A., and Thadani, P. V. (1980): Neurochemical teratology of drugs of abuse. In: *Advances in the Study of Birth Defects, Vol. 4, Neural and Behavioral Teratology*, edited by T. V. N. Persaud, pp. 199–234. University Park Press, Baltimore.
126. Sloviter, R. S., Drust, E. G., and Connor, J. D. (1978): Specificity of a rat behavior model for serotonin receptor activation. *J. Pharmacol. Exp. Ther.*, 206:339–347.
127. Smart, J., and Dobbing, J. (1971): Vulnerability of the developing brain. II. Effects of early nutritional deprivation on reflex ontogeny and development of behavior in the rat. *Brain Res.*, 28:85–95.
128. Sobotka, T. J., Spaid, S. L., Brodie, R. E., and Reed, G. (1981): Neurobehavioral toxicity of ammoniated glycyrrhizin, licorice component, in rats. *Neurobehav. Toxicol. Teratol.*, 3:37–44.
129. Spear, L. P. (1979): The use of psychopharmacological procedures to analyze the ontogeny of learning and retention: Issues and concerns. In: *Ontogeny of Learning and Memory*, edited by

N. A. Spear and B. A. Campbell, pp.135–155. Lawrence Erlbaum Associates, Hillsdale, New Jersey.

130. Spear, L. P., Shalaby, I. A., and Brick, J. (1979): Chronic administration of neuroleptic drugs during development: Behavioral and psychopharmacological effects. Cited in Spear (129).

131. Spyker, J. (1975): Assessing the impact of low level chemicals on development: Behavioral and latent effects. *Fed. Proc.*, 34:1835–1844.

132. Spyker, J. (1975): Behavioral teratology and toxicology. In: *Behavioral Toxicology*, edited by B. Weiss and V. G. Laties, pp. 311–349. Plenum Press, New York.

133. Spyker, J. M. (1976): Assessing the impact of low level chemicals on development: Behavioral and latent effects. In: *Behavioral Pharmacology: The Current Status*, edited by B. Weiss and V. G. Laties, pp. 161–180. Plenum Press, New York.

134. Stanley, W. C., Cornwell, A. C., Poggiani, C., and Trattner, A. (1963): Conditioning in the neonatal puppy. *J. Comp. Physiol. Psychol.*, 56:211–214.

135. Stebbins, W. C. (1970): *Animal Psychophysics: The Design and Conduct of Sensory Experiments.* Appleton-Century-Crofts, New York.

136. Stehouwer, D. J., and Campbell, B. A. (1978): Habituation of the forelimb-withdrawal response in neonatal rats. *J. Exp. Psychol. [Anim. Behav.]*, 4(2):104–119.

137. Stelzner, D. J., (1971): The normal postnatal development of synaptic endfeet in the lumbosacral spinal cord and of responses in the hindlimb of the albino rat. *Exp. Neurol.*, 31:337–357.

138. Sykes, S. E., and Cheyne, J. A. (1976): The effects of prenatal and postnatal protein malnutrition on physical and motor development in the rat. *Dev. Psychobiol.*, 9(3):285–296.

139. Tanimura, T., Ema, M., and Kihara, T. (1980): Effects of combined treatment with methylmercury and polychlorinated biphenyls (PCB's) on the development of mouse offspring. In: *Advances in the Study of Birth Defects, Vol. 4, Neural and Behavioral Teratology*, edited by T. V. N. Persaud, pp. 163–198. University Park Press, Baltimore.

140. Tapp, J. T., Zimmerman, R. S., and DiEncarnacao, P. S. (1968): Intercorrelation analysis of some common measures of rat activity. *Psychol. Rep.*, 23:1047–1050.

141. Thompson, R. F., and Glanzman, D. L. (1976): Neural and behavioral mechanisms of habituation and sensitization. In: *Habituation: Perspectives from Child Development, Animal Behavior, and Neurophysiology*, edited by T. J. Tighe and R. N. Leaton, pp. 49–93. Lawrence Erlbaum Associates, Hillsdale, New Jersey.

142. Thompson, R. F., and Spencer, W. A. (1966): Habituation: A model phenomenon for the study of neuronal substrates of behavior. *Psychol. Rev.*, 73:1643.

143. Tilney, F., and Kubie, L. S. (1931): Behavior in its relation to the development of the brain. *Bull. Neurol. Inst. N. Y.*, 1:229–313.

144. Tilson, H. A., Cabe, P. A., Ellinwood, E. H., and Gonzalez, L. P. (1979): Effects of carbon disulfide on motor function and responsiveness to d-amphetamine in rats. *Neurobehav. Toxicol.*, 1:57–63.

145. Tilson, H. A., Mitchell, C. L., and Cabe, P. A. (1979): Screening for neurobehavioral toxicity: The need for and examples of validation of testing procedures. *Neurobehav. Toxicol. [Suppl.]*,1:137–148.

146. Volokhov, A. A. (1959): Comparative physiological investigation of conditioned and unconditioned reflexes during ontogeny. *Pavlov J. Higher Ner. Activ.*, 9:49–60.

147. Vorhees, C. V., Brunner, R. L., and Butcher, R. E. (1979): Psychotropic drugs as behavioral teratogens. *Science*, 205:1220–1224.

148. Vorhees, C. V., Brunner, R. L., McDaniel, C. R., and Butcher, R. E. (1978): The relationship of gestational age to vitamin A-induced postnatal dysfunction. *Teratology*, 17(3):271–276.

149. Vorhees, C. V., Butcher, R. E., Brunner, R. L., and Sobotka, T. G. (1979): A developmental test battery for neurobehavioral toxicity in rats: A preliminary analysis using monosodium glutamate, calcium carrageenan and hydroxyurea. *Toxicol. Appl. Pharmacol.*, 50:267–282.

150. Walsh, R. N. (1980): Comment: On the necessity for a shift in emphasis from means-oriented to problem-oriented research in developmental psychobiology. *Dev. Psychobiol.*, 13:229–231.

151. Walsh, R. N., and Cummins, R. A. (1976): The open field test: A critical review. *Psychol. Bull.*, 83:482–504.

152. Weiss, B. (1975): Effects on behavior. In: *Principles for Evaluating Chemicals in the Environment*, pp. 198–216. National Academy of Sciences/National Research Council, Washington.

153. Weiss, B., and Laties, V. G. (1979): Assays for behavioral toxicity: A strategy for the Environmental Protection Agency. *Neurobehav. Toxicol. [Suppl.]*, 1:213–215.

154. Werboff, J., Goodman, I., Havlena, J., and Sikov, M. R. (1961): Effects of prenatal X-irradiation on motor performance in the rat. *Am. J. Physiol.*, 201:703–706.
155. Wilson, J. G. (1973): *Environment and Birth Defects.* Academic Press, New York.
156. Winne, D. (1968): Zur Planung von Versuchen: Wieviel Versuchseinheiten? *Arzneim. Forsch.*, 18:1161.
157. Woodworth, R. S., and Schlosberg, H. (1954): *Experimental Psychology.* Holt, Rinehart and Winston, New York.
158. Yanai, J., and Ginsburg, B. (1976): Long-term effects of early ethanol on predatory behavior in inbred mice. *Physiol. Psychol.*, 4:409–411.
159. Zenick, H. (1976): Evoked potential alterations in methylmercury chloride toxicity. *Pharmacol. Biochem. Behav.*, 5:253–255.
160. Zimmerman, E., Sonderegger, T., and Bromley, B. (1977): Development and adult pituitary–adrenal function in female rats injected with morphine during different postnatal periods. *Life Sci.*, 20:639–646.

*Developmental Toxicology*, edited by
C. A. Kimmel and J. Buelke-Sam. Raven Press,
New York © 1981.

# Regulatory Requirements for Reproductive Toxicology: Theory and Practice

## A. K. Palmer

*Huntingdon Research Center, Huntingdon, Cambridgeshire PE18 6ES, England*

In earlier commentary (16), it was stated that low opinions of screening tests for safety evaluation more often than not reflected deficiencies in knowledge and attitudes of critics, assessors, legislators, and investigators rather than the deficiencies of the test systems. Since then, the impact of further legislation appears to have increased the divergence among the various governmental, academic, and industrial interests involved. In direct form, the additional legislation has involved traditional areas such as screening of new drugs and has also embraced areas such as the working environment to which extensive toxicological screening is a virtual novelty. Indirectly, resources for safety screening have been further burdened by peripheral legislation such as the introduction of codes for Good Laboratory Practices (GLP) (7). The deisrability of these extensions to the scope of toxicological screening is unquestionable in principle, but the manner of their operation often gives cause for concern. Without correct balance, flexibility, and understanding, application of the rules may be self-defeating or at the very least mislead the populace to believe that they are afforded greater protection than is the case.

Toxicology is a subject where all things are relative rather than absolute; to quote Paracelsus: "All substances are poisons, there is nothing that is not poisonous; only the dose determines that a substance does not poison." Thus, to state in "absolute" terms that a material is teratogenic, carcinogenic, or mutagenic, etc., can be meaningless, as the more important factor is whether the circumstances in which such activity occurs would be encountered in practical use. This, however, requires a multidisciplinary approach for which mastery of all aspects is impossible and in which errors will be inevitable. All involved, therefore, must appreciate that alternative test systems may be equally valid and above all should retain an open balanced approach. If regulations are applied rigidly, then investigators perform tests by rote rather than by utilizing their knowledge of the test material to find the best way to investigate potential hazards. To avoid denying themselves this contribution, regulatory agencies should take positive action to prevent guidelines from becoming mandatory. Conversely, if guidelines are too vague, then studies of such variety may be performed that assessors have difficulty in finding common ground to make comparisons between different materials.

259

With these thoughts in mind, the following chapter has been based more on the unpublished or unpublishable aspects of practical performance of over 1,100 reproductive toxicity studies. These have included reproduction studies (fertility, multigeneration, multiple breeding, and dominant lethal assays), embryotoxicity, and teratogenicity studies (in rabbits, rats, mice, pigs, and primates), and peri- and postnatal studies of a standard or nonstandard format.

## SAFETY EVALUATION OF DRUGS

Before a new drug can be marketed, most countries require that it be examined with respect to its potential to affect all aspects of reproduction through maturation of the gonads, mating, gestation, parturition, lactation, and in some cases through to the development and maturation of the filial generation (8,11). The system required by countries constituting the major world markets for drugs consists of a three-segment design similar to, but not necessarily identical with, that introduced by the United States Food and Drug Administration in 1966 and briefly involves the following.

1. A fertility/general reproductive study in which one species (usually the rat) is dosed prior to and through mating and early gestation (Japan) or even through to weaning of reared offspring (U.K., U.S.A.); for drugs intended for long-term continuous or intermittent use, it may be recommended that offspring be reared (untreated) to maturity and examined for possible adverse effects on later development, behavior, and reproductive capacity.

2. Teratology studies in two species (usually rats and rabbits) are recommended. The test material is administered to pregnant females during organogenesis, and the animals are killed just prior to parturition for determination of litter values and examination of fetuses for abnormalities. The Japanese authorities recommend that a proportion of females in each group be allowed to rear their young to weaning, and also, "where necessary," some young are reared to maturity.

3. A peri- and postnatal study in at least one species (usually the rat) is required by most countries and consists of administering the test compound to pregnant females during late gestation and throughout lactation. In some countries (Japan, Italy), it is recommended that a proportion of offspring from each group be reared to maturity.

For all segments, most authorities recommend that, wherever possible, the test material be administered by the intended clinical route(s) and at three dosages, the highest of which should induce a minimal toxicity in the parent animal or be the maximum practical or tolerated dosage. Almost all original documentation also contains statements that, for special cases, alternative or additional investigation may be required. In practice, additional investigations are frequently welcomed, but there is often great reluctance to accept alternative methodology.

Set against the overall similarity of premarketing requirements, differences are minor. Nevertheless, these differences cause great difficulty in amalgamating segments for different agencies, particularly when they are performed piecemeal. The latter often arises because of the less stringent requirements of some countries prior to clinical trial. In the current international situation, it is debatable whether the advantages of early investigation in man outweigh the subsequent problems in arriving at an internationally acceptable package of reproductive studies. An even greater risk is that clinical trials will be performed with a material that causes an adverse effect on fertility (particularly of males) or some other aspect of reproduction that would not be covered by the performance of a teratogenicity test.

### Fertility and General Reproductive Studies (Segment 1)

#### *Early Designs*

Regulatory tests of this type can be traced back to the FDA's "two-litter test" (Fig. 1) which was originally intended for the safety evaluation of pesticides and food additives. Following the thalidomide disaster, the test was pressed into use for the safety evaluation of drugs and was the main form of test required by the United States from 1961 to 1966. Although no longer in use, the two-litter test deserves some mention, since many of its "deficiencies" (11) were the result of its performance in isolation. With the increased skills and awareness available today and the support of the other two segments, the basic simplicity of the design affords many advantages so that it could now be more useful than the designs that replaced it.

The two-litter test used one control and two test groups, each containing 20 male and 20 female rats. The test material was administered, usually in the diet, for 60 days prior to mating and through two cycles of mating, pregnancy, and lactation. At the time, however, interest was almost exclusively centered on the detection of thalidomide-like malformations, and in this respect it rapidly became apparent that, in the two-litter test, the recovery rate of malformed offspring was extremely low. This was a source of concern, and the fact that the primary objectives of any screening test could be fulfilled by demonstration of an alternative adverse effect tended to be overlooked. For example, the selective adverse effect of thalidomide

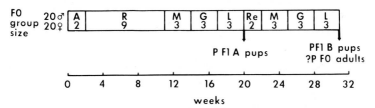

**FIG. 1.** FDA two-litter test. Abbreviations for all figures are: A, acclimatization; R, rearing or premating period; M, mating; G, gestation; L, lactation; Re, rest/regroup; P, macroscopic examination (brief); D, litter values *in utero* mid-pregnancy; T, litter values *in utero* day 20 of pregnancy, fetal weights and detailed examination of fetuses; B, behavioral testing; C, cessation (withdrawal) of treatment; O, organ weight analysis; H, histology; S, spermatogenesis check; ?, ill-defined or no instructions.

was demonstrated by significant reductions in the numbers of litters born, litter size at birth, and neonatal survival (11).

This pattern of response, rather than the occurrence of malformations, is a likely consequence of the administration of any teratogenic or embryotoxic agent, since the prolonged dosing period violates the basic teratological principle that malformations are induced by the application of a precise dosage at a precise time (20). That similar patterns of response are also the most likely consequences of a variety of drug actions such as interference with hormonal balance either directly (e.g., oral contraceptives), or indirectly (e.g., haloperidol or sulpiride-like drugs), or even by impairment of ejaculation (e.g., some guanethidine-like hypotensives) caused confusion when the two-litter test was performed in isolation. Nowadays, this would be considerably alleviated by the concurrent performance of other segments.

## Current Designs

It would be gratifying to believe that the change to the three-segment design would have resolved the majority of problems encountered with the two-litter test, but unfortunately many of them remain (11), particularly in the design of the fertility and reproductive segment.

The first of the current designs introduced by the FDA (Fig. 2A), includes one control group and three (originally two and now three by common usage) test groups, each containing 10 males and 20 females. The long premating treatment period (60 days) is retained for the males, the explanation being that it covers the spermatogenic cycle of the rat. The reduction from 20 to 10 males per group was certainly intended to be economical and suggests that emphasis is still on the female of the species. Also, for convenience, the premating treatment of females is reduced to 14 days to cover one or two estrous cycles, it being impossible to cover female gametogenesis since this occurs prenatally. Treatment of both sexes is continued through a 2- or 3-week mating period to determine whether there are effects on libido, fertilization, and ovum transport and through gestation and lactation of females to determine whether there are effects on implantation, embryogenesis, or fetal and neonatal development. Ten females in each group, presumably one of the pair mated to each male, are sacrificed in midpregnancy, corpora lutea are counted, and uterine contents are examined to determine numbers of live and dead (resorbing) embryos. This procedure is intended to alleviate one of the problems of the two-litter test in that it enables distinction between the apparent nonpregnancy due to embryotoxicity and/or dominant lethal effects (mutagenesis) and real nonpregnancy due to other causes. The remaining females are allowed to give birth and rear their young to weaning. At weaning, dams and offspring are killed and examined for abnormalities.

Major differences in this design have been introduced by the British authorities (Fig. 2B) who recommend that the interim sacrifice of females be performed on day 20 of pregnancy. This allows detection of mutagenic (dominant lethal) or embryonic effects as well as fetal examination similar to conventional teratogenic

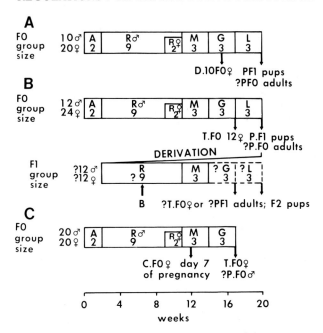

**FIG. 2. A:** FDA fertility and general reproduction study. $F_0$ males are treated 9 weeks prior to mating; $F_0$ females are treated only 2 weeks prior to mating. Female group size is reduced 50% by the interim sacrifice (D). **B:** United Kingdom fertility and general reproduction study. $F_0$ males are treated 9 weeks prior to mating; $F_0$ females are treated only 2 weeks prior to mating. Female group size is reduced 50% by the interim sacrifice (T). The $F_1$ generation receives no direct treatment. The *dotted lines* indicate options to be used by investigators to clarify observations in the main sections. **C:** Japanese fertility study. $F_0$ males are treated 9 weeks prior to mating; $F_0$ females are treated only 2 weeks prior to mating. Abbreviations as in Fig. 1.

studies. It is also recommended that, for drugs with an intended continuous or intermittent use for periods of about 6 months, some offspring be reared (untreated) to maturity and mated to assess their reproductive capacity. It is also recommended that the development of offspring to maturity be monitored and that assessment of auditory and visual function and of possible alterations in behavior be made. One control and three test groups are recommended with the highest dosage intended to be minimally toxic or the maximum tolerated. For both the interim sacrifice and the rearing phase, a minimum of 12 females per group is required, and conventionally a minimum of 12 male and 12 female offspring are reared to maturity. The U.K. authorities also recommend that pharmacokinetic studies with pregnant animals be performed although not necessarily within the reproductive study.

The recommendation that some offspring be reared untreated to maturity for evaluation of development, auditory and visual function, behavior, and capacity to reproduce is made primarily by the United Kingdom and Japan, and in both cases, requirements are nebulous. For the United Kingdom, derivation from the general reproduction study is preferred on the grounds that it will cover the possible effects of treatment from premating through to postnatal development. For Japan, the $F_1$ generation is derived from the peri- and postnatal and/or rat teratology studies, perhaps because there is no rearing of offspring in the Japanese fertility study. Current guidelines also contain no specific recommendations as to the age at which $F_1$ animals are to be mated or the exact procedures to be followed, nor are there any specifications as to the methods to be employed for determination of auditory or visual function or behavioral testing. Perhaps the lack of specific requirements is advisable as, currently, the validity of available test methods and their interpretation is questionable, particularly within the framework of regulatory requirements.

Recommendations issued by the European Economic Community are broadly similar to those of the United Kingdom and additionally recommend that separate male and female studies be performed, i.e., treated males are mated with untreated females and vice versa. However, from practical experience, the necessity to perform separate studies for males and females would occur in less than 1% of cases. More often than not, this would provide clearer elucidation of the overall biological profile of the test compound rather than its effect on reproduction per se.

For Japan, the study differs from both the United Kingdom and the United States in that it is essentially a fertility study rather than a reproductive study (Fig. 2C). The specification for one control and three test groups is similar to that of the United Kingdom and, although a slightly longer (3 months) premating treatment period for males is requested, the premating dosing period in the United States and the United Kingdom is generally acceptable. Less readily accepted is the use of unequal numbers of males and females per group, since there is a stated preference for at least 20 male and 20 female rats or mice per group (slightly lower group size may be accepted if the test is performed in another species), and monogamous mating is preferred. Treatment by the intended clinical route continues through mating for both sexes, and up to and including day 7 of gestation for females. Thereafter treatment is withdrawn, and all females are killed on day 20 of gestation; corpora lutea (except in mice) and live and dead (resorbing) fetuses are counted. Fetuses are then weighed and examined for external, skeletal, and visceral abnormalities as required for teratogenic (Segment 2) tests.

At an international level, to fulfill the major requirements of Japan, the United Kingdom and the United States, a Segment 1 study would require one control and three test groups, each composed of 20 males and 54 females, or a total of 80 males and 216 females, compared with a minimum of 30 males and 60 females for the basic FDA study. This investigation would take twice as long, given the necessity to rear $F_1$ offspring to maturity, and two sets of detailed fetal examinations would be required. The comparison with the U.K. and Japanese designs is similar if less extreme and points to an enormous waste of resources. Even so, the compromise would not meet the sugggestions for separate studies recommended by the European Economic Community.

Although it is not possible to detail all the arguments, this waste would appear to be unnecessary. Manufacturers do not deliberately set out to develop highly potent mutagens or teratogens. Consequently, the occurrence of embryolethality is a rare event, and insistence on performance of an interim sacrifice at 13 or 20 days or both, in general, is meaningless. Most compounds provide negative or equivocal results even at dosages causing minimal maternal toxicity. The "equivocal" nature of many results is often a by-product of the study design and, in particular, of the practice of mating one male to two females. Especially for all-or-none results, which occur quite frequently, valid comparisons can be made only with respect to the number of males in a study or the number of females in one phase of the study (i.e., those killed during pregnancy or those allowed to rear young).

Contingency analysis is the approved method of dealing with all-or-none responses, but unfortunately with low numbers, efficiency is extremely poor. Even when all males or all females of one phase of the FDA study can be legitimately included for intergroup comparisons, statistical significance ($p < 0.05$ exact test) is attained only when there is a 40 to 50% difference between groups. It must be emphasized that in safety evaluation, clear-cut differences, so common to the literature and to those working with highly potent agents, rarely occur and cause no problem if they do. Instead, the chief concern is with the interpretation of differences around the limits of normal variation. In this respect, the validity of current reproduction studies can be seriously compromised by the coincidental or treatment-related death or infertility of an occasional male or by less than ideal (100%) mating performance and pregnancy rate, thus requiring even larger differences before the $p < 0.05$ level is reached. Faced with this situation in the early stages of experimentation, the investigator must run the risk of obtaining too few litters in both sacrificed and reared components or must introduce a bias (Table 1) into the study to save one aspect at the expense of the other. Either way, this can lead to an unacceptable or unsatisfactory study requiring intuitive interpretation which may differ for the eager manufacturer versus the cautious investigator or assessor.

As to the respective merits of the sacrifice at midpregnancy (U.S.A.) or just prior to parturition (U.K.), sacrifice of females at day 20 of gestation affords several advantages over sacrifice on day 13. These include accuracy of estimating mating performance, onset of pregnancy, and the duration of gestation. Perhaps of greater

TABLE 1. *Effect of biased selection of an $F_1$ generation: rat reproduction study with an anti-ulcer agent*

| $F_0$ generation dosage (mg/kg) | Untreated $F_1$ generation performance | |
| --- | --- | --- |
| | Precoital time (days) | Pregnancy rate (%) |
| 0 | 3.5 | 92 |
| 2.5 | 2.5 | 92 |
| 25 | 2.5 | 92 |
| 250 | 7.0[a] | 69[a] |

[a]Difference due to mating of one infertile male to three females, compared with 1 : 1 mating for other groups. Insufficient $F_1$ males were available as only three litters weaned because of treatment effects on $F_0$ generation.

importance is that, in practice, the occurrence of adverse fetal or maternal effects during the perinatal period is more frequently encountered than the rare event of early embryotoxicity. In such situations, sacrifice on day 20 of gestation affords greater discrimination between direct and indirect fetal effects and for more accurate determination of the time of increased sensitivity. In addition, sacrifice on day 20 of pregnancy provides more useful information on intrauterine growth, because fetal weights, as well as the assessment of malformations, can be compared with those obtained in teratology studies. However, it is seldom that the same dosages can be employed in reproductive and teratogenic tests. Commonly, one has to employ lower dosages in the former to avoid undue maternal toxicity or total litter loss.

Detailed examination of fetuses for malformations would appear to be of debatable value in the U.K. design and meaningless in the Japanese fertility study, since treatment is withdrawn on day 7 of gestation (i.e., before organogenesis). Mistiming of pregnancy and the time of withdrawal of treatment can lead to problems in interpretation of the eventual results. However, the use of 20 males and 20 females per group, 1 : 1 mating, and the restriction to investigation of prenatal events alone allows the Japanese fertility study to avoid many of the problems that arise in the U.K. and FDA general purpose studies. The study integrates neatly with its corresponding teratology and peri- and postnatal studies so that when all three are performed and interpreted correctly, the package provides good cover for all aspects of reproduction. Unfortunately, the different segments are not always compatible with Western designs, and this often frustrates an international approach.

## An Alternative Approach

In view of the problems associated with current general reproductive studies, consideration of a simple alternative would be worthwhile. Practical experience shows that truly selective effects are rare and that, in any event, the ability to investigate these can be hampered by the more commonly occurring effects on pregnancy rate and peri- and postnatal survival. The purpose of screening tests is the detection of unwanted effects elicited by relatively unknown materials. Assurance that an effect has been elicited takes precedence over determination of the precise nature of the effect. The latter can be elucidated by further investigation once an effect has been demonstrated.

Important elements of a simple general purpose reproductive test (Fig. 3) would include the use of one control and three test groups with the high dosage causing either minimal maternal (or paternal) toxicity or being the highest practical dosage attainable. Within reason, the material would be administered by the intended clinical route; gavage would be preferable to dietary administration for the oral route. Rats, and to a slightly lesser extent, mice would be the most practical species. Each group would consist of equal numbers of each sex to insure subsequent 1 : 1 mating. Empirically, 20 animals of each sex per group would appear adequate and, in the absence of treatment-related effects, would be expected to provide not less

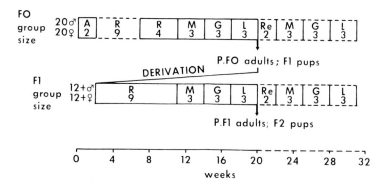

**FIG. 3.** Proposed fertility and general reproduction study for drugs, pesticides, and industrial chemicals. *Dotted lines* indicate options to be used by investigators to clarify observations in the main sections and may take forms other than those indicated. Either 9 or 4 weeks premating treatment may be used for the $F_0$ generation, depending on the nature of the test compound. The $F_1$ generation is preferably untreated, but could be dosed for pesticides. P could be delayed where necessary, and also extended to preserve tissues from all adults and one male and one female weanling per litter as a contingency for subsequent histopathological examination if warranted. Abbreviations as in Fig. 1.

than 15 litters at weaning, thus allowing choice of one male and one female from not less than 10 to 12 litters to form the basis of an evenly balanced untreated $F_1$ generation. These numbers should be considered minimal, and an initial group size of 30 per sex would appear optimal.

The duration of the premating treatment period must inevitably remain a compromise. Experience suggests that a 4-week premating period for both sexes is reasonable in the vast majority of cases. Treatment would continue through a 2- to 3-week mating period, gestation, and lactation for both sexes. For males, this is insurance in case of the need for further investigation. During mating, procedures such as daily examination of vaginal smears, regular weighing of females (daily or every second day and/or at specified days of pregnancy) would be employed to provide accurate estimates of mating performance, precoital time, pregnancy rate, and the duration of gestation.

At birth and daily during lactation, offspring should be counted and examined to enable accurate monitoring of development. Offspring and parent females should be weighed at least at weekly intervals through lactation, as important changes that may occur at peak lactation around days 8 to 12 postpartum may be missed by the common practice of recording only at 4 and 21 days. At or shortly after weaning (day 21 postpartum), one male and one female per litter weaned (or a minimum of 10 to 12 litters) should be selected to form the basis of the $F_1$ generation when required (most times). Surplus offspring would be killed, and all subjected to thorough macroscopic examination. Histopathological examination would not be required routinely, although a sensible investigator will know when to process a particular animal through this procedure for "diagnostic" purposes.

In the majority of studies, i.e., unequivocally negative or even unequivocally positive, parent animals will also be killed and subjected to thorough macroscopic investigation but not routine histology. Obviously, greater attention will be given to the reproductive tract and, for the occasional, apparently infertile male, histopathological examination of testes would be common sense. Similarly, for females killed at 21 days post-partum, close examination of the reproductive tract and in some cases, counting of the number of implantation site scars would be of value. For apparently nonpregnant females, the uterus would be immersed in ammonium sulfide for the detection of early embryonic deaths. With equivocal results, instead of being sacrificed, $F_0$ males and females could be remated for further investigations while the $F_1$ generation is being reared.

Although there might appear to be a slight loss of precision by omission of an interim sacrifice, this is more than compensated for by: (a) the ability to continue the study, as even with a 40% loss of litters to weaning, a useable balanced $F_1$ generation could be selected from the remaining 12 litters; and (b) the facility to conduct a second mating and institute procedures specifically designed to answer any questions raised by the initial procedure either in the reproduction study or as a cross reference to other segments.

Distinction between selective effects on either sex, if not immediately evident, can be clarified (or verified) at a second mating by cross-mating controls and test animals, by remating the treated males to a fresh group of untreated females, or by withdrawal of treatment. The ability to perform a second mating would be facilitated by the shorter premating period which allows animals to be mated at an earlier age (9 to 10 weeks of age for females and 10 to 12 weeks of age for males appears to be the optimum for first mating rats of Sprague–Dawley origin).

## Tests for Selective Embryotoxicity (Segment 2)

### General Factors

Being introduced to regulatory safety evaluation as a consequence of the thalidomide disaster, these tests are commonly, and in many ways unfortunately, referred to as teratogenic tests. All countries require the use of two test species, one being a "nonrodent." Pregnant females are dosed with the test compound during organogenesis and killed prior to parturition. The uterus is examined, litter values recorded, and fetuses examined for external, visceral, and skeletal anomalies.

The design of studies owes much to the demonstration of the effect of thalidomide in NZW rabbits (18). With this study, Somers created an essential bridge between previous academic investigations of teratogenicity and safety evaluations by employing a more practical (for screening) repeated daily-dosing technique. There has been little change in the design used by Somers. That requirements of all countries are basically the same and that the design has withstood criticism for 17 years suggests that it is essentially correct and that improvement lies in increasing skills of performance and interpretation.

Much of the confusion caused by the relatively frequent occurrence of low incidences of malformation in a narrow range of dosages and often contradictory results arise from the popular belief that the capacity of materials to induce abnormal development is an absolute but rare characteristic. However, the same pattern of results also can be explained by a more valid biological concept: materials commonly induce abnormal development that is manifest only under limited conditions. The concept is also more in accord with the toxicological dictum that "all substances are poisons," which, in teratology, is represented by Karnofsky's law (10): any material may be teratogenic if given to the right species, at the right dosage, at the right time. That this concept is only rarely demonstrated derives from the fact that malformations can be viewed as catastrophies in an objective (mathematical) sense (22) as well as an emotive one.

## Species

Authorities require initial screening tests to be performed in rats and rabbits; mice may be used as an additional or alternative species. These are used because they are available, economical, and relatively easy to manage (2,16); their consequent widespread use has provided an accumulation of knowledge of their reactions to a wide variety of chemical entities which allows results to be put into perspective. This latter aspect is of tremendous importance and often outweighs theoretical reasons (e.g., similarity in metabolism or physiology) in favor of an alternative exotic species.

Almost without exception, exotic species such as nonhuman primates, pigs, etc., are best used for confirming positive results recorded with common species; as an example, the use of primates to demonstrate the action of thalidomide or pigs to demonstrate the effects of hypovitaminosis A. Using unconventional species to demonstrate negative results is akin to playing Russian roulette. Anyone failing to recognize that "negative" results merely reflect operation of the laws of chance will be lulled into a false sense of security. Conversely, sooner or later, a coincidental malformation will occur in a test group and, because of the mystique attached to species such as primates, the manufacturers will have to abandon an expensive investment, and the medical profession will fail to acquire a valuable new drug.

## Dosages

In principle (21), tests should involve the use of three dosages for which: (a) the highest dosage should cause minimal maternal toxicity; (b) the lowest dosage should cause the clinically intended effect in the test species or be a low multiple of the intended human dosage; and (c) the intermediate dosage (or dosages) should be logarithmically spaced between high and low dosages.

The best way to select dosages (12,17) is to establish first the highest dosage by performance of a specific dose range study in females of the intended test species, for the intended duration, by the intended route. Lower dosages are then selected in a descending sequence using two- or threefold and not more than fivefold intervals. Final dosages may be adjusted to provide a close match with those employed in other similar studies for purposes of comparison. Without prior knowledge that the test material is embryotoxic, is an abortifacient, or is considerably more toxic in pregnancy, it is cheaper, quicker, more convenient, just as accurate, and more prudent to use nonpregnant animals.

A convenient marker of minimal maternal toxicity, such as a 10% reduction in weight gain, is extremely useful but cannot always be attained; prolonged sedation or interference with hormonal balance (direct or indirect) are obvious examples of effects that may disturb the maternal economy without reducing weight gain. Conversely, irrevocable individual responses such as sudden death may precede general responses such as retarded weight gain; in such cases, it is better to choose a maximum tolerated dosage that can be shown to be meaningful by reference to other studies. Sometimes it is impossible to provoke a pharmacological or toxicological response at the maximum dosage that can be administered practically (12) in which case pharmacokinetic studies may be required to demonstrate the validity of the test system.

Additionally, it is important to consider dosage form. Even before GLPs, it was important to ensure the quality and consistency of the test material, as many of the "negative" results obtained with thalidomide may be attributed to its hydrolysis (17) when dissolved in sodium hydroxide. The herbicide 2,4,5-T might not have been branded as a dangerous teratogen (3) had the investigators appreciated the extremely toxic nature of the dioxin contaminant. Subtle to profound differences in results can arise from differences in vehicle, dose volume, and concentration employed.

### Controls

It is surely unnecessary to stress the need for a negative control group in each study or the value of historical control values for interpretation of the relevance of low-frequency events such as malformation. It would also appear unnecessary to specify that concurrent controls should be selected, treated, and handled in an identical manner to test group animals except for the administration of the test material. In certain cases it may also be prudent to add a completely untreated control group where the vehicle may induce effects or where the dosing procedure may be traumatic, e.g., inhalation and some forms of topical application.

Positive control groups are of value only when the new test material can be expected to produce adverse effects and the positive control can be called a *comparative* control (16). Thus, aspirin is a useful comparative control only when testing another salicylate in rats, or dexa- or betamethasone in any species only when testing a new fluorinated corticosteroid. It is naive to assume that the ability to detect large numbers of obvious malformations such as craniorachischisis, cleft palate, etc., induced by positive controls provides assurance that an investigator is capable of detecting and interpreting the more subtle forms of response that will occur with the far more frequent, less potent materials encountered in drug screening.

*Route of Administration*

It is quite logical that test materials should be administered by the intended route or routes to be used in man since it does not always follow that the route allowing the highest rates of administration always causes the greatest effect. Of course, administration by unusual routes can be problematical (12), topical application and instillation into body orifices frequently limiting the amount that can be administered. To compensate for these problems, it may be necessary to perform supportive studies with more practical routes of administration such as gavage, subcutaneous, or intravenous administration. Such extensions should also include comparative pharmacokinetic and/or pharmacological tests to insure correct extrapolation of results.

*Frequency of Dosing*

For regulatory screening tests, the day of observing plugs or spermatozoa in vaginal smears of rats and mice or of coitus in rabbits and hamsters is considered to represent day 0 of pregnancy. Test materials are then administered once daily during and including days 6 to 15 of pregnancy for rats and mice and days 6 to 18 of pregnancy for rabbits for the majority of countries. The difference from classic single-dose techniques is important because: (a) drugs are rarely administered as single doses; (b) repeated dosing may lead to accumulation of test material, metabolites, or effects; (c) the whole period of organogenesis must be covered; and (d) there can be no assumption as to which period of organogenesis may be the most susceptible.

When physical aspects of the dosing technique limit the amount that can be administered or when compounds with a short half-life are investigated, then more than one daily dosage should be considered. Conversely, for long-acting materials or depot preparations, intervals of 2 to 3 days between doses may be more appropriate. For pronounced enzyme induction or cumulative toxicity, it may also be more appropriate to reduce the total dosing period to a few days and perform two to three studies.

*Observations*

Compared with those of academic teratologists, the observations made by investigators in safety evaluation are generally broader in scope and more extensive as a consequence of the different aims and methods employed. In particular, greater attention has to be paid to maternal parameters so that results may be put in perspective with those of other studies; this allows determination of whether a selective effect has been obtained. Objective distinction between induced and coincidental abnormalities in safety evaluation is difficult because of: (a) the aim of establishing the lowest dosage causing an adverse effect rather than establishing an optimum dosage for induction of malformations; (b) the generally low teratogenic potential of the materials tested; (c) the relatively unknown potential of the test material; and (d) the necessity to use repeated dosing to cover all stages of organogenesis.

Since obvious malformations are unreliable indicators of teratogenic activity in isolated initial screening tests, the investigator must examine and record other parameters that often associate with teratogenicity, that occur more frequently and consistently, and that, consequently, are more readily analyzable (15,16), e.g., number of live and dead young, litter and fetal weights, and examination of fetuses for subtle structural changes in skeletal and visceral tissues. It can be useful to distinguish between early and late intrauterine deaths, since potent teratogens more frequently increase the incidence of the former, whereas late fetal deaths are more often a secondary consequence of maternal toxicity. It is useful to estimate numbers of corpora lutea for rats or rabbits as insurance against accidental attribution of reduced litter size to treatment.

For routine screening, recording of uterine position of dead and abnormal offspring and individual fetal weights is generally a useless exercise. The purpose of such procedures is to enable correlation of different findings. In practice, the information is rarely reported in a way that suits this purpose and perhaps represents a degree of sophistication beyond the scope of first-stage screening. For second-stage investigations, such procedures may be very valuable. Occasional abnormally sized (large or small) or externally abnormal fetuses can be weighed separately to provide continuity with subsequent examinations.

There are a variety of recommendations, regulatory and otherwise, concerning the means by which these examinations may be made. Logically, the investigator should choose the methods he or she can use confidently and consistently to examine the maximum number of tissues in the maximum number of fetuses. The fraction (two-thirds or one-half) of rat fetuses examined for skeletal or visceral defects is irrelevant, provided sufficient numbers from each litter are examined.

For visceral examination of rats and mice, Wilson's hand sectioning technique (20), at its very best, may be slightly better than microdissection and as effective as serial sectioning with a microtome. Such a high level of competence on the Wilson technique, however, is very difficult to achieve, since it requires regular examination of large numbers of fetuses. For many investigators, the more natural microdissection (1) may be a safer technique as adequate proficiency can be attained and retained more readily. Microdissection has the added advantage that when small numbers of litters or fetuses have to be examined, it can be performed on fresh unfixed specimens allowing individual fetuses to be examined for both visceral and skeletal effects.

## Organization of Results

Increased efficiency of examination inevitably leads to higher background incidences of structural changes, and it is important that this does not lead to confusion (14,15). Results quoted as percentages should also be supported by absolute values as the implications of a 10% incidence can be totally different if this is 1/10 or 10/

100. In particular, results should always be presented so that the number of litters and fetuses with one or more effects is accurately portrayed. Bearing in mind the importance attached to low-frequency events, presentation of results by types of abnormality recorded frequently leads to artificial magnification of the degree of effect. A single fetus with multiple effects or a single litter containing several anomalous fetuses tends to be counted more than once.

It is also advisable to categorize structural changes either in terms of their severity or in terms of their natural frequency (14,15). It is important that serious irreversible changes such as exencephaly, gastroschisis, etc., are not masked by more frequent minor and often reversible changes such as unossified sternebrae. One of the most important facets of categorization is the paradox that it is difficult to maintain when a positive response occurs. Significant increases in the incidence of subtle changes are almost invariably present at dosages lower than those at which obvious malformations are evident. These subtle changes provide evidence that the system is under stress and approaching the critical point at which a catastrophic event (malformation) may occur.

*Analysis of Results*

Analysis of several hundred tests have shown that the litter, not the individual fetus, is the only valid sample unit for statistical analyses (9,13,19) and that litter values are not normally distributed (β-binomial, and Poisson distributions are the most common). For litter values, nonparametric methods of analysis tend to be more applicable but, like all statistical methods, are not infallible and should be used only as a guide to reaching a judgment and not the sole criterion for judgment. As far as major malformations are concerned, statistical analysis may as well be forgotten as authorities view with suspicion incidences of abnormality well below those that would be required for valid demonstration of statistical significance. Group sizes of 60 or more (i.e., at least three times standard group sizes of current screening tests) would be required to establish, with reasonable certainty, the statistical significance of a 100-fold increase in malformation rate if the basic incidence were 0.1%. As an actual example, to investigate one particular anomaly (microphthalmia) it was necessary to use 1,000 to 1,500 rats (i.e., 250–300 per group) to validly demonstrate the statistical significance of a slight increase in the normal incidence. Obviously, studies of such dimensions would be untenable for routine screening and can be carried out only when a selected specific and previously known endpoint is to be examined.

It is fortunate that teratogenic action will always cause other effects such as embryonic death, reduced fetal weight, and increased incidences of minor changes at, or more importantly, below dosages at which major malformations occur. However, it must be remembered that whereas induction of malformations is always accompanied by more subtle structural changes (that may be reversible) or effects on parameters such as embryonic death or fetal weight, the reverse is not always applicable, and subtle changes (or effects on fetal growth) do not always herald the presence of marked or moderate teratogenic activity.

## Peri- and Postnatal Studies (Segment 3)

The simplest study of the three-segment design is the peri- and postnatal study. For most countries, 20 pregnant female rats are dosed daily from day 15 of gestation through parturition, lactation, and to weaning (day 21 postpartum). Parturition is observed, and litter values from birth through lactation to weaning are recorded as in general reproductive studies. For Japan, treatment is initiated on day 17 of pregnancy and, at weaning, an $F_1$ generation is selected "where necessary" (see General Reproductive Studies above). Principles of choice of dosages and route of administration are similar to those employed for general reproductive and fertility studies.

The virtues of the peri- and postnatal study appear to be vastly underrated (14). In earlier discussion of fertility, it was mentioned that most problems arise in the perinatal period, and these can be investigated in a more controlled manner in a peri- and postnatal study since confounding variables resulting from effects on pregnancy rate and sequence of mating are avoided. Quite often, more pronounced effects on parturition and immediate postnatal development are recorded in peri- and postnatal studies compared with general reproductive studies. Most likely, this is due to the occurrence of enzyme induction or developing tolerance with the longer premating treatment period in the reproductive studies. Most certainly, many of the problems and difficulties that arise in general reproductive studies (Segment 1) could be avoided if peri- and postnatal studies were performed prior to the general reproductive study. This is particularly so in the case of nonsteroidal antiinflam-matory agents, drugs affecting cholinergic and adrenergic receptors, progestogens, synthetic endomorphins, neuroleptics, or hypnotics affecting the neurohormonal axis. The simplicity and shorter dosing period of the peri- and postnatal study confers a flexibility which is most useful and, with small modifications, the design can readily be transferred to a variety of species ranging from mice and hamsters to pigs and primates.

Cross-fostering studies can usually be done more readily than in the general reproductive studies. There is also a great deal of favor of deriving an $F_1$ generation from a peri- and postnatal study (as required by Japan and Italy) rather than from the current forms of general reproductive study; e.g., control of selection is better because of the greater numbers of litters and offspring available. Also, for rats and mice, which are relatively immature at birth, the perinatal period would appear to offer scope for induction of neural effects, leading to deficits in behavior, and for induction of effects on secondary sexual characteristics, leading to reproductive deficiencies.

To date, the majority of behavioral testing reported in the literature has been performed in conjunction with a teratogenic study base and more often than not using highly potent agents (e.g., lead, methylmercury, hydroxyurea, etc.). These studies have shown that behavioral deficits can be induced during organogenesis, and selective effects have been claimed. However, the question as to whether the dosage regimes operative during the peri- and postnatal or general reproductive studies would provide even greater information cannot be answered until such time as more equal proportions of the various types of dosage regimes are employed and until such time as a greater variety of potent and less potent materials have been examined.

## SAFETY EVALUATION OF PESTICIDES, FOOD ADDITIVES, AND NEW FOODS

The situation pertaining to the development of pesticides, food additives, or novel food materials is infinitely more complex and political than the safety evaluation of drugs. Internationally, requirements vary from the overdetailed and restrictive through the nebulous to the nonexistent. The more likely losers in the resulting confusion are the underdeveloped countries for which avoidance of the small or hypothetical risks attached to the use of pesticides or irradiation of food stuffs may only increase the certainty of contracting vector-born disease, dysentery, and schistosomiasis from natural pollution or the deficiency disease of malnutrition.

### Tests Required

Reproductive tests currently required for pesticides or food additives include a multigeneration study, usually in rats, and investigation for teratogenicity either within the multigeneration study or as a separate teratogenicity test in one or possibly two species. The inclusion of a teratogenicity test is, of course, a conditioned response to the thalidomide disaster, whereas the origin of the multigeneration study can be traced to the two-litter test from which the three-segment design for drugs evolved.

Several explanations may be given as to why testing should have evolved along a different pathway from safety evaluation of drugs. The explanation with most merit is that exposure to pesticides and food additives differs from exposure to drugs in many respects: (a) materials are administered to whole populations rather than to individuals; (b) populations of all age groups are exposed for long continuous periods, albeit at low dosages; (c) individuals have little or no choice (and often no knowledge) as to whether or not they are exposed to the material; (d) in socially developed countries, individuals generally derive little direct benefit from the administration of the test material; benefits arise indirectly in the form of improved standards of living and social development; (e) a small proportion of the population (e.g., factory workers, spray operations) may be exposed for shorter periods at relatively high dosages, often by routes not applicable to the general population; they may also be exposed to more toxic intermediates in a manufacturing process.

It is only in recent years that attention has been directed towards the latter group through regulations such as those promulgated by EPA and OSHA in the United States and HSWA in the United Kingdom.

### Food and Drug Administration Multigeneration Study

The most widely used multigeneration study is that employed by the FDA. Originally, it was intended for the testing of both intentional food additives (e.g., sweeteners, coloring agents) and unintentional food additives (e.g., pesticides, veterinary products that may persist as residues in meat).

In its usual form, the FDA multigeneration study (Fig. 4A) involves the use of 10 male and 20 females per group. One control and two test groups are required, but in recent years most investigators have employed three test dosages. Treatment continues for at least 60 days prior to mating for each generation and continues throughout to termination. Each generation is required to produce two litters, the first of which is discarded at weaning. From second litters, 10 males and 20 females are selected to form the basis of the next generation while surplus young and adults are killed. The procedure is repeated until young from the second litters of the third generation are weaned, at which time histopathological examination, organ weight analysis, and sometimes skeletal examination of 10 male and 10 female offspring per group are added to the list of observations.

Most of the criticisms applicable to the two-litter test and the general reproductive studies of drugs can be transferred directly to the multigeneration study, i.e., those related to the prolonged premating treatment period, the unequal numbers of males and females, and the limited group size (11). Admittedly, the common practice of administering test compounds in the diet is more justifiable, as this is the way the general population will be exposed, and, in general, the inaccuracy is less critical because of the wider safety margins and wider intervals between dosages usually employed. In this respect, a ± 10 to 20% error in dosage has less impact with 10-fold intervals between dosages and a 100- or 1,000-fold margin between the lowest dosage and the anticipated human exposure level. However, in situations where dietary concentration of 1,000 ppm (0.1%) or dosage intervals less than 5-fold are involved, the inaccuracy of dietary administration may reach critical levels, and administration by gavage would be preferable. At the other end of the scale, the administration of very high dietary concentrations of 5 to 20% or more of diet necessary for artificial sweeteners or novel foods (e.g., microbial proteins, irradiated products) may limit the intake of necessary nutrients, vitamins, and trace elements if the diet is not balanced. Offspring are particularly vulnerable, as during the immediate preweaning and postweaning periods their intake in milligrams-material per kilogram of body weight may be three to four times greater than that of the adult at the same dietary concentration. With many agents it may be advisable to reduce dietary concentrations during this period.

One of the least recognized consequences of dietary imbalance is that promotion of weight gain can reduce reproductive capacity of rats, as body weight is a more

---

**FIG. 4. A:** FDA multigeneration study. **B:** Japanese multigeneration study. There is a reduced number of females during lactation (L) because of the interim sacrifice (T). **C:** EPA multigeneration study, 1979. This interpretation differs from that provided by the EPA which differs from their textural comments. Certain illogical requests such as histopathology on 25 adult $F_1$ females (see group size) have been ignored, as has the request for investigation of spermatogenesis on bred males of the $F_2$ generation. In the second derivation, animals would have to be regrouped at weaning to avoid accidental pregnancies which could occur around 7 weeks of age. Abbreviations as in Fig. 1.

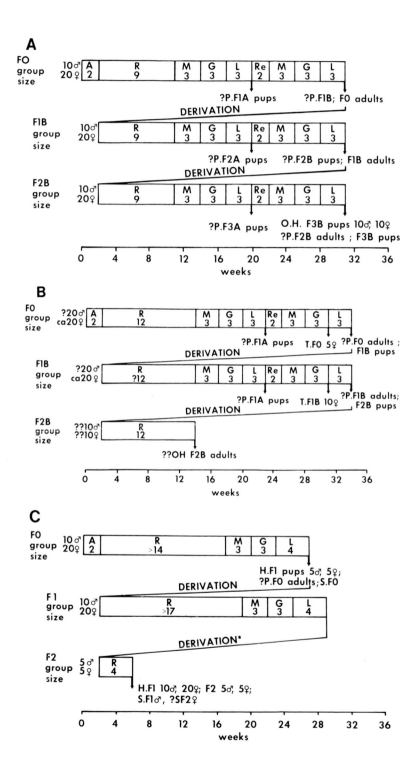

critical factor than age in the determination of reproductive capacity. One example (of many) is briefly illustrated in Table 2. In the first study employing the prolonged premating period required by the FDA, the low pregnancy rate and poor survival of offspring among controls precluded continuation beyond the first generation. In the second study, continuation through three generations was obtained by reducing the premating period to achieve mating at a more appropriate body weight.

The insistence by authorities that derivation of filial generations should be from second litters is a prime example of the application of fact out of context. In the widest context, the view that more problems occur with first litters is true when immatures are included; however, in multigeneration and reproductive studies the long premating treatment period ensures that animals are fully mature at the first mating. In consequence, first matings are as successful and often more successful (two times out of three in our laboratories) than second matings in terms of pregnancy rate (Table 2), litters available at weaning, and litter size.

Use of two or more litters per generation more frequently confuses rather than clarifies results as does routine extension to a third generation (11). When effects on reproduction occur, they are usually progressive or cumulative so that a combination of prolonged treatment and several matings can lead to such low numbers of litters and offspring at weaning that continuation of the study (Table 2) or interpretation of results can be seriously jeopardized. In particular, the possibility of increased manifestation of a latent natural defect never seems to be considered. Actual examples of such events are illustrated in Tables 1 and 3 whereas the theoretical situation pertaining to the increasing influence of an anomalous genome is illustrated in Table 4. In the latter, the transmission is minimized because a 100% pregnancy rate, maximum dispersion, and transmission of the original genetic pool are assumed, but this is seldom achieved in practice. The reverse situation of natural or accidental selection of a population resistant to the test material could also occur as not more than 10% of young born will be continued into a subsequent generation.

Organ weight analysis and histopathological examination of 10 males and 10 females of the final $F_3$ generation is of questionable value (11). Considering the number of confounding variables that could have influenced the study from the initial $F_0$ generation through to the $F_3$ generation and that during the study 900 to 1,200 young per group would have been born, the adequacy of a sample size of 20 per group is extremely debatable.

## Japanese Multigeneration Study

The multigeneration study required for Japan (Fig. 4B) improves on the FDA design by the use of equal numbers of each sex per group with subsequent 1 : 1 mating and mating for only two ($F_0$ and $F_1$) generations. However, these improvements are negated by the requirement for a longer premating period (at least 12 weeks) which makes the animals that much older at the first mating and beyond their peak at the second mating. This is compounded by the requirement that at the

TABLE 2. Body weight and pregnancy rate of rats (CD): studies with sweeteners[a]

| | Study 1 ($F_0$ generation only) | | | | | | Study 2 ($F_0$ + $F_1$ + $F_2$ generations) | | | | | | |
| | Male 1 | | | Male 2 | | | Male 1 | | | Male 2 | | | Grand average/ pregnancy rate (%) |
| Treatment | No. females | Body weight (g) | Pregnancy rate (%) | No. females | Body weight (g) | Pregnancy rate (%) | No. females | Body weight (g) | Pregnancy rate (%) | No. females | Body weight (g) | Pregnancy rate (%) | |
|---|---|---|---|---|---|---|---|---|---|---|---|---|---|
| Control | 40 | 355 | 55 | 30 | 389 | 37 | 60 | 243 | 95 | 60 | 328 | 93 | 329/70 |
| Sucrose | 39 | 361 | 56 | 30 | 407 | 27 | 60 | 254 | 95 | 60 | 342 | 83 | 341/65 |
| Sweetener A | 158 | 348 | 66 | 119 | 383 | 55 | 240 | 244 | 95 | 240 | 329 | 96 | 326/78 |
| Sweetener B | 40 | 333 | 73 | 30 | 362 | 63 | 60 | 242 | 92 | 60 | 313 | 98 | 313/82 |

[a]All diets were isocalorific. Animals in Study 2 were younger and lighter at mating and had higher pregnancy rate. Pregnancy rate at first mating generally higher than at second mating. Grand average shows inverse correlation of pregnancy and body weight irrespective of age and parity.

TABLE 3. *Effects of a recessive gene[a]* in a rat multigeneration study

| Treatment | incidence (%) of litters containing offspring with locomotor incoordination | | |
| | $F_0$ generation | $F_1$ generation | $F_2$ generation |
| --- | --- | --- | --- |
| Control | 0.0 | 2.6 | 0.0 |
| Low dosage | 0.0 | 0.0 | 8.2 |
| Intermediate dosage | 13.0 | 2.7 | 6.7 |
| High dosage | 0.0 | 6.8 | 7.1 |

[a]On the average, there were 30 or more litters per generation. Demonstration that the increased incidence of abnormal offspring in $F_1$ and $F_2$ generations was not due to treatment but to inheritance of a recessive gene was achieved by maintenance of derivation records through the three generations.

TABLE 4. *Increased influence of a genome through successive generations[a]*

| Generation | | | |
| 1 | 2 | 3 | 4 |
| --- | --- | --- | --- |
| A | Ab | Abcd | Abcdefgh |
| b | bc | bcde | bcdefghi |
| c | cd | cdef | cdefghij |
| d | de | defg | defghijA |
| e | ef | efgh | efghijAb |
| f | fg | fghi | fghijAbc |
| g | gh | ghij | ghijAbcd |
| h | hi | hijA | hijAbcde |
| i | ij | ijAb | ijAbcdef |
| j | jA | jAbc | jAbcdefg |
| 10%[b] | 20%[b] | 40%[b] | 80%[b] |

[a]To avoid brother and sister matings, animals derived from first mating pair A are mated to second mating pair b and hence have A and b factors. At the third generation mating, an animal could inherit factors from four of the original mating pairs, and at the fourth generation from eight of the original mating pairs.
[b]This represents the proportion of genotypes containing A, an undesirable genome.

second mating, five $F_0$ females and 10 $F_1$ females be killed prior to parturition. Some of the last generation are reared for 3 months to detect latent effects (including carcinogenicity!). Exactly how many offspring should be reared, how they should be selected, and the observations that should be performed are not stated. Rearing of one male and one female from each of the 10 reared litters of the second mating of the $F_1$ generation seems acceptable. At 3 months of age, the $F_{2B}$ are generally subjected to organ weight analysis and histopathological examination, again without specifics as to how this should be performed.

## Environmental Protection Agency Multigeneration Study

The most recent design (Fig. 4C) for multigeneration studies has been provided by the EPA in connection with the registration of pesticides (5) and the Toxic Substances Control Act (6). Only a single mating from each of two generations is required, and no interim sacrifice is required as embryotoxicity and teratogenicity are investigated by means of concurrent tests in two species. The value of this simplification in procedure is unfortunately nullified by retention of a group size of 10 males and 20 females and the consequent problems of analysis following a 1 : 2 mating (see reproductive studies for drugs). The duration of the premating treatment period has been increased to 100 days for the $F_0$ generation and 120 days for the $F_1$ generation, again extending beyond the optimum breeding age for rats. With respect to timing, the EPA also offers no explanation as to why rats should be weaned at 30 days of age when, internationally, weaning at 21 days (3 weeks) of age is more common. Nor are reasons given as to why $F_0$ adults and their offspring ($F_1$) should be subjected to pathological examination 30 days after birth whereas $F_1$ adults and their offspring ($F_2$) are to be subjected to pathological examination 30 days after weaning, i.e., 60 days after birth. Specifically, there appears to be no reason why similar investigations performed at 21 days post-partum for both generations are not equally valid.

In suggesting the use of one control and three test dosages, the highest of which should cause minimal maternal (or paternal?) toxicity, the EPA has taken a step in the right direction. However, this is then confused by the suggestion that effects on reproduction should be induced at the intermediate dosage. Since wide safety margins and wide intervals between dosages are a common feature of studies with pesticides, this presumes that all compounds will show a selective action on reproduction, which is contrary to past experience. Surely, the whole purpose of using intermediate (and low) dosages is to determine whether or not a selective effect occurs.

Since dosages are now based on the same criteria as those adopted for prolonged toxicity and carcinogenicity studies (including those involving *in utero* exposure), the requirements for extensive histopathological examinations of all $F_1$ adults and some $F_1$ and $F_2$ offspring would appear to provide expensive, time-consuming duplication of information available in other studies. Moreover, they can be considered inadequate in that failure to add the supportive evidence of organ weight analysis, failure to examine the $F_0$ adults, restriction in the numbers of weaning (or near weaning) animals examined (five male, five female per group), and differences in age at the time of examination of young animals (30 days of age for $F_1$, 60 days of age for $F_2$) could all add uncertainty to interpretation of different patterns of results. If histopathological examination is considered relevant in these studies, it would seem advisable to include supportive organ weight analysis, examine $F_0$ as well as $F_1$ adults, and examine corresponding numbers (i.e., one male, one female per litter) of offspring at the same age (i.e., weaning).

In the same vein, the requirements for investigation of spermatogenesis should also be rationalized. The exact methodology is not specified, and it is difficult to imagine how examination of bred males at the same age can be attained for $F_0$, $F_1$, and $F_2$ animals when the latter are not bred and are killed at an earlier age. For the $F_0$ and $F_1$ generation, the fact that a male was capable of inducing a successful pregnancy would be adequate. For unsuccessful males, further mating and ultimately histological examination (on an individual diagnostic basis) should be sufficient. If $F_2$ animals have to be examined, this could be achieved by histopathological examination but on a more adequate sample than the five males per group suggested.

Amidst all the detail, reduced concentration on the main purpose of the study is evident in the failure to define the mating period, to recommend recording of vaginal smears and regular weighing of adults and offspring during pregnancy and lactation (weekly or twice weekly, would be preferable), and failure to determine precoital time and duration of gestation.

## An Alternative Multigeneration Study

As in the case for reproductive studies for drugs, different national requirements for pesticides and food additives force complex, unwieldy designs that are unnecessary given that all have the same basic aim. Again, practical experience with different designs suggests that simplification at the initial screening stage provides the solution. At this juncture, it would be fair to mention that the most satisfactory multigeneration studies we have performed have been those following a design originally suggested by the EPA (Fig. 5).

In this design, one control and three test groups each containing 20 male and 20 female rats were treated for 60 days prior to mating and through mating, gestation,

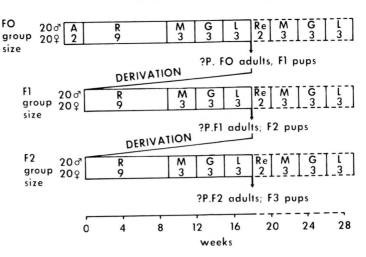

**FIG. 5.** EPA multigeneration study, 1966. *Dotted lines* indicate options to clarify equivocal findings. Abbreviations as in Fig. 1.

and lactation. The study continued until three generations had produced litters. The simplicity of the design allowed "negative" materials to be screened economically and quickly, and the flexibility allowed competent investigators to extend the study, without disruption of the flow, to clarify equivocal results. Why this design was abandoned in favor of the unworkable designs suggested in 1975 (4) remains a mystery.

Current multigeneration studies could be replaced by the simple design recommended for safety evaluation of drugs (Fig. 3). Bearing in mind the different exposure conditions of the general public, there would be a better case for a longer (9 weeks) premating treatment of the $F_0$ generation and for treatment of the $F_1$ generation. Conversely, for the smaller selected industrial population, a case can be made for using the shortest form of test available, i.e., 4 weeks premating dosing, and termination at weaning of first generation animals. This would allow the use of higher dosages and alternative routes of administration to match the more likely conditions and exposure in industrial situations.

## Environmental Protection Agency Teratogenicity Studies

The EPA requires performance of an embryotoxicity/teratogenicity test separately rather than as an interim sacrifice with a multigeneration study. However, initiation of treatment at or just before implantation and continued through pregnancy to termination to some extent nullifies the advantage of performing a separate test. As the test will be performed in conjunction with a multigeneration study, the use of a dosing period similar to that employed in drug testing would be equally and, perhaps, even more meaningful.

Several minor suggestions make the EPA recommendations less economical and do not provide important information in a screening context. These include: (a) the provision of nesting materials when animals may be caged in groups and will be killed prior to parturition; (b) the inclusion of positive controls; (c) the induction of an effect on fetuses at the intermediate dosage (presumptive); and (d) weighing of the gravid uterus, measurement of crown–rump length, and examination of dead fetuses for abnormalities.

In a primary screen, attention should be directed to the determination of more important factors such as fetal viability, fetal weight, and incidence of abnormalities in live young. In contrast to the concern for detail in some aspects, it is recommended that animals be weighed only at the start of dosing and termination. Experience suggests that females should be weighed regularly (at least twice weekly), and dosages adjusted according to body weight up to day 15 for rats and day 18 for rabbits.

The EPA requirements in all their ramifications and detail are certainly more extensive than required internationally and are considered by many to be excessive. For materials to which portions of the general public will be exposed for long periods (e.g., pesticides), these types of studies may be appropriate. With respect to occupational safety, however, the claim that EPA requirements are excessive is more justifiable. In the occupational situation, relatively restricted populations may be exposed to a wide, extensive range of untested basic materials and their intermediates, with short-term accidental exposure to very high dosages likely to present a much greater hazard than for the general public. In this situation, the adoption of shorter, simpler, and more economic tests coupled with an appreciation that these constitute a priority selection system would afford greater protection. Concentration on the use of teratogenic tests for occupational hazards is dangerous in that it will provide virtually no protection to the vast majority of the work force, the predominant male population. Performance of a simple reproductive study, as suggested earlier for drug testing, or even a combined subacute toxicity/reproduction study would provide far greater cover for all aspects of male and female reproduction. Moreover, with correct interpretation of the results, this broader cover can be accomplished without in any way increasing the risk of teratogenesis in pregnant females. With respect to the latter, it must be remembered that: (a) the first priority of a screening test is to determine the lowest dosage at which any adverse effect occurs; (b) teratogens almost invariably induce associated effects at and below dosages causing frank malformations; and (c) these associated effects often preclude use of teratogenic dosages in a reproductive study. In application, exposure levels will be set well below those causing any adverse effect and, therefore, well below those likely to induce malformations.

## CONCLUSION

In summary, the safety evaluation of chemicals has led to a proliferation of complex legislative requirements that not only tie up valuable resources in unnecessary duplication but may also defeat the objective of such legislation. The extreme multidisciplinary nature of safety evaluation extends intellect to the limit and sometimes beyond. The ghost of thalidomide leads to consistent requirements for teratogenicity tests when objectively and historically alternative hazards may be of greater priority. Scientists in authority may persist with old themes in the face of contradictory fact, examples being retention of prolonged premating treatment periods, derivation of animals from second litters, insistence on interim sacrifices at a specific day of pregnancy, and belief that in-depth investigation of a few (notably in histopathology or behavioral testing) will provide protection in areas where low-frequency events may predominate. Perhaps it is fear or lack of confidence in the scientific community that leads to legislation and to demands by the general public for guarantees of safety that are unattainable and out of proportion with the natural hazards of life.

Resolution of the complex situations pertaining to safety evaluation is unlikely to be achieved by increasing the complexity of screening tests. There is a limit to the amount of information they provide. Whether one uses the most complex, time-consuming, and expensive designs or the most simple, inexpensive tests, the difference in the amount and fidelity of the information is negligible compared with the variation and permutation of exposure in man.

Experience with various test methods suggests that it would be of greater benefit to: (a) establish simple initial screening tests that will provide clear answers, albeit to limited questions; (b) accept that these tests provide a starting point rather than an endpoint in safety evaluation; (c) become more aware of the degree and limitations of extrapolation that can be made from these studies; and (d) learn to use the same results from the same tests in different risk/benefit estimations. With respect to the latter, in medicine, greater risks are accepted for life-saving drugs (e.g., antitumor agents) than for antiemetics on an individual basis. In relation to industrial hygiene, pesticides, food additives and the like, it is, therefore, logical that a country or agency should accept greater or lesser degrees of risk on a population basis.

The three-segment design as currently employed for safety evaluation of drugs but with the simpler form of reproductive study previously suggested (Fig. 3) could well be applied to the safety evaluation of pesticides, food additives, new food materials, and industrial chemicals. It would have to be recognized, of course, that the different components may have different values in different areas of legislative control. For example, teratogenic and peri- and postnatal studies would appear to be more pertinent for drug evaluation than for safety at work. Nevertheless, if the population as a whole believes that teratogenic tests should be performed, then it is as equally valid to include peri- and postnatal studies. As is the case with drug testing, there would also be a practical value to performing peri- and postnatal studies and teratogenic studies in the initial stages of the safety evaluation of pesticides or industrial chemicals, for pregnant and lactating animals are frequently more sensitive to general toxic effects. It is certainly worthwhile establishing whether such problems may arise early in the scheme of things using relatively inexpensive tests rather than disrupting a longer, more expensive reproduction study at a late stage.

In the industrial situation with its backlog of minimally investigated materials and likely exposure to high dosages for short periods (e.g., accidents), a short general reproductive study would appear to provide a greater cover and, therefore, be a greater priority than performance of teratogenic tests and/or a "dominant lethal assay" (for male fertility). One would generally choose the shortest format, i.e., dosing for 4 weeks prior to mating and through mating and gestation to lactation for 21 days post-partum or even a combined general toxicity/reproductive study. At the very least, the study would provide preliminary data for selection of dosages for subsequent more widely applicable investigations.

For pesticides and food additives, compared with drugs and industrial chemicals, use of a longer reproductive study (i.e., continuing until the second generation had reared their young to weaning) might perhaps be justifiable (Fig. 3), considering that the general public would be exposed for long periods with little opportunity for individual control of dosage. It would also be more appropriate to limit pathological examinations to thorough macroscopic examination of all adults and offspring within a study. If considered necessary, tissues from all adults ($F_0$, $F_1$) and from one male and one female weanling per litter born ($F_1$ and $F_2$ generations) could be preserved against the contingency of histopathological examination. With proper evaluation and cross reference to other studies, it is unlikely that this extension will be necessary in the majority of cases, but when it is required, the pathologist will have available a more meaningful sample on which to make interpretation.

In whatever sequence these tests may be performed for the different legislative areas, the key factor is to consider each segment not in isolation but as part of an integrated unit. The integrated results in turn must be consolidated with other toxicological and pharmacological results (14). Only then can the overall toxicological (or biological) profile of a test material begin to take shape and provide the point at which cautious extrapolation outside the test species can begin. In some cases, secondary investigations will be required to provide a clearer profile, although in many, it will be sufficiently clear to determine whether or not use in humans would be a justifiable risk.

Justifiable risk will vary from compound to compound. For pesticides, food additives, and some other materials the benefit/risk ratio could be expected to differ in different countries. Guarantee of absolute safety should never be given, and, during the early years of use, there should be careful monitoring, particularly for idiosyncratic responses that could never be detected in animal tests.

## NOTE ADDED IN PROOF

Since the preparation of this article, evidence has come to light of a strong movement to harmonize regulations through the auspices of the OECD (Organization for Economic and Commercial Development) and the IRLG (Interagency Regulatory Liaison Group). Although only at a draft stage and as yet unpublished, the proposed studies for the investigation of reproductive toxicity follow closely the alternative methodology suggested by the author.

## REFERENCES

1. Barrow, M. V., and Taylor, W. J. (1969): A rapid method for detecting malformations in rat fetuses. *J. Morphol.*, 127:291–306.
2. Brown, A. M. (1963): Matching the animal with the experiment. In: *Animals for Research*, edited by W. Lane-Petter, pp. 261–285. Academic Press, London.
3. Courtney, K. D., Gaylor, D. W., Hogan, M. D., Falk, H. L., Bates, R. R., and Mitchell, I. (1970): Teratogenic evaluation of 2,4,5-T. *Science*, 168:864–866.
4. Environmental Protection Agency (1975): Proposed rules: Methods for study of reproductive and teratogenic toxicity. *Federal Register*, 40:26898–26899.
5. Environmental Protection Agency (1978): Proposed guidelines for registering pesticides. *Federal Register*, 43:37336–37403.
6. Environmental Protection Agency (1979): Proposed health effects test standards for toxic substances control act. *Federal Register*, 44:44054–44093.
7. Food and Drug Administration (1978): Good laboratory practices regulations. *Federal Register*, 43:59986–60025.
8. Frohberg, H. (1977): An introduction to research in teratology. In: *Methods in Prenatal Toxicology*, edited by D. Neubert, H.-J. Merker, and T. E. Kwasigroch, pp. 1–13. Georg Thieme, Berlin.
9. Haseman, J. K., and Hogan, M. D. (1975): Selection of the experimental unit in teratology studies. *Teratology*, 12(2):165–171.
10. Karnofsky, D. A. (1965): Mechanisms of action of certain growth inhibiting drugs. In: *Teratology: Principles and Techniques*, edited by J. G. Wilson and J. Warkany, pp. 185–193. University of Chicago Press, Chicago.

11. Palmer, A. K. (1972): Some thoughts on reproductive studies for safety evaluation. In: *Proc. ESSDT, International Congress Series, No. 288*, Vol. 14, pp. 79–80. Excerpta Medica, Amsterdam.
12. Palmer, A. K. (1974): Problems associated with the screening of drugs for possible teratogenic activity. In: *Experimental Embryology and Teratology 1*, edited by D. H. M. Woollam and G. M. Morriss, pp. 16–33. Paul Elek, London.
13. Palmer, A. K. (1974): Statistical analysis and choice of sample units. *Teratology*, 10(3):301–302.
14. Palmer, A. K. (1976): Assessment of current test procedures. *Environ. Health Perspect.*, 18:97–104.
15. Palmer, A. K. (1977): Incidence of sporadic malformations, anomalies and variations in random bred laboratory animals. In: *Methods in Prenatal Toxicology*, edited by D. Neubert, H.-J. Merker, and T. E. Kwasigroch, pp. 52–71. Georg Thieme, Berlin.
16. Palmer, A. K. (1978): The design of subprimate animal studies. In: *Handbook of Teratology, Vol. 4*, edited by J. G. Wilson and F. C. Fraser, pp. 215–253. Plenum Press, New York.
17. Schumacher, H., Blake, D. A., Gurian, J. M., and Gillette, J. R. (1968): A comparison of the teratogenic activity of thalidomide in rabbits and rats. *J. Pharmacol. Exp. Ther.*, 10(1):189–197.
18. Somers, G. F. (1962): Letter to the editor. *Lancet*, 1:28:4.
19. Staples, R. E., and Haseman, J. K. (1974): Selection of appropriate experimental units in teratology. *Teratology*, 9(3):259.
20. Wilson, J. G. (1965): Embryological considerations in teratology. In:*Teratology: Principles and Techniques*, edited by J. G. Wilson and J. Warkany, pp. 251–277. University of Chicago Press, Chicago.
21. World Health Organization Scientific Group (1967): *Principles for the Testing of Drugs for Teratogenicity, Technical Report No. 364*. World Health Organization, Geneva.
22. Zeeman, E. C. (1977): *Catastrophe Theory: Selected Papers 1972–1977*. Addison-Wesley, Reading, Massachusetts.

*Developmental Toxicology*, edited by
C. A. Kimmel and J. Buelke-Sam. Raven Press,
New York © 1981.

# Epidemiology and Developmental Toxicology

## J. David Erickson

*Bureau of Epidemiology, U.S. Public Health Service, Department of Health and Human Services, Center for Disease Control, Atlanta, Georgia 30333*

This chapter describes the uses of epidemiology, particularly as they apply to developmental toxicology, and is divided into two major sections. The first deals with definitions of epidemiology, indicates its scope, describes its uses, and explains some general problems that are encountered in doing epidemiologic research. The second describes the methods of epidemiology, indicating the strengths and weaknesses of each approach.

## EPIDEMIOLOGY: DEFINITIONS AND USES

MacMahon and Pugh (13) define epidemiology as "...the study of the distribution and determinants of disease frequency in man." To many persons who consider themselves epidemiologists, this definition is too narrow. There are those who evaluate health services without necessarily searching for the determinants of the disease. Veterinary epidemiologists may study the distribution and determinants of disease, but not in man. But despite these and other arguments that might be raised about this definition, it will well suit our purposes here, if we also note that epidemiology is concerned with finding means for preventing disease. Epidemiology is as much a group of methodologies as it is a distinct scientific discipline. It grew in response to the great epidemic diseases. But now, more and more epidemiologists devote their energies to chronic and noninfectious diseases, including the problems of abnormal development.

The definition used here implies two major phases of inquiry, one of describing the distribution of disease and the other of searching for determinants. The first phase is often called descriptive epidemiology, and the second, analytic epidemiology. The descriptive phase may be thought of as a form of medical demography to document the variations of disease with such factors as age, race, or sex. This description may itself provide clues as to the causes of disease, and it is useful in defining normative values. Simply knowing how often a disease occurs and which subsets of the population are at highest or lowest risk is an important initial step towards understanding the disease. Disease does not occur randomly in a population; some who are exposed to a noxious agent will develop disease, and some will not. Descriptive epidemiology seeks to define the characteristics of those who do and do not become ill. Analytic epidemiology seeks to discover which of those characteristics are actually responsible for the disease.

Analytic epidemiology is much like many other types of health-related research in that it aims to discover disease determinants. But it differs from other sciences in that it deals with populations rather than with individuals. It is further set apart in that it often operates on a relatively simple mechanistic basis. Developmental toxicologists are used to thinking in rather detailed and sophisticated mechanistic terms, being concerned about specific enzymatic reactions, and so on. The simple mechanistic approach of epidemiology can nevertheless be useful; often, prevention can be achieved without a sophisticated understanding of causal mechanisms. A classic example derives from John Snow's work on cholera in London during the last century (17). Snow was able to demonstrate that the occurrence of cholera was associated with the consumption of drinking water from some location, and he was able to prevent the disease by restricting the use of that water. He did this without understanding that a cholera *Vibrio* contaminated the water, without understanding the physiological and biochemical disturbances that accompany the infection, without understanding the ecology of the *Vibrio*, and so on. In other words, he operated on a simple mechanistic basis and yet was able to prevent disease successfully. The same principle applies today.

A primary motivation for doing medical and biologic research is to improve human health. For this reason, epidemiology occupies a central role in all health research, including developmental toxicology. Laboratory work with nonhuman animals provides us with an opportunity to learn about pathogenetic mechanisms and offers clues that can be followed up in studies of humans and can be done relatively quickly and cheaply. But we must not ignore our primary motivating force and need to give proper emphasis to the study of humans.

Although epidemiology plays a central and imperative role in learning about developmental toxicology as it affects humans, there are problems involved. It is often time consuming and expensive. This is especially true if one is dealing with rare disease states, and most diseases that could conceivably result from developmental toxicity are rare. We shall return to this problem in a later section, but one aspect of it needs to be addressed here. The scientific and lay literature are replete with articles saying that a particular chemical or environmental pollutant causes some type of developmental disturbance. These accusations are often based on no more than anecdotes, but they do generate considerable public concern. The task of confirming or refuting the accusation often falls to the epidemiologist; his is frequently an unenviable task, since it is logically impossible to prove a lack of an association. It is not possible to assert that an agent does not have some particular effect. One can only say that, within the limitations of a particular study, no effect was observed. Such a negative result always needs to be considered in terms of the study's sensitivity, since a null finding from an insensitive study has no utility. We may consider a not so extreme example that will help to clarify this point. Suppose that a chemical is thought to cause an increase in the frequency of a certain congenital malformation. Further, suppose that (a) the malformation normally occurs once in every 1,000 births, (b) the chemical increases the frequency to 2 per 1,000 in the offspring of exposed women, and (c) 10% of pregnant women are exposed. If we study the offspring of 1,000 women (no small accomplishment), we would expect to find 100 exposed women and 0.2 affected children. Since we cannot observe 0.2 and 0.9 affected, we might find 1, or more probably 0, affected among the exposed and 0, or more probably 1, affected among the unexposed.

The outcome of such a study would show no difference between exposed and unexposed, and some might be tempted to term it a negative study indicating no effect of exposure. In truth, the only valid interpretation of such a study would be an agnostic one—the results would tell us almost nothing. This is a bit of an overstatement. We do learn something about the unknown state of nature. From such a study, we would learn that the risk associated with the chemical could not be 1,000-fold the normal, not 100-fold, and so on. Thus, the study would allow us to put some upper limit on the risk due to the chemical, but it would not allow us to be very precise about that limit.

We should also give consideration to the strength of the inferences that can be drawn from epidemiological studies from another point of view. Epidemiological studies can also be categorized as either experimental (interventional) or observational. The intervention study, exemplified by the vaccine field trial, is very much like the classical experiment familiar to the developmental toxicologist. A key feature of experimental studies is the random assignment of the experimental units to treatments. In the vaccine trial, study subjects are randomly assigned to the new vaccine regimen or to a standard or placebo regimen. Through the agency of this randomization, the investigator ensures, in a certain probabilistic sense, that the two groups will differ only in their vaccine regimen. Other characteristics that might influence the susceptibility to disease will be equal in the two groups. Thus, inferences about the efficacy of the vaccine can be relatively firm.

In observational studies, the investigator looks at what has happened in two groups without any intervention, without any random assignment of subjects to treatments. An observational study of the vaccine problem would consist of the observation of disease occurrence among persons who just happened to be vaccine recipients and a contrasting of their experience with a group who just happened not to be vaccinated. If a difference in disease rates between the two groups is observed, how does one know that it is due to the vaccine and not to some other factor (or factors) which predicts both for the susceptibility or resistance to disease and the propensity or reluctance for a person to be a vaccine recipient (epidemiologists call such factors confounding variables)? For example, perhaps persons who are relatively resistant to the disease through the agency of better health care, a more salubrious lifestyle, etc., also happen to be recipients of the vaccine. If such a situation were obtained, one would be hard pressed to know how much of a reduced incidence of disease was due to the vaccine and how much to other factors that confer disease resistance. Sometimes, the investigator can use descriptive studies to determine likely confounding variables and can then design an observational study so as to nullify their effects. At other times, the investigator is able to correct for them statistically. But even if he is able to identify and account for some confounding variables, he can never be sure that account has been made of all factors that influence disease occurrence. There must, therefore, be some residual uncertainty about how much of the differences noted result from the treatment.

As discussed above, one of the effects of the randomization in an experiment is to give the study "balance," to help insure that confounders are equally distributed in the experimental and control groups. It should be noted, however, that randomization does not offer a guarantee that this will happen; sometimes randomization will "fail." Thus, even with the experimental approach, there will be some residue of uncertainty when inferences are made. In summary then, the randomization approach will, on the average, yield a picture that is free of confounding effects, but in any particular instance, we cannot know if there has been a clouding of that picture by confounding variables. Because, on the average, randomization will "work," we can feel somewhat more secure in drawing inferences from an experimental than an observational study. But it is obvious that it is not an all-or-none situation, and making judgments about the results of any study must be done cautiously.

Because there is always some uncertainty about the meaning of the results of even the best designed and executed study, the making of causal inferences is part art. This uncertainty injects an element of the subjective into what we would prefer to be a completely objective process. In this regard, it is useful to recall a well known aphorism: correlation (statistical association) does not necessarily imply causation. Since statistical associations are all that we can obtain from any kind of study, this aphoristic statement also implies an element of subjectivity. A number of attempts have been made to codify this subjective process, and one of the best was set forth by the 1964 Surgeon General's Advisory Committee on Smoking and Health (18). Briefly, the Committee suggested the consideration of the following points.

1. Do diverse methods of study yield similar results?
2. Is the observed association strong?
3. How specific is the association?
4. Does the putative cause temporally precede the effect?
5. Is the association coherent with known facts about the natural history and biology of the disease?

## METHODS IN EPIDEMIOLOGY

Much of the day-to-day practice of epidemiology involves the application of the principles of mathematical statistics to the analysis of medical data. No general discussion of these principles is presented here, and the interested reader is referred to one of the standard texts on applied statistics or biometry. As noted above, we search for and evaluate associations between putative agents and disease. Of the several ways in which such associations can be quantified, that of relative risk appears throughout the epidemiologic literature but is not widely discussed in statistical texts. Therefore, some of its fundamental properties will be presented here.

The relative risk is the ratio of two disease rates and is occasionally termed the rate ratio. Since disease rates are sometimes considered as being some indication of disease risk, the term "risk ratio" is also sometimes applied to this quantity. In Table 1, data dealing with the thalidomide tragedy appear (14); for the purposes of all discussion that follows, we will consider these data to represent a complete population of births.

Thalidomide was marketed as a seemingly innocuous drug but was later discovered to be a developmental toxin, resulting in limb reduction deformities in the children of women who took the drug in early pregnancy. There were a total of 24 mothers who had been exposed to thalidomide 0 to 8 weeks after conception, and 10 of their babies had skeletal limb defects. Thus, the rate (or risk) of defects after exposure was 0.4167 (10/24), and the rate in the absence of exposure was 0.0024 (51/21,485). The relative risk, that is, the risk after exposure relative to the risk after no exposure, was 173.6 (0.4167/0.0024). This quantity indicates very strong association between thalidomide exposure and limb defects.

The odds ratio is often used in epidemiology as a surrogate for the relative risk. It is ratio of two odds—the odds of having the defect given exposure relative to the odds of having the defect given no exposure. From the data in Table 1, the former odds is 0.7143 (10/14), the latter is 0.0024 (51/21,434), and the odds ratio is 297.6 (0.7143/0.0024). The odds ratio is useful because an important new statistical approach to data analysis deals with associations in terms of the odds ratio; it is also useful for another reason that will be discussed below.

The major study designs that are useful in investigating human developmental disturbances are discussed below as well. These are studies of group characteristics, cohort studies, case-control studies, and intervention studies. Population surveillance is also considered.

## Studies of Group Characteristics

The approach here is to compare group levels of putative toxins with group levels of disease. For example, one might gather information on a group basis about the

TABLE 1. *Limb reduction deformities and thalidomide exposure*[a]

| | Numbers with and without limb reduction defects | | | Defect Rate per 1,000 |
|---|---|---|---|---|
| Thalidomide | With | Without | Total | |
| Exposed | 10 | 14 | 24 | 416.7 |
| Not exposed | 51 | 21,434 | 21,485 | 2.4 |
| Total | 61 | 21,448 | 21,509 | 2.9 |
| Percent exposed | 16.4 | 0.1 | | |

[a]Derived from McBride (14).

sales of some drug and about the frequency of some congenital malformation. The correlation between the level of sales and the frequency of the malformation is then assessed. If the drug is a cause of the defect, then one would expect that higher rates of malformation occurrence would be found in the groups with higher sales levels and vice versa.

This study approach has not been widely used in developmental toxicology but has found wide application in cancer (7) and cardiovascular epidemiology (5). In these latter studies, the groups used have often been defined by some political unit. Since appropriate data are often available on a national basis, many studies of this genre involve international comparisons. In the United States, data are often available for cities, counties, or states, and many studies have used these political divisions to form groups. While political divisions are commonly used to form comparison groups, a variety of criteria can be used.

The data in Table 2 are derived from a Center for Disease Control study of this type (3). It was suggested that the noise associated with major airports might be a cause of an increased frequency of birth defects (8). We explored this hypothesis using data gathered in metropolitan Atlanta. The rates of defect occurrence were compared in several groups defined on the basis of average community noise level.

A variant of the line of reasoning used in these studies can be seen in the data presented in Fig. 1. The sales of thalidomide in West Germany are plotted along with the frequency of the occurrence of limb defects. The defect curve follows the sales curve with approximately an 8-month lag. Thus, women who were in their early stages of pregnancy during the periods when drug sales were low had relatively few babies with defects, whereas those who were at the same stage when drug sales were high had larger numbers of affected babies.

This form of study is perhaps the most primitive type used in epidemiology (this does not necessarily imply that they are easy to do) and is especially susceptible to what has been termed the "ecological fallacy" (19); i.e., an association that holds for groups may not hold for the individuals in the groups. Suppose that it is found that there is a positive association between group level of a drug's sales and group level of malformation occurrence. Further study might reveal that among the individuals within each group there is no association between drug exposure and

TABLE 2. *Airport noise and neural tube defects*[a]

|  | Numbers with exposure to noise $\geq 65$ L$^{dn}$ | | |
|  | Exposed | Not exposed | Percent exposed |
| --- | --- | --- | --- |
| Neural tube defects | 28 | 263 | 9.62 |
| No defect | 7,736 | 74,440 | 9.41 |
| Defect rate per 1,000 | 3.61 | 3.52 | |

[a]Derived from Edmonds et al. (3).

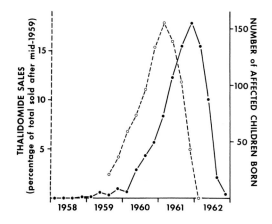

**FIG. 1.** Quarterly thalidomide sales *(interrupted line)* and births of children with defect syndrome *(solid line)* in West Germany, excluding Hamburg (12).

malformation frequency. Thus, the association apparent at a group level could not be attributed to the drug but would have its origin in other causes.

## Cohort Studies

The cohort study usually begins with the assembly of a sample of people who are exposed to a suspected toxin and a sample of those who are not exposed. The groups are then followed to ascertain the subsequent disease experience in each group. Since the cohort study is forward-looking, proceeding from suspect cause to disease, it is sometimes termed prospective. The cohort study is much like the experiment, with the primary difference being that the investigator does not manipulate the exposure but simply observes what happens. Because of the prospective nature of these studies, it is possible to compute disease rates, and, therefore, the relative risk may also be derived. This feature is a major advantage of the cohort approach. From a logical and temporal point of view, the cohort study directly answers the question of interest: does exposure to the suspect agent increase the occurrence of the disease? Another major advantage is that it is possible to study any of the effects of exposure to the agent. However, since the typical cohort study begins with samples of exposed and nonexposed, it is usually not possible to compute exposure rates. A typical study might begin with samples of equal numbers of exposed and nonexposed subjects, and it is obvious that the exposure rate derived from such a study (i.e., 50%) would not necessarily reflect the true exposure rate in the population from which the samples were drawn. This is, however, a minor disadvantage.

The cohort study also has the advantage that it is free from certain types of bias in ascertaining information about exposure. This is so because exposure information is gathered before information about the occurrence of disease is obtained. There is, however, a possibility of biases occurring in the ascertainment of disease occurrence in some situations. These issues will be discussed further in the next section.

The main disadvantage of the cohort study is the expense that is often incurred in its execution and the time that is required for its completion. The expense of a cohort study is, in part, proportional to the frequency of the disease under consideration. If the disease is rare, as are many developmental disturbances, then one must follow a large number of study subjects to ascertain even a few cases. To be concrete, suppose we are primarily interested in studying the effects of some agent on a particular congenital malformation that occurs normally at the rate of one in every 1,000 births. Obviously, in order to ascertain more than a handful of cases, several thousand pregnancies must be studied.

The time required for a cohort study depends on how long it takes for the disease to become manifest. If interest centers on developmental defects that are detectable at birth and if the exposure of interest occurs during pregnancy, considerations of time are of little consequence. On the other hand, if interest is about diseases that occur or are detectable only later in life, the time element becomes an important consideration; the same holds if the exposure of interest occurs some time before pregnancy. Examples of these difficulties in developmental work include such outcomes as mental growth or childhood or adult cancer and such exposures as irradiation of pregnant women or even the effects on the baby or irradiation of the mother while she herself is *in utero*.

Despite the decided advantages of cohort studies, the time and expense involved sometimes make them infeasible. In such instances, the case-control study is often the approach followed.

## Case-Control Studies

In case-control studies, one assembles a group of cases and a comparison ("control") group and contrasts their histories of exposure to the suspect toxic agent. Since the case-control study is backwards-looking, starting out with the presence or absence of disease and searching for evidence of prior exposure, it is often termed retrospective. As was noted in the section on cohort studies, the question of interest generally is: does the agent increase the frequency of the disease? The case-control study directly answers the converse question: is there a history of increased exposure among those with the disease? The cohort study provides direct estimates of disease rates and, hence, a direct estimate of the relative risk. This is not possible with a case-control study. A typical case-control study might begin with an equal number of cases and controls. The disease frequency computed from such a study would be 50% and would be meaningless, since it would be dictated solely by the study design. The case-control study, then, does not provided a direct estimate of the relative risk, the ratio of the disease rates in the exposed and unexposed. On the other hand, a case-control study does provide direct estimates of the exposure rates.

Even though case-control studies do not provide direct estimates of disease rates, it has been shown that they can provide indirect estimates of the relative risk. The use of the case-control study to make this indirect estimate involves the logic of Bayes' theorem and generally an assumption that the disease is rare (2). It turns out that the application of these principles yields the odds ratio (which was presented earlier as being a surrogate for the relative risk) as the proper indirect estimate.

To illustrate some of these ideas, let us suppose that we do a case-control study of the thalidomide episode, using the data in Table 1 to derive our samples of cases and controls. In this hypothetical situation, we have studied all 61 cases with limb reduction deformities, and we choose 20 controls for every case. From the data in Table 1, we note that the rate of thalidomide exposure among those without defects was 0.007 (14/21,448). Thus, among 1,220 controls, we would expect 0.85 to have been exposed to thalidomide. Since this is an unobservable outcome, we simplify the situation by assuming that we observe 1 exposure. These hypothetical data are presented in Table 3. Suppose that we do compute disease "rates" from these data. There are a total of 11 exposed and 1,170 not exposed. Then the disease "rate" in the exposed would be 0.9091 (10/11) and 0.0436 in the unexposed. These "rates" obviously do not agree with the disease rates computed from the population in Table 1, 0.4167 (10/24) in the exposed and 0.0024 (51/21,485) in the unexposed. On the other hand, the exposure rates computed from the data in Table 3 correspond to those computed from Table 1. The odds ratio computed from Table 3 (i.e., the odds of exposure given the defect, 10/51, relative to the odds of exposure given no defect, 1/1,119) is 219.4 and constitutes a reasonable estimate of the relative risk computed from the population, 173.6. In general, the odds ratio and relative risk will correspond more closely. In this particular instance, the very high rate of defects among the exposed causes the odds ratio to be somewhat higher than the relative risk.

A major problem of case-control studies involves biases in determining exposures. Sometimes a relatively reliable history of prior exposure may be obtained. Often, however, the history must be derived from the questioning of diseased persons or their relations. Persons who are affected by the disease may have a tendency to provide a distorted picture of their exposure history. We feel that the potential for this distortion is very great in case-control studies of birth defects. In the metropolitan Atlanta area, we question women about first-trimester exposures 3 to 6 months after their children are born. Since the time lag is great and because we feel that the mother of a defective child will tend to embroider her memory, we do not compare their accounts with those of normal babies. Instead, we compare the

TABLE 3. *Results of a hypothetical case-control[a] study of thalidomide and limb defects*

| Limb defect | Exposed | Not exposed | Percent exposed |
|---|---|---|---|
| With | 10 | 51 | 16.39 |
| Without | 1 | 1,119 | 0.09 |

[a]Derived from data in Table 1; see text.

exposure history of mothers of babies with one particular defect with the history of mothers of babies of all other types of defects (15). This approach is illustrated in Table 4 which shows an association between diazepam exposure and cleft lip. Note that this approach would fail if some agent raised the frequency of all types of malformations. However, most known human teratogens induce specific malformations or patterns of them; results of experiments with animals also generally support this point of view.

Despite the major concern with bias and the fact that case-control studies approach the question of interest indirectly, they have several very significant advantages. And it is reemphasized that they are often the only feasible way of approaching some problems. Usually the case-control study can be done more quickly than the cohort study, since one obtains a history of exposure after occurrence of disease rather than waiting for disease to develop subsequent to exposure. Case-control studies are also much more economical when the disease in question is rare and where the exposure of concern is moderately frequent.

## Intervention Studies

The data from the thalidomide study shown in Fig. 1 have the flavor of an intervention study, in that after the drug was withdrawn from the marketplace, it was observed that the frequency of the defect subsequently fell. However, the manipulation of exposures on a pilot basis has rarely been done in the field of human developmental toxicology. The various rubella vaccine field trials certainly fit the mold of the intervention process.

## Surveillance

The surveillance of populations and the monitoring of trends in disease occurrence are not widely used epidemiologic tools for many chronic diseases. But surveillance and monitoring of some forms of developmental disturbances, notably congenital malformations, are practiced in many parts of the world (6), and the procedures deserve emphasis here. The rationale for these surveillance programs rests on the thalidomide episode. There is a presumption that, if the occurrence of birth defects had been subject to surveillance and trends monitored, the epidemic of limb defects would have been detected earlier. A further presumption is that, if the epidemic had been discovered earlier, the causal connection would have been made sooner.

TABLE 4. *Diazepam and cleft lip with or without cleft palate[a]*

|  | Exposed | Not exposed | Total |
|---|---|---|---|
| Cleft lip | 7 | 42 | 51 |
| All other defects | 9 | 220 | 229 |

[a]Derived from Safra and Oakley (15); odds ratio is 4.07.

Surveillance programs for birth defects usually operate on some variant of the following scheme. A target population is defined and the numbers of babies with various types of defects are ascertained on a timely basis. The total numbers of births that occur in the same population are also determined, and using these, malformation occurrence rates are computed. Because of the completeness of ascertainment of the occurrence of defects varies from program to program, each makes comparisons of current defect rates with its own base-line or "normal". If an increase in the frequency at which a defect occurs is noted, one of the first lines of investigation involves an attempt to learn if it might have resulted from some artifact of the reporting system. If the increase cannot readily be attributed to an artifact, other studies are often mounted (e.g., 1,9).

The Center for Disease Control administers two birth defects surveillance and monitoring programs, the Metropolitan Atlanta Congenital Defects Surveillance Program and the quasi-national Birth Defects Monitoring Program (BDMP). The Atlanta program has a population base of about 25,000 births per year, and cases are ascertained during regular staff visits to local hospitals. The BDMP's method of case ascertainment involves using computer-coded discharge forms provided by about 1,200 hospitals around the U.S.; the population of births under surveillance numbers about 1,000,000 per year. The data gathered in Atlanta are of a higher quality than are the national data, although the Atlanta program is numerically and geographically limited. Thus, the two systems complement each other in many respects.

Our experience with ventricular septal defect (VSD) illustrates several aspects of surveillance and monitoring procedures; unfortunately, it is a problem for which we have not yet reached a solution. Both the BDMP (Fig. 2) and the Atlanta data have shown a substantial upward secular trend in VSD occurrence, and the BDMP data revealed that the increase is nationwide. Since the increase has been noted in data gathered by two different surveillance programs, it is unlikely that the increase can be attributed to some administrative change in reporting (1). However, because VSD can range from a mild, often not apparent lesion to a massive, life-threatening

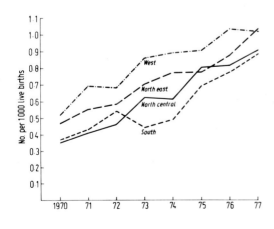

**FIG. 2.** Incidence of ventricular septal defect in the United States, Birth Defects Monitoring Program hospitals, 1970 to 1977, by region (9).

defect, the completeness with which it is reported could vary considerably with pediatric acuity or fashion. It is also possible that changes in pediatric practice, such as the recent establishment of newborn intensive-care centers, have resulted in an increased survival of high-risk babies. The natural history of VSD indicates that many lesions, particularly the smaller ones, resolve spontaneously. To investigate the possibility that the statistical increase is due to an increase in the diagnosis of minor lesions that will eventually resolve, we compared data from the early 1970s with data from the later years of the decade. We sought to determine the rate of spontaneous closure during the first year of life in each of the two time periods. We found that there had not been an increase of spontaneous closure of the lesions diagnosed in the later years (9). Thus, the increase in VSD frequency may be "real." A case-control study looking for causal associations is the logical next step to be taken in seeking the cause of this epidemic.

Data gathered as a part of surveillance programs are useful for a variety of other purposes as well. They can serve as the base for descriptive studies (1,11,16), as a source of cases for case-control studies (10,15), or as the starting point for other types of analytic studies (4).

## REFERENCES

1. Anderson, C. E., Edmonds, L. D., and Erickson, J. D. (1978): Patent ductus arteriosus and ventricular septal defect. Trends in reported frequency. *Am. J. Epidemiol.*, 107:281–289.
2. Cornfield, J. (1951): A method of estimating comparative rates from clinical data. Applications to cancer of the lung, breast and cervix. *J. Natl. Cancer Inst.*, 11:1269–1271.
3. Edmonds, L. D., Layde, P. M., and Erickson, J. D. (1979): Airport noise and teratogenesis. *Arch. Environ. Health*, 39:243–247.
4. Erickson, J. D. (1979): Down syndrome and paternal age. *Am. J. Hum. Genet.*, 31:489–497.
5. Fabsitz, R., and Fenleib, M. (1980): Geographic patterns in county mortality rates from cardiovascular diseases. *Am. J. Epidemiol.*, 111:315–328.
6. Flynt, J. W., and Hay, S. (1979): International clearinghouse for birth defects monitoring systems. *Contrib. Epidemiol. Biostatist.*, 1:44–52.
7. Hoover, R., Mason, T. J., McKay, F. W., and Fraumeni, J. F. (1975): Geographic patterns of cancer mortality in the United States. In: *Persons at High Risk of Cancer*, edited by J. F. Fraumeni. Academic Press, New York.
8. Jones, F. N., and Tauscher, J. (1978): Residence under an airport landing pattern as a factor in teratism. *Arch. Environ. Health.*, 38:10–12.
9. Layde, P. M., Dooley, K., Erickson, J. D., and Edmonds, L. D. (1980): Is there an epidemic of ventricular septal defect in the United States? *Lancet*, 1:407–408.
10. Layde, P. M., and Erickson, J. D. (1980): Maternal fever and neural tube defects. *Teratology*, 21:105–108.
11. Layde, P. M., Erickson, J. D., Falek, A., and McCarthy, B. J. (1980): Congenital malformations in twins. *Am. J. Hum. Genet.*, 32:69–78.
12. Leck, I. (1974): Paediatric aspects of epidemiology—insights into the causation of disorders of early life. In: *Scientific Foundations of Paediatrics*, edited by J. A. Davis and J. Dobbing, pp. 727–757. W. B. Saunders, Philadelphia.
13. MacMahon, B., and Pugh, T. F. (1970): *Epidemiology Principles and Methods*. Little, Brown, Boston.
14. McBride, W. G. (1965): *Personal communication*, cited in: T. H. Ingalls and M. A. Klingberg (1965): Congenital malformations: Clinical and community considerations. *Am. J. Med. Sci.*, 249:316–344.
15. Safra, M. J., and Oakley, G. P. (1975): Association between cleft lip with or without cleft palate and prenatal exposure in diazepam. *Lancet*, 2:478–480.

16. Safra, M. J., Oakley, G. P., and Erickson, J. D. (1976): Descriptive epidemiology of small bowel atresia in metropolitan Atlanta. *Teratology*, 14:143–149.
17. Snow, J. (1855): *On the Mode of Communication of Cholera, second edition*. Churchill, London. Reproduced in *Snow on Cholera*. Commonwealth Fund, New York, 1936. Reprinted by Hafner, New York, 1965.
18. Surgeon General's Advisory Committee Report on Smoking and Health (1964): *USPHS Publication 1103*. United States Government Printing Office, Washington.
19. Susser, M. (1973): *Causal Thinking in the Health Sciences*. Oxford University Press, New York.

*Developmental Toxicology*, edited by
C. A. Kimmel and J. Buelke-Sam. Raven Press,
New York © 1981.

# Embryo Explants and Organ Cultures in Screening of Chemicals for Teratogenic Effects

## D. M. Kochhar

*Department of Anatomy, Jefferson Medical College, Thomas Jefferson University, Philadelphia, Pennsylvania 19107*

There has been a resurgence of interest in designing *in vitro* methods for screening environmental chemicals that could augment and refine currently available methods using pregnant animals. Teratogenesis, the process of abnormal development, is one of the important manifestations of toxicity induced *in utero* by chemicals, and in this regard, it should be as amenable to *in vitro* testing as are other aspects of toxicity, e.g., carcinogenesis and mutagenesis. Unlike other testing systems, however, *in vitro* testing for teratogenesis presents certain special circumstances, since the target is a rapidly growing embryo whose tissues are simultaneously embarked on divergent pathways of organogenesis. This chapter outlines some advantages of a few presently available *in vitro* testing systems and discusses their limitations and future prospects. The discussion is limited to systems that employ mammalian embryos and embryonic tissues in culture, and instances from our own work on limb bud organ cultures are used to illustrate the feasibility of these approaches to the study of teratogenesis.

## LIMITATIONS OF TERATOLOGICAL TESTING IN ANIMALS

Preclinical screening of new drugs and chemicals for teratological activity is conducted on pregnant laboratory animals such as mice, rats, rabbits, and, in certain rare instances, on nonhuman primates. The procedure involves daily administration of the compound during the period of organogenesis followed by examination of the near-term fetuses for skeletal, visceral, and external anomalies. With a decade or so of experience with this procedure, a certain degree of confidence has been generated that seems to lull investigators into complacency and lack of trust in new approaches. The procedure itself is beset with problems, foremost among which is extrapolation of data gathered in one species of animals to another, namely, man, where direct monitoring is impractical. Another is the cost of animal testing. In addition, the procedure allows no assessment as to whether the administered drug influences the embryo directly or through one of its metabolites; the drug and/or metabolites may even alter maternal or placental metabolism and thereby indirectly influence the developing embryo. With no buildup of historical data about the mechanism of action of drugs previously tested, each new drug is an entity by itself and can only be evaluated using a "blind" pregnancy test.

These are certainly not the only reasons why investigators would seek other ways of monitoring teratogenicity. Apart from new therapeutic drugs and chemicals, there are chemical agents already present in our environment—and still others being introduced every day—about which we know very little regarding the potential hazard they present to the embryo. It is estimated that there are about 60,000 chemicals in common use today. If these chemicals and those that are yet to come are to be tested, they present a formidable task that will prove impossible to meet in the foreseeable future with the pregnant animal-testing procedures currrently in use (76).

## POTENTIAL OF TISSUE CULTURE TECHNIQUES

A number of advantages to toxicity testing are offered by tissue culture methodology, and a variety of *in vitro* test systems are being utilized in carcinogenesis and mutagenesis studies (4,5,16,32). The following features make tissue culture methods particularly relevant to studies on teratogenesis (36,37,63).

1. Embryonic cells and tissues are made accessible to direct observation.
2. The stage of development of the target organ or tissue at the time of exposure can be precisely determined.
3. Variability in tissue response is reduced or eliminated by direct control over the experimental conditions.
4. Replicate samples can be obtained from the same litter or even from the same embryo.
5. Control over the duration of exposure of the target cells and tissues to the agent can easily be exercised.
6. Maternal/placental metabolism of the drug is circumvented; hence, rather precise assessment of the active form of the chemical agent can be made.

In general, these advantages are offered by all types of *in vitro* systems whether they involve monolayer cell cultures or employ tissue culture of whole embryos or embryonic organs. The usefulness of cell cultures in studies on teratogenesis, however, is limited by the fact that cells grown as monolayers or as colonies cannot be considered representative of the complex developmental events encountered in embryogenesis. Tissue interactions, differential patterns of cell proliferation and cell death, morphogenetic cell movements, and all other similar events require some degree of tissue organization that the monolayer cell cultures cannot provide. In spite of this fact, a few *in vitro* teratology-monitoring systems that utilize cultured cells have recently been proposed (12,74), and these will be discussed in a following section.

## WHOLE EMBRYO EXPLANT

The most successful methods of culturing mammalian embryos have been devised by New and co-workers (17,55–57). To prepare the postimplantation rat or mouse embryo for culture, the whole conceptus is removed from the uterus and transferred to a dish of sterile saline. The decidua are removed with forceps, and the underlying Reichert's membrane is then torn open and also removed except for the portion around the periphery of the developing placenta. The embryo, now surrounded only by its amnion and the visceral yolk sac, is placed in tubes or bottles containing the nutrient medium to which the test substance is added. The tube is thoroughly flushed with a suitable gas mixture enriched in oxygen and put on a rotating disk or rollers in a 37°C incubator. The rotation promotes oxygenation of the medium and thus facilitates more efficient gaseous exchange for the floating embryo. A further modification in the method provides a continuous rather than intermittent flow of gas during culture (58).

A number of investigators have exposed cultured embryos to various chemical and physical agents to assess teratogenicity. In general, the results show that the chemicals known to be teratogenic *in vivo* produce deformities of similar nature in cultured embryos. One of the first chemicals investigated was trypan blue. Trypan blue was applied in various concentrations to rat embryos cultured on plasma clots (72). A majority of the embryos showed a decreased rate of development and had other abnormalities commonly found after *in vivo* treatment such as enlarged pericardium, edema, and swelling of the head folds. Similarities between *in vivo* and *in vitro* teratogenic effects was shown by 6-aminonicotinamide, a nicotinamide antimetabolite, and by excess vitamin A (49,73). Vitamin A (retinol or retinoic acid) caused maldevelopment of brain and pharyngeal arches, reduced overall growth, a failure of blood circulation, and a number of ultrastructural changes similar to those found in rat embryos after maternal hypervitaminosis A (50).

The unique opportunity provided by embryos in culture was used to advantage in studies on the direct effects of hyperglycemia and hyperthermia, two factors that, through conflicting evidence, had previously been linked with teratogenesis. Cockroft and Coppola (18) found that D-glucose has a direct teratogenic effect on rat embryos exposed *in vitro* to eight to 10 times the normal glucose concentration of rat serum. The teratogenic glucose level of 12 mg/ml is in the same range found in the serum of severely diabetic patients (25). The major abnormality was an unusual fusion between anterior and posterior parts of the neural folds; also found were microcephaly, edema, and eye malformations. Mouse embryos cultured at early somite stages in the serum of streptozotocin-induced diabetic rats frequently developed exencephaly (62). The effects of hyperthermia were examined by simply raising the incubation temperature of the cultured embryos above 37°C (19). The embryos cultured at 40.5°C were all malformed, with the major malformations being microcephaly and pericardial edema. When more precise measurements were made of certain dimensions of the developing brain, even the embryos cultured at 40°C were found to be microcephalic. These results are comparable to those of studies where either the pregnant uterus or the whole animal is subjected to hyper-thermia (20,65); reduced brain weight and cephalic deformities were also common among embryos *in vivo*.

Studies such as these give assurance that the potential teratogenic activity of certain chemical and physical agents can be determined using a good embryo culture system and that the activity corresponds well to what is known of these agents in other testing situations. So far, however, only a very few agents have been tested in this manner, and those tested were known beforehand to be potent teratogens. Hence, they produced grossly visible changes in the embryo that were identifiable using the usual morphological criteria. It is certain that other criteria will have to be developed if the full potential of the test system is to be realized in the screening of unknown agents, some of which may possess low or mild teratogenic activity.

In a recent study, Brown et al. (13) used a comprehensive morphological scoring system to evaluate the effects of ethanol on rat embryos *in vitro*. Causation of congenital malformations in human fetuses by maternal chronic alcoholism is now well established (66). However, it is unknown if the developmental anomalies in what is now termed "fetal alcohol syndrome" are the result of a direct action of ethanol or its metabolites, or if they are associated with other factors such as maternal nutrition and metabolic dysfunction. Rat embryos were cultured on day 9.5 of gestation in rat serum and continuously exposed for 2 days to 150 or 300 mg/100 ml ethanol. No gross defects were apparent in the exposed embryos, but there was a dose-dependent reduction in several of their growth parameters such as crown–rump length, total DNA and protein contents, and the number of somites. As mentioned above, it is difficult to assign a great deal of significance to the finding of growth retardation in cultured embryos, since any number of adverse culture conditions could also have produced the same effect. However, Brown et al. (13) contend that their observations were based on a sensitive cumulative scoring system that took into account a number of morphometric parameters (14). Using this system, the authors were able to demonstrate that ethanol-treated embryos were not only growth-retarded but also had a further disproportionate reduction in head length. Reduced head length would result in microcephaly which usually accom-panies mental retardation, one feature of the fetal alcohol syndrome (66).

One major shortcoming of many *in vitro* systems is that they lack the drug-metabolizing enzymes of the intact animal. Hence, the teratogenic activity of a test chemical may not be apparent unless such enzyme preparations are added to the culture system. The major activation (or detoxification) of drugs is carried out by a multicomponent, membrane-bound complex of enzymes called mixed-function oxygenases (MFO). Metabolism occurs when the drug, in the presence of molecular oxygen and NADPH, is oxidized by MFO enzymes. Recently, Fantel et al. (21) have combined cultured rat embryo with a preparation of MFO obtained from rat liver and have shown that cyclophosphamide undergoes bioactivation and expresses teratogenicity *in vitro*. These authors reported that cyclophosphamide, in concen-trations as high as 250 μg/ml, was innocuous if either the hepatic microsomal fraction or the necessary cofactors were omitted from the medium of 10-day cultured rat embryos. In the presence of these additives, cyclophosphamide, at concentrations ranging from 6.25 to 25 $\mu$g/ml, produced a number of changes in developmental parameters such as somite number, crown–rump length, and total protein content. A high proportion of embryos were also malformed, exhibiting hypoplastic brain vesicles and visceral arches, axial and limb deformations, and blunted tails.

It is probable that the preparation and application of enzymatically active drug-metabolizing microsomal fraction are impractical for routine work. Particularly, the methodology may be considered too laborious for preliminary screening of teratogens, or the microsomal fraction may produce nonspecific cytotoxicity (46). Another approach to developing a crude bioassay would be to employ *in vivo* activation of the parent compound. The feasibility of this approach was recently demonstrated by Klein et al. (33). These authors collected serum from rats at various time intervals after an injection of cyclophosphamide and added it to rat embryos explanted in culture at the head-fold stage. One-hour serum was embryo-lethal, but 4-hr serum permitted survival of embryos which developed exencephaly and were growth-retarded. The embryos were otherwise resistant to a direct action of cyclophosphamide at levels up to 800 $\mu$g/ml of medium.

Chatot et al. (15) have taken the rat embryo culture system further to the screening of human sera for the presence of teratogenic factors. They selected five subjects undergoing cancer chemotherapy and six subjects receiving anticonvulsants. Sera withdrawn from these patients were either embryo-lethal or teratogenic for the cultured embryo. Sera from normal subjects, male or female, and serum samples from a subject who had discontinued chemotherapy permitted adequate growth and virtually normal development of the cultured rat embryo.

These are very preliminary studies, and the authors have found a good deal of variability in the growth and development permitted by sera from even normal subjects. This approach, however, can be valuable in determining the "persistent" teratogenic activity of a drug. By using sera collected at different times after injecting animals with a suspected teratogen, it should be possible to determine how long after the initial injection the drug remains "teratologically active."

Only a very few of the previous studies have monitored the metabolic responses of the cultured embryo to teratogens. The question is an important one, since concordance between *in vitro* and *in utero* development at the metabolic level will justify our reliance on the embryo culture system for screening purposes. In my laboratory, we have studied the behavior of certain teratogenic antimetabolites regarding their effects on embryonic DNA synthesis *in vitro* and compared it to *in utero* effects. Drugs such as cytosine arabinoside (ara-C), hydroxyurea, and ribavarin produced dose-dependent inhibition of DNA synthesis whether the embryos were exposed indirectly *in utero* or directly in the culture medium (35,41,42).

We also compared the inhibitory effects of ara-C and hydroxyurea to test the efficacy of the culture system in reflecting basic differences in metabolic effects of the two drugs. From pharmacokinetic studies in other systems, it is known that hydroxyurea has a shorter half-life in the body and produces cytotoxicity more rapidly than ara-C. Eleventh-day mouse embryos were removed from the dams 2 hr after the dams had been injected with equivalent teratogenic doses of ara-C (25 mg/kg) or hydroxyurea (1 gm/kg), and the embryos were cultured in a drug-free medium for a period of 24 hr. The rate of DNA synthesis was monitored at intervals during this period by exposing embryos to [$^3$H-]thymidine for 1 hr. Results were compared with control embryos from untreated dams cultured and labeled under identical conditions. Both drugs initially produced a virtual shutdown of DNA synthesis which was followed by a period of recovery in the attainment of normal metabolic functions. The inhibitory profiles of the effects of the two drugs were, however, different from each other reflecting what has already been observed in other systems. Hydroxyurea produced its maximal inhibitory response not only earlier than did ara-C, but the recovery process was also faster (37). We are now using the cultured embryo routinely in our studies on biosynthesis and the role of extracellular macromolecules such as collagen and proteoglycans in embryogenesis and cell differentiation (43). Much further work on various other metabolic pathways is still needed.

## ORGAN EXPLANTS

Techniques of embryonic organ culture are well established and are in use in several laboratories for investigation on developmental mechanisms (40,54,61,63). Organ explants have been of great use in teratological studies where they have contributed to an understanding of complex morphogenetic events such as in the development of face, palate, tooth, sense organs, sex organs, kidneys, and limbs (29,31,36,39,51,63,68,69). Despite these efforts, no definitive testing system for teratogens has yet emerged. Concerted and systematic efforts in standardizing and defining potential advantages and limitations of organ culture systems are now needed. The following is a summary of our work dealing with the use of embryonic limb buds in an organ culture screening system.

### Limb Bud Organ Culture

Limb bud organ culture has several theoretical and practical advantages over the culture of other organs. Only minor manipulations are needed in excising limb buds from the embryo once the extraembryonic membranes are removed, i.e., no delicate microsurgery is required. Staging of embryonic age is easy using the size and shape of the limb bud; in fact, usual staging systems depend on limb bud development as an important criterion (30,67). A large body of literature already exists showing that the vertebrate limb, during its normal development, goes through a number of well-characterized morphological and biochemical events common to most other embryonic organs and tissues. Cultured limb buds progress through similar processes of cell differentiation and tissue organization. In final form, the explanted organ possesses most of its normal complement of skeletal parts such as shoulder or pelvic girdle, long bones, and digits, having differentiated in proper proximodistal sequence (7,36,39).

The first attempts at cultivating limb buds in organ culture were made in chick embryos (10,22). In 1970, two reports appeared using mouse embryos as limb bud donors (34,64). Our technique was based on the method of Trowell (71) and employed a partial chemically defind medium. The potential of this technique in embryological and teratological investigations was quickly realized, and, as a result, these methodologies have now been adopted by a number of other laboratories (47,54,78). Over the years, the technique has undergone some minor modifications (1,3,7,39,44). The major highlights of this technique are the following.

1. Cultures can be initiated from embryos at stages in which they are undergoing critical organogenetic phases, such as days 11 to 13 of gestation, and maintained for extended periods of time, usually 6 to 9 days.
2. The test compound can be introduced into the culture medium at any time, and the duration of treatment can easily be regulated by simply transferring the culture to a control medium.
3. Any detrimental effects on growth and differentiation of the organ can be monitored quickly in a preliminary screening, after which more precise qualitative and quantitative studies can be designed.

The major advantages of this technique stem from the flexibility and ease with which it can be combined with other *in vivo* and *in vitro* methods, reproducibility of results, and the fact that only small quantities of the test chemical are needed for initial screening. The last point is important in circumstances where a number of unknown metabolites or pollutants are to be monitored during drug development and industrial processing, respectively.

### Assessment of Teratogenic Effects

After exposure to the test agent, the cultured limbs are scored not only visually for abnormal morphology but also quantitatively by measurement of the total amount of cartilaginous skeleton formed (7,38,39). We have obtained satisfactory dose–response relationships with several well-known teratogenic agents (1,38,41).

For such studies, it is essential that, for a given developmental stage of donor embryos (measured in terms of somite pairs), the extent of growth and differentiation of limbs under normal culture conditions be constant and reproducible and that any specific drug treatment produce replicable effects. To meet these requirements, one needs a method to quantify the amount of cartilage in the cultured limbs that is simple, quick, and applicable to individual cartilages of the limb to determine if a treatment differentially affected one region of the limb more than another. This led to the introduction of cartilage area units (CAU) for the purpose of quantifying limb growth. The essentials of this technique are described below (for review see 1,2).

Limbs are stained with toluidine blue, cleared, and then photographed under low magnification. After being processed, the photographic slides are projected onto graph paper of uniform squares. The outline of the cartilage is drawn on the graph paper, and various cartilage zones (scapula, humerus, radio–ulna, and digits) are delimited. The number of graph paper squares occupied by each cartilage is counted, and this number is referred to as the area unit for that particular cartilage. Alternatively, area can be measured by planimetry and expressed as $mm^2$. Such an approach to quantifying the amount of cartilage has certain built-in errors. In organ culture, the various cartilages of the limb grow in a three-dimensional aspect rather than in a two-dimensional aspect as in photographic records. Sometimes two cartilages overlap or some parts (especially scapula and humerus) bend downwards in the growing cultures. In most cases, these errors can easily be rectified by comparing the enlarged outline against the original stained limb. The data obtained are very reproducible, and the cartilage area units in the limb explants of similarly staged and treated embryos are found to be quite similar and with only small variation. In a few cases, where variation is large (e.g., when the standard error is more than 10 to 15% of the mean value), the experiment is repeated one or more times to collect a larger sample so as to obtain a statistically valid mean value. All measurements are made on toluidine blue-stained preparations. When no metachromasia is detected, a complete suppression of chondrogenesis is presumed to have occurred (8). We have found this quantification technique very useful in a number of studies. An alternate, semiquantitative method is now also available (52). Even though the measurements are not absolute, our method has the advantage of being simple and quick.

## Concordance Between *in Utero* and *in Vitro* Teratogenesis

Before a great deal of effort is put into devising an efficient and effective *in vitro* system for routine screening of chemicals, drugs, and environmental pollutants for teratological effects, it is essential to show that *in vivo* results can be duplicated *in vitro*. For example, in our system, if limbs at a certain developmental stage are sensitive or resistant to a particular agent *in vivo*, they should be equally sensitive or resistant to the same agent in the *in vitro* situation. To satisfy this requirement, we have tested a number of compounds to ascertain the extent of parallelism. The results of a few such studies are summarized below.

### Cytosine Arabinoside and All-Trans-Retinoic Acid

Detailed teratological studies with two drugs in our laboratory have established that at appropriate doses both are able to induce a very high incidence (virtually 100%) of limb defects in fetuses from dams that had received a single dose of either compound. Analyses of the missing limb bones revealed that for any given developmental stage, the pattern of limb malformations was highly specific for each drug (3,41). For example, retinoic acid (R.A.) injected on day 12 of gestation (embryos having 41 ± 2 somites) produced phocomelia. The only bones present were those of the girdle and the paw; all the intermediate long bones (humerus, radius, ulna) were missing. A similar treatment with ara-C also malformed the limbs, but this treatment resulted in missing digits (adactyly) with relatively unaffected long bones.

Two types of experiments involving limb buds in organ culture confirmed the efficacy of those two drugs in eliciting a similar response in tissue culture as they did *in utero*. In one series of experiments, limb buds of day-12 embryos from untreated dams were excised and cultured in the presence of either 1 µg/ml of R.A. or 1.4 µg/ml of ara-C, concentrations that were deemed effective in a preliminary study. After 24 hr, the drug was removed, and the cultures were supplied with fresh control medium. After 6 days of culture, the patterns of missing or deformed cartilages were assessed in toluidine blue-stained specimens. In a second series of studies, 12-day embryos were cultured in the presence of effective concentrations of either drug for 24 hr, after which their limbs were excised and cultured in the drug-free medium for 6 days as above. In both instances, the susceptibility of proximal limb regions to R.A. and of distal limb regions to ara-C, was observed, resulting in malformations depicting phocomelia and adactylia, respectively.

## 5-Bromo-2'-deoxyuridine

The thymidine analog 5-bromo-2'-deoxyuridine (BudR) is a known teratogen, but its effect on limb development is highly stage dependent. Maximum limb malformations occur if the analog is administered late on the 10th or on the 11th day of gestation, moderate effects are seen in 12-day embryos, and by day 13 of pregnancy, the drug has no deleterious effect on limb morphogenesis. Exactly the same pattern of drug sensitivity was observed when either limb buds or whole embryos were exposed to BudR *in vitro* (1,2).

Limbs at an early stage of development (early day-11 embryos, somite stage 26–29) were extremely sensitive to the analog. Treatment with low levels (2–4 µg/ml) and for a relatively short period of time in culture (2–3 days) completely and irreversibly suppressed chondrogenesis in the explants. Limbs from older embryos (somite stage 40 and up) were found to be much less sensitive to the inhibitory effect of the drug. A prolonged exposure to a much higher dose (100–150 µg/ml) resulted in incomplete suppression of chondrogenesis. Finally, only a 20% inhibition was observed in the cultures of limbs from mid-13-day mouse embryos.

The increasing resistance to BudR was not exclusive to forelimbs of the older embryos. The forelimbs of 11-day mouse embryos during the course of their development in culture also became increasingly refractory to the drug. Whereas treatment on the third day of culture resulted in 78% reduction in total cartilage area units, similar treatment carried out on the fifth day of *in vitro* growth showed only a modest depression (35%) of cartilage development. The maximum effect on chondrogenesis was observed if the limb explants were exposed to BudR during the early part of their culture history. Once the limbs were allowed to grow and differentiate in control medium for 3 to 6 days (simulating the *in vivo* growth of embryos), the analog, at least in concentrations of up to 25 µg/ml, failed to inhibit chondrogenesis at all. This time of total resistance came earlier in older limbs: after

3 and 6 days in culture for the limbs of 13th- and 12th-day embryos, respectively. The limbs of day-11 embryos were still sensitive to BudR after a growth of 6 days in culture, although the effect was now confined to the distal elements (radio–ulna) only.

In another study, a combination of whole-embryo culture and organ culture techniques was adopted to expose postimplantation mouse embryos to BudR and to evaluate the effects of long-term treatment on subsequent differentiation of limb buds. Early- and mid-11-day mouse embryos were exposed to various concentrations of BudR for 12 or 24 hr. Forelimbs of the treated embryos were then cultured in drug-free medium, and the extent of cartilage development in the explants examined. Exposure of embryos to 50 to 150 μg/ml of BudR for 24 hr resulted in significant inhibition of chondrogenesis in subsequent limb cultures, and the effect was dose related. After treatment with 150 μg/ml of the drug, the forelimbs of the early-day-11 embryos (somite stage 26–29) showed an almost complete lack of cartilage, whereas the limbs of mid-11-day embryos (somite stage 32–34) were not nearly as sensitive and exhibited about 50% reduction in the amount of cartilage development. This led to the conclusion that, if embryos in which limb development is at a very early stage are exposed to BudR, the future course of limb differentiation is permanently and irreversibly damaged, resulting in a partial or even complete suppression of chondrogenesis in the organ. As both the dose and perhaps also the duration of treatment were found to be critical, we further suggested that the rather low frequency of reported limb malformations after *in vivo* injection of teratogenic doses of BudR may result from only a small amount of the chemical reaching the embryos.

## Drug Metabolism *in Vitro*

The importance of drug-metabolizing enzymes, collectively called cytochrome P-450-mediated monooxygenases, has been appreciated in other toxicological testing systems. For example, it is well established that although many environmental carcinogens are inactive per se, their activated derivatives are highly carcinogenic (48). Similarly, it has been shown (26) that mammals can convert nonmutagenic chemicals (promutagens) to highly mutagenic metabolites.

In most experimental animals, typical P-450 enzymes are believed not to develop until the late prenatal or even the neonatal stage (23,24,60; see also W. Klinger et al., *this volume*). In contrast, P-450 enzymes are present in liver microsomes of human fetuses as early as 8 to 15 weeks of gestation (59,77). This would mean that activation of compounds may not occur in fetuses of laboratory animals, whereas human fetuses are perfectly capable of such activation. Therefore, development of an efficient and reproducible *in vitro* activation system would be a very useful advance for *in vitro* teratological testing.

Microsomal fractions obtained from livers of phenobarbital-injected animals are commonly used for drug activation in other *in vitro* systems such as the Ames test for mutagenesis (5). In limb bud culture systems, however, Manson and Simons

(46) found that the liver microsomal preparation as such was toxic to the limb bud. These authors have developed another approach that has been successful with at least one tested drug, cyclophosphamide. Cyclophosphamide is teratogenic in a number of mammalian species including man (6,27,70); however, added directly to the culture medium, it produced no deformities in the explanted limb bud (9,46). The addition of certain metabolites of cyclophosphamide did result in deformation and lack of normal differentiation in limb bud cartilage (9,46). To generate the metabolism of cyclophosphamide in the limb bud culture system, Manson and Simons (46) used monolayers of hamster embryo cells (HEC) as the source of MFO enzymes. Hamster embryo cells were grown for 6 days at the bottom of tissue culture dishes and treated with phenobarbital. Limb buds were set up in the same plates, and cyclophosphamide introduced into the medium. Limb bud development was abnormal in this instance, indicating that teratologically active metabolites were generated by this method. These are preliminary findings, and there is some question regarding the authenticity of the metabolites formed *in vitro*. Yet this has indicated that the organ culture system is reliable enough to distinguish between teratogens and nonteratogens.

## CELL CULTURE

Among various types of *in vitro* methodologies, cell culture is perhaps the most widely used system in physiological/pharmacological investigations. The fact that cell culture can mimic only a very limited spectrum of events in embryological development makes it a poor model to choose for teratogenic testing. There is, however, one important advantage. Cells can be grown in mass quantities, and established cell lines from animal and even human tissues are available from various sources. Thus, labor-intensive steps in obtaining timed embryos and other manipulations required for explanting whole embryos or organs are avoided.

Braun et al. (12) have recently formulated a simple test system that allows monitoring the property of cell attachment exhibited by certain cell types in culture. The authors assume that the attachment of cells to a lectin-coated plastic substratum reflects a measure of the cells' ability to interact with other cells, a property known to play a key role in embryogenesis. Any agent that interfered with cellular attachment and, hence, with cellular interactions would be considered a potential teratogen.

The procedure involves *in vivo* labeling of mouse ascitic ovarian tumor cells with tritiated thymidine, after which the cells are incubated *in vitro* with the test drug. Small polyethylene disks coated with the plant lectin concanavalin A are submerged in the cell suspension. After a 20-min incubation period at room temperature, the disks are removed, washed in saline, and counted in a scintillation counter.

It was found that the tumor cells attached to lectin-derivatized disks within 5 min at room temperature (12). A wide variety of drugs were tested for their inhibitory effect on cell attachment, including anesthetics, tranquilizers, and antiinflammatory agents. With the exception of a few well-known teratogens such as thalidomide, methotrexate, vinblastine, colchicine, actinomycin D, and trypan blue, all others inhibited cell attachment. The frequency of such false-negative findings, i.e., known teratogens that did not inhibit attachment, was 36%. In a subsequent study (11), thalidomide was found to inhibit attachment if certain of the incubation conditions were modified, i.e., cells were incubated with thalidomide in a mouse liver microsomal activation system, and the mixture was maintained at 37°C for more than 30 min.

There are several problems that need to be resolved in this assay. The mechanism by which any of the tested compounds interfere with attachment is not known. This is an important aspect, since a number of teratogens were without any effect. Nucleic acid antimetabolites are generally strongly teratogenic, yet they would not be expected to interfere with cell attachment, and in this system they did not. In such a short-term assay (50 min of drug–cell interaction), only those agents capable of physical interference with the cell surface would be identified. Even with our inadequate knowledge of teratogenic mechanisms, indications suggest that there are a number of embryonic cellular events besides cell–cell adhesion that are sensitive to teratogens. Hence, it is not surprising that several teratogens had no effect on cell attachment. In the words of Wilson (76), a test system that gives many false negatives is "worse than useless."

Two other cell culture systems have recently been used to monitor the effects of chemicals on cell differentiation (74). These are chick embryo neural crest cells and limb bud mesenchymal cells. Cranial neural crest cells obtained from early chick embryos differentiate either into neuron-like cells or into pigment cells depending on the types of sera used in the culture medium (28). Cultures are exposed to the test chemical for 24 hr on the third day following subculture, and 5 days later development is assessed by phase contrast microscopy. Primary cultures are employed in the case of limb bud mesenchyme. Here, drugs are added to fresh medium on days 1 and 3 or on day 1 only. The cultures are terminated on day 4 and observed for evidence of chondrogenesis under a phase microscope; estimation of chondrogenesis is obtained by staining the cultures with alcian blue for sulfated proteoglycan content. To achieve activation of drugs such as cyclophosphamide, Wilk et al. (74) used the method of Madle and Obe (45) in which the drug and activation system are combined in a dialysis bag and the bag added to the culture medium.

A total of 14 compounds were tested including some known potent teratogens. A positive correlation between teratogenic activity and inhibition of cell differentiation was observed. Some of the other effects associated with teratogens were detachment of cells from the substratum, apparent decrease in cell multiplication, and changes in cell morphology. The only parameter, however, that was quantifiable to any degree was the extent of chondrogenesis as judged by alcian blue-staining. From this preliminary study, it is not possible to assign any positive or negative significance to the degree of suppression of chondrogenesis with regard to teratogenesis.

## LIMITATION OF *IN VITRO* SCREENING

Since teratogenicity of drugs and chemicals is initially tested in species other than man, one of the limitations we currently face involves the extent of extrapolation between different species. A similar limitation may hold for any of the *in vitro* systems discussed above. The question is: if an agent produces detrimental effects on embryonic cells and tissue *in vitro*, can it be labeled a "teratogen" simply on that basis?

In view of the diversity and sensitivity of developmental events encountered during organogenesis, it can be assumed that the embryo is likely to be influenced by any agent that is pharmacologically active. Wilson (75) stated that "to maintain that any drug or other chemical agent is devoid of embryotoxic potential in man is foolhardy." Even after extensive testing in pregnant animals, the best that can be said about a "safe" drug is that at a given dosage and under the circumstances of the experiment, it produced no teratogenicity in the selected species of animals. In whole-animal testing, the dosage must be kept well below the adult lethal dose so that, in some cases, there is no opportunity to titrate for a possible teratogenic dose.

Tissue culture systems allow for precise determination of the dose–response relationship provided that an adequate endpoint is selected for monitoring. This information alone, however, will not permit the investigator to classify drugs into "safe" or "unsafe" categories. It does give the investigator a powerful measuring instrument by which to screen a number of related analogs and metabolites for their relative embryotoxic potential.

The chief drawback of the "direct assay" (i.e., one in which an agent is added directly to the culture medium) is that, even though the parent compound under investigation may be inactive, it remains possible that an "activated" form of the compound may be teratogenic. Various efforts to generate metabolic activation *in vitro* have been summarized above (11,21,45,46,53,74). The success and feasibility of these approaches for *in vitro* teratogenesis remain to be explored further.

## CONCLUSIONS

A selective survey of mammalian tissue culture systems being utilized by investigators in teratology studies has been presented. A few potentially useful systems that could lead to the development of an adequate initial screening device are available. Before this occurs, however, a considerable effort is required to validate such systems through exhaustive comparisons between *in vitro* effects of a variety of agents and the responses shown by mammalian embryos *in utero*.

## ACKNOWLEDGMENTS

The studies in the author's laboratory were supported by N.I.H. grant HD-10935-03. I am indebted to my colleague Dr. N. D. Agnish for assistance in the preparation of this manuscript.

# REFERENCES

1. Agnish, N. D., and Kochhar, D. M. (1976): Direct exposure of post-implantation mouse embryos to 5-bromodeoxyuridine *in vitro* and its effects on subsequent chondrogenesis in the limbs. *J. Embryol. Exp. Morphol.*, 36:623–638.

2. Agnish, N. D., and Kochhar, D. M. (1976): Direct exposure of mouse embryonic limb buds to 5-bromodeoxyuridine *in vitro* and its effect on chondrogenesis: Increasing resistance to the analog at successive stages of development. *J. Embryol. Exp. Morphol.*, 36:639–652.

3. Agnish, N. D., and Kochhar, D. M. (1977): The role of somites in the growth and early development of mouse limb buds. *Dev. Biol.*, 56:174–183

4. Ames, B., Durston W. E., Yamasaki, E., and Lee, F. D. (1973): Carcinogens are mutagens: A simple test system combining liver homogenates for activation and bacteria for detection. *Proc. Natl. Acad. Sci. U.S.A.*, 70:2281–2285.

5. Ames, B. N., Lee, F. D., and Durston, W. E. (1973): An improved bacterial test system for the detection and classification of mutagens and carcinogens. *Proc. Natl. Acad. Sci. U.S.A.*, 70:782–786.

6. Ashby, R., Davis, L., Dewhurst, B. B., Espinol, R., Penn, R. N., and Upshall, D. G. (1976): Aspects of teratology of cyclophosphamide. *Cancer Treat. Rep.*, 60:477–482.

7. Aydelotte, M. B., and Kochhar, D. M. (1972): Development of mouse limb buds in organ culture: Chondrogenesis in the presence of proline analog, L-azetidine-2-carboxylic-acid. *Dev. Biol.*, 28:191–201.

8. Aydelotte, M. B., and Kochhar, D. M. (1975): Influence of 6-diazo-5-oxo-L-norleucine (DON), a glutamine analogue, on cartilaginous differentiation in mouse limb buds *in vitro*. *Differentiation*, 4:73–80.

9. Barrach, H. J., Bauman, I., and Neubert, D. (1978): The applicability of *in vitro* systems for the evaluation of the significance of pharmacokinetic parameters for the induction of an embryonic effect. In: *Role of Pharmacokinetics in Prenatal and Perinatal Toxicology*, edited by D. Neubert, H. J. Merker, H. Nau, and J. Langman, pp.323–336. Georg Thieme, Stuttgart.

10. Bradley, S. J. (1970): An analysis of self-differentiation of chick limb buds in chorio–allantoic grafts. *J. Anat.*, 107:479–490.

11. Braun, A. G., and Dailey, J. P. (1980):Thalidomide metaboite inhibits tumor cell attachment to lectin coated surfaces. *Teratology*, 21:29A.

12. Braun, A. G., Emerson, D. J., and Nichinson, B. B. (1979): Teratogenic drugs inhibit tumor cell attachment to lectin-coated surfaces. *Nature*, 282:507–509.

13. Brown, N. A., Goulding, E. H., and Fabro, S. (1979): Ethanol embryotoxicity: Direct effects on mammalian embryos *in vitro*. *Science*, 206:573–575.

14. Brown, N. A., Goulding, E. H., and Fabro, S. (1980): A morphological scoring system for rat embryonic development. *Teratology*, 21:30A.

15. Chatot, C. L., Klein, N. W., Piatek, J., and Pierro, L. J. (1980): Successful culture of rat embryos on human serum: Use in the detection of teratogens. *Science*, 207:1471–1473.

16. Chu, E. H. Y., and Malling, H. V. (1968): Mammalian cell genetics. II. Chemical induction of specific locus mutation in Chinese hamster cells *in vitro*. *Proc. Natl. Acad. Sci. U.S.A.*, 61:1306–1312.

17. Cockroft, D. L. (1977): Post-implantation embryo culture. In: *Methods in Prenatal Toxicology*, edited by D. Neubert, H. J. Merker, and T. E. Kwasigroch, pp. 231–240. Georg Thieme, Stuttgart.

18. Cockroft, D. L., and Coppola, P. T. (1977): Teratogenic effects of excess glucose on head-fold rat embryos in culture. *Teratology*, 16:141–146.

19. Cockroft, D. L., and New, D. A. T. (1978): Abnormalities induced in cultured rat embryos by hyperthermia. *Teratology*, 17:277–284.

20. Edwards, M. J. (1969): Congenital defects in guinea pigs: Prenatal retardation of brain growth of guinea pigs following hyperthermia during gestation. *Teratology*, 2:329–336.

21. Fantel, A. G., Greenway, J. C., Juchau, M. R., and Shepard, T. H. (1979): Teratogenic bioactivation of cyclophosphamide *in vitro*. *Life Sci.*, 25:67–72.

22. Fell, H. B., and Landauer, W. (1935): Experiments on skeletal growth and development *in vitro* in relation to the problem of phokomelia. *Proc. R. Soc. Lond. [Biol.]*, 118:133–154.

23. Fouts, J. R. (1973): Microsomal mixed-function oxidases in the fetal and newborn rabbit. In: *Fetal Pharmacology*, edited by L. Boreus, pp. 305–320. Raven Press, New York.

24. Fouts, J. R., and Adamson, R. H. (1959): Drug metabolism in the newborn rabbit. *Science*, 129:897–898.

25. Fulop, M., Rosenblatt, A., Kreitzer, S. M., and Geratenhaber, B. (1975): Hyperosmolar nature of diabetic coma. *Diabetes*, 24:594–599.
26. Gabridge, M. G., and Legator, M. S. (1969): A host-mediated microbial assay for the detection of mutagenic compounds. *Proc. Soc. Exp. Biol. Med.*, 130:831–834.
27. Gibson, J. E., and Becker, B. A. (1968): The teratogenicity of cyclophosphamide in mice. *Cancer Res.*, 28:475–480.
28. Greenberg, V. H., and Schrier, B. K. (1977): Development of choline acetyltransferase activity in chick cranial neural crest cells in culture. *Dev. Biol.*, 61:86–93.
29. Greene, R. M., and Pratt, R. M. (1977): Inhibition by DON of rat palatal glycoprotein synthesis and epithelial cell adhesion *in vitro*. *Exp. Cell Res.*, 105:27–37.
30. Hamburger, V., and Hamilton, H. L. (1951): A series of normal stages in the development of the chick embryo. *J. Morphol.*, 88:49–82.
31. Johnston, M. C., and Pratt, R. M. (1975): The neural crest in normal and abnormal craniofacial development. In: *Extracellular Matrix Influences on Gene Expression*, edited by H. C. Slavkin and R. C. Greulich, pp. 773–777. Academic Press, New York.
32. Kao, F., and Puck, T. T. (1969): Genetics of somatic mammalian cells. IX. Quantitation of mutagenesis by physical and chemical agents. *J. Cell. Comp. Physiol.*, 74:245–258.
33. Klein, N. W., Vogler, M. A., Chatot, C. L., and Pierro, L. J. (1980): The use of cultured rat embryos to evaluate the teratogenic activity of serum: Cadmium and cyclophosphamide. *Teratology*, 21:199–208.
34. Kochhar, D. M. (1970): Effects of azetidine-2-carboxylic acid, a proline analog, on chondrogenesis in cultured limb buds. In: *Metabolic Pathways in Mammalian Embryos During Organogenesis and Its Modification by Drugs*, edited by R. Bass, R. Beck, H. J. Merker, D. Neurbert, and B. Randham, pp. 475–482. Georg Theime, Stuttgart.
35. Kochhar, D. M. (1975): Assessment of teratogenic response in cultured post-implantation mouse embryos: Effects of hydroxyurea. In: *New Approaches to the Evaluation of Abnormal Embryonic Development*, edited by D. Neubert and H. J. Merker, pp. 250–276. Georg Thieme, Stuttgart.
36. Kochhar, D. M. (1975): The use of *in vitro* procedures in teratology. *Teratology*, 11:273–288.
37. Kochhar, D. M. (1980): *In vitro* testing of teratogenic agents using mammalian embryos. *Teratogen. Carcinogen. Mutagen.*, 1:63–74.
38. Kochhar, D. M. (1981): Teratogenesis testing *in vitro*. In: *Toxicity Testing in Vitro*, edited by R. M. Nardone. Academic Press, New York (*in press*).
39. Kochhar, D. M., and Aydelotte, M. B. (1974): Susceptible stages and abnormal morphogenesis in the developing mouse limb, analyzed in organ culture after transplacental exposure to vitamin A (retinoic acid). *J. Embryol. Exp. Morphol.*, 31:721–734.
40. Kochhar, D. M., Aydelotte, M. B., and Vest, T. K. (1976): Altered collagen fibrillogenesis in embryonic mouse limb cartilage deficient in matrix granules. *Exp. Cell Res.*, 102:213–222.
41. Kochhar, D. M., Penner, J. D., and Knudsen, T. B. (1980): Embryotoxic, teratogenic and metabolic effects of ribavirin in mice. *Toxicol. Appl. Pharmacol.*, 52:99–112.
42. Kochhar, D. M., Penner, J. D., and McDay, J. A. (1978): Limb development in mouse embryos: II. Reduction defects, cytotoxicity and inhibition of DNA synthesis produced by cytosine arabinoside. *Teratology*, 18:71–92.
43. Kochhar, D. M., Penner, J. D., McDay, J. A., and Knudsen, T. B. (1980): Expression of the mutant gene *cmd* (cartilage matrix deficiency) during prenatal development. *Teratology*, 21:51A.
44. Kwasigroch, T. E., and Neubert, D. (1978): A simple method to test chondrogenic and myogenic tissues for differential effects of drugs. In: *The Role of Pharmacokinetics in Prenatal and Perinatal Toxicology*, edited by D. Neubert, H. J. Merker, H. Nau, and J. Langman, pp. 621–630. Georg Thieme, Stuttgart.
45. Madle, S., and Obe, G. (1977): *In vitro* testing of an indirect mutagen (cyclophosphamide) with human leukocyte cultures: Activation with liver microsomes and use of a dialysis bag. *Mutat. Res.*, 56:101–104.
46. Manson, J. M., and Simons, R. (1979): *In vitro* metabolism of cyclophosphamide in limb bud culture. *Teratology*, 19:149–158.
47. Manson, J. M., and Smith, C. C. (1977): Influence of cyclophosphamide and 4-ketocyclophosphamide on mouse limb development. *Teratology*, 15:291–300.
48. Miller, E. C., and Miller, J. A. (1974): Biochemical mechanisms of chemical carcinogenesis. In: *The Molecular Biology of Cancer*, edited by H. Busch, pp. 377–402. Academic Press, New York.

49. Morriss, G. M., and Steele, C. E. (1974): The effect of excess vitamin A on the development of rat embryos in culture. *J. Embryol. Exp. Morphol.*, 32:505–514.
50. Morriss, G. M., and Steele, C. E. (1977): Comparison of the effects of retinol and retinoic acid on post-implantation rat embryos *in vitro*. *Teratology*, 15:104–120.
51. Neubert, D., and Barrach, H. J. (1977): Significance of *in vitro* techniques for the evaluation of embryotoxic effects. In: *Methods in Prenatal Toxicology: Evaluation of Embryotoxic Effects in Experimental Animals*, edited by D. Neubert, H. J. Merker, and T. E. Kwasigroch, pp. 202–209. Georg Thieme, Stuttgart.
52. Neubert, D., Hinz, N., Baumann, I., Barrach, H. J. and Schmidt, K. (1978): Attempt upon a quantitative evaluation of the degree of differentiation of or the degree of interference with development in organ culture. In: *Role of Pharmacokinetics in Prenatal and Perinatal Toxicology*, edited by D. Neubert, H. J. Merker, H. Nau, and J. Langman, pp. 337–349. Georg Thieme, Stuttgart.
53. Neubert, D., Merker, H. J., Nau, H., and Langman, J. (1978): *Role of Pharmacokinetics in Prenatal and Perinatal Toxicology*. Georg Thieme, Stuttgart.
54. Neubert, D., Merker, H. J., and Tapken, S. (1974): Comparative studies on the prenatal development of mouse extremities *in vivo* and in organ culture. *Naunyn-Schmiedebergs Arch. Pharmacol.*, 286:251–270.
55. New, D. A. T. (1967): Development of explanted rat embryos in circulating medium. *J. Embryol. Exp. Morphol.*, 17:513–525.
56. New, D. A. T. (1976): Techniques for assessment of teratologic effects: Embryo culture. *Environ. Health Perspect.*, 18:105–110.
57. New, D. A. T. (1978): Whole-embryo culture and the study of mammalian embryos during organogenesis. *Biol. Rev.*, 53:81–122.
58. New, D. A. T., and Cockroft, D. L. (1979): A rotating bottle culture method with continuous replacement of the gas phase. *Experientia*, 35:138–139.
59. Pelkonen, O., Jouppila, P., and Karki, N. T. (1973): Attempts to induce drug metabolism in human fetal liver and placenta by administration of phenobarbital to mothers. *Arch. Int. Pharmacodyn. Ther.*, 202:288–297.
60. Rane, A., Berggren, M., Yaffee, S., and Ericsson, J. L. E. (1973): Oxidative drug metabolism in the perinatal rabbit liver and placenta. *Xenobiotica*, 3:37–48.
61. Rutter, W. J., Pictet, R. L., Harding, J. D., Chirgwin, J. M., McDonald, R. J., and Przybyla, A. E. (1978): An analysis of pancreatic development: Role of mesenchymal factor and other extracellular factors. In: *Molecular Control of Proliferation and Differentiation*, edited by J. Papaconstantinou and W. J. Rutter, pp. 205–227. Academic Press, New York.
62. Sadler, T. W. (1980): Effects of maternal diabetes on early embryogenesis: 1. The teratogenic potential of diabetic serum. *Teratology*, 21:339–347.
63. Saxen, L., Karkinen-Jaasklainen, M., and Saxen, I. (1976): Organ culture in teratology. In: *Current Topics in Pathology*, edited by A. Gropp and K. Benirschke, pp. 123–143. Springer-Verlag, Berlin.
64. Shepard, T. H., and Bass, G. L. (1970): Organ cultures of limb buds from riboflavin-deficient media. *Teratology*, 3:163–167.
65. Skreb, N., and Frank, Z. (1963): Developmental abnormalities in the rat induced by heat shock. *J. Embryol. Exp. Morphol.*, 11:445–447.
66. Streissguth, A. G., Landesman-Dwyer, S., Martin, J. C., and Smith, D. W. (1980): Teratogenic effects of alcohol in humans and laboratory animals. *Science*, 209:353–361.
67. Theiler, K. (1972): *The House Mouse: Development and Normal Stages from Fertilization to 4 Weeks of Age*. Springer-Verlag, New York.
68. Thesleff, I. (1976): Differentiation of odontogenic tissues in organ culture. *Scand. J. Dent. Res.*, 84:353–356.
69. Thesleff, I. (1977): *In vitro* development of oral tissues. In: *Methods in Prenatal Toxicology*, edited by D. Neubert, H. J. Merker, and T. E. Kwasigroch, pp.252–262. Georg Thieme, Stuttgart.
70. Toledo, T. M., Harper, R. C., and Moser, R. H. (1971): Fetal effects during cyclophosphamide and irradiation therapy. *Ann. Intern. Med.*, 74:84–91.
71. Trowell, D. A. (1954): A modified technique for organ culture *in vitro*. *Exp. Cell Res.*, 6:246–248.
72. Turbow, M. M. (1966): Trypan blue induced teratogenesis of rat embryos cultivated *in vitro*. *J. Embryol. Exp. Morphol.*, 15:387–395.

73. Turbow, M. M., and Chamberlain, J. G. (1968): Direct effects of 6-aminonicotinamide on the developing rat embryo *in vitro* and *in vivo*. *Teratology*, 1:103–108.
74. Wilk, A. L., Greenberg, J. H., Horigan, E. A., Pratt, R. M., and Martin, G. R. (1980): Detection of teratogenic compounds using differentiating embryonic cells in culture. *In Vitro*, 16:269–276.
75. Wilson, J. G. (1977): Embryotoxicity of drugs in man. In: *Handbook of Teratology, Vol. 4*, edited by J. G. Wilson and F. C. Fraser, pp. 309–355. Plenum Press, New York.
76. Wilson, J. G. (1978): Review of *in vitro* systems with potential for use in teratogenicity screening. *J. Environ. Pathol. Toxicol.*, 2:149–167.
77. Yaffe, S. J., Rane, A., Sjoqvist, F., Boreus, L. O., and Orrenius, S. (1970): The presence of a monooxygenase system in human fetal liver microsomes. *Life Sci.*, 9:1189–1200.
78. Yasuda, Y. (1977): Digital anomalies of mouse limbs induced by treatment with urethan *in vitro*. *Teratology*, 15:89–96.

*Developmental Toxicology*, edited by
C. A. Kimmel and J. Buelke-Sam. Raven Press,
New York © 1981.

# A Profile of Developmental Toxicity

## Carole A. Kimmel

*Perinatal and Postnatal Evaluation Branch, Division of Teratogenesis Research,
National Center for Toxicological Research, Jefferson, Arkansas 72079*

Current methods for assessing developmental and reproductive toxicity have been described in detail by A. K. Palmer (*this volume*) and reflect the imprecise nature of our ability to evaluate and predict developmental toxicity. At present, every new drug, pesticide, or food additive must be evaluated in a test protocol (in some cases in more than one species) using a rather arbitrary exposure regimen and observing a limited range of endpoints. Estimations of the lowest effective dose and the choice of the appropriate model to use for risk estimation (threshold versus nonthreshold) are difficult or impossible to make and further demonstrate our limited knowledge about the nature of the phenomena that we study.

Our focus on the study of endpoints in developmental toxicity has resulted in the proliferation of a number of individual tests that are often conducted and interpreted in isolation. For example, in a teratology study, acute and chronic toxicity data may be used to select doses and species. Information on mutagenic and carcinogenic potential, organ specificity, and pharmacokinetics may be considered, but such information is rarely correlated among animals or groups of animals in the same study or laboratory. In addition, there is little or no attempt to determine commonality in the events leading to a response across types of endpoints, across different agents giving the same endpoint, or the dose–effect relationship among endpoints examined. And too often, there is a tendency to require that the animal model mimic exactly the human manifestations rather than to interpret a disruption in the animal model as indicative of a potential for developmental toxicity in man. There is little or no justification for such assumptions until we know more about mechanisms of action and subsequent developmental pathogenetic events across species.

There are no simple solutions to these problems, but we must acknowledge the limitations and set about to address the gaps in our knowledge in a concerted fashion. If our primary task is to predict and thereby minimize human developmental toxicities, then an alternate course, one that may be more difficult and costly at first, must be taken.

Kretchmer (17) has indicated the importance of considering research in teratology as a continuum from the molecular and cellular aspects to organismal studies to preventive health care. Smithells (21) pointed to certain "challenges" of teratology, the first of which is to recognize its interdisciplinary nature, a fact noted by the earliest teratologist, Isidore Geoffroy St. Hilaire. These concepts recognize that there is more to understanding developmental toxicity than is evident from current approaches; however, they can provide a philosophical framework for focusing on improved methods of assessing developmental toxicity.

## A PROFILE OF DEVELOPMENTAL TOXICITY

If we seek to predict human developmental toxicities more accurately, then we must consider what types of information will enhance the predictabiltiy of the animal models that we use. Accepting the challenge of an interdisciplinary approach may allow the definition of a profile of developmental toxicity for a given chemical. This profile would include all data necessary to describe the exposure pattern for an agent, its interaction with the developing system, and the deleterious outcome. From such a profile, it would then be possible to predict effects to other species, including man, or to explain differences among species in terms of differences in some aspect of the profile.

Development is a continual and constantly changing process from conception to death as represented by the smooth curve at the top of Fig. 1. The stage sensitivity of the developing organism during prenatal and early postnatal life represents a unique and much more complex system with which to work than the adult organism. The straight line represents stages of development with specific events indicated; currently-used toxicity testing procedures are noted below. Endpoints measured using these test procedures are often evaluated in isolation with little regard for effects on other systems. However, in order to delineate a complete profile of developmental toxicity, we must integrate information on endpoints, pharmacokinetics, mechanisms of action, and subsequent developmental alterations (pathogenesis). These elements could be considered key correlates of a developmental toxicity profile. These are represented at the bottom of Fig. 1 and discussed as follows.

The first line represents a period of exposure that can occur either acutely or any time throughout this period (thus the dotted line) from before conception through early postnatal life. The study of pharmacokinetics and of mechanisms would be carried out during this period around the time of toxicant exposure.

The second line represents the evaluation of developmental pathogenesis subsequent to exposure and action; this would include altered morphogenetic as well as biochemical development that could directly influence the final manifestation of the toxicant.

The third line, representing the longitudinal evaluation of functional capacity, would allow determination of the various morphological, physiological, behavioral, or biochemical effects of a toxicant in the same animal or group of animals in a longitudinal fashion, i.e., over time. In this way, an estimation could be made of primary versus secondary effects and the dose–response relationships.

The overlap of these three lines is intentional and also implies the overlap or integration necessary among the contributing correlates in evaluating a develop-

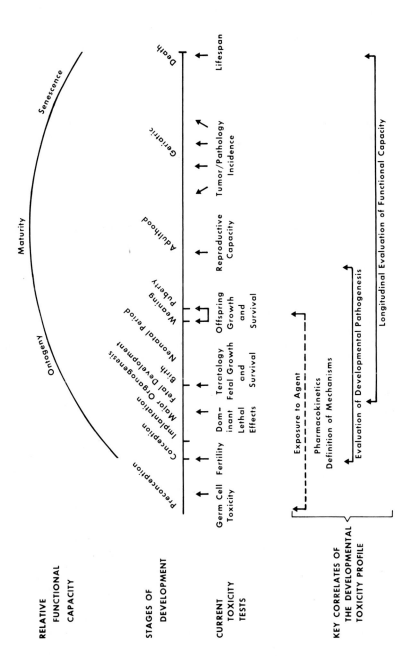

**FIG 1.** Basic components of functional development, current toxicity tests, and approximate timing and overlap among the key correlates of a developmental toxicity profile.

mental toxicant. Hicks and D'Amato (10) emphasized the importance of such integration in their review and evaluation of the effects of X-irradiation. For purposes of improved predictability, increased accuracy would be gained by collection and integration of information from pharmacokinetic or mechanistic studies together with endpoint evaluations. However, the greatest degree of predictability would come from knowledge in all relevant areas.

Such an effort obviously will require a team approach, involving investigators from many disciplines with a common goal for delineating the developmental toxicity profile. Comparison of data on the key correlates in individual animals should be made where possible so that subtle patterns or associations are not obscured by the averaging of data. Profiles should be established for several species, and data should be gathered for man when possible, thus providing an accurate basis for the estimation of risk.

## DESIGN CONSIDERATIONS IN DEVELOPMENTAL TOXICITY STUDIES

Factors to be considered in any developmental toxicity study include choice of species or strain, range and number of doses, controls, route of exposure, time of exposure, and endpoints to be assessed. Choice of the factors concerned with species, dose, and route of exposure can be determined much more easily if pharmacokinetic data are available, especially comparative human and laboratory animal data. If not, other background information, e.g., the most common route for human exposure and available acute or subchronic toxicity information, may influence these choices.

Two aspects of study design that are extemely important are the establishment of a dose–response relationship and the longitudinal evaluation of functional capacity. The dose–response pattern for the developmental toxicity of a chemical is important not only for detecting the lowest effective dose level but also for distinguishing specific or primary toxicity from that which may be secondary to more generalized toxicity. A longitudinal evaluation of functional systems must be included to allow evaluation of maturational patterns, latency to onset of abnormal functions, and rate of occurrence or increasing severity of functional alterations or lesions in particular systems.

An integrated study on developmental lead toxicity will be used to illustrate important points to be considered in experimental design (4,5,8,14,15,18,25). This study was carried out by a group of collaborators and employed a multidisciplinary approach to evaluate the full range of potential endpoints and related lead exposure levels.

The evaluation of chronic developmental lead toxicity was approached in a stepwise fashion by determining a dose–response for: (a) gross toxicity (morbidity and mortality) in the maternal animal; (b) prenatal embryotoxic and teratogenic effects; (c) alterations in early postnatal physical and behavioral development; (d) alterations in adult behaviors; and (e) altered functional capacities (e.g., immunologic, renal, reproductive) (15).

Maternal animals were exposed to lead in drinking water (0.5 to 250 ppm lead) from 21 days of age through gestation and lactation, and their offspring were subsequently exposed to the same levels and followed for a maximum of 9 months of age. Pups were culled to 10 per litter at birth and 8 per litter at 4 days of age with $4 \pm 1$ of each sex. Equalization of litter size and sex ratio is extremely important in any developmental toxicity study because of interaction of litter size with nutrition and growth of offspring (12).

Table 1 is a composite summary of the data from this study. Comparison of the dose–response for each of these endpoints revealed that adult toxicity was expressed as retarded weight gain when females were exposed to lead from weaning. Growth retardation in the neonate was altered at the same exposure levels as those that affected maternal weight gain. This effect on growth was then used as the standard against which all other toxic signs were compared to determine whether these other effects were specific to lead exposure or were secondary to growth retardation. The functional systems indicated in Table 1 were chosen for examination from available information that indicated their potential sensitivity to lead. The relative specificity of effects on these or other functional systems may vary depending on the agent or class of agents being studied. As indicated in Table 1, delays in age at vaginal opening, learning in a T-maze task, impairment of cell-mediated and humorally-mediated immune competence, and altered renal morphology and weights were found at exposure levels below those associated with growth retardation (<50 ppm lead). Although these same effects were seen in animals at higher exposure levels, their occurrence as a possible direct effect of lead exposure could not be deduced without the dose–response evaluation. In addition, effects on renal morphology were noted only after 9 months of exposure (6-month evaluations did not reveal any changes) and therefore would not have been detected without this longitudinal approach. Tissue lead levels were also measured longitudinally and confirmed that animals were exposed in a dose-related manner in this study. The last column in Table 1 integrates information from all the endpoints examined in this study and indicates the lowest effective exposure level of lead. As indicated, 5 ppm cannot be concluded definitely to be a toxic level, but it certainly should be considered suspect. Detailed presentations of these data may be found elsewhere (4,5,8,14, 18,25).

## ELEMENTS OF A DEVELOPMENTAL TOXICITY PROFILE: CURRENT STATE OF THE ART

Although only a few chemicals have been studied in an integrated fashion [e.g., X-irradiation (10) and methylmercury (23)], there has been a tremendous proliferation of reports in specific areas that will help to define better methods for delineating a profile of developmental toxicity. For example, we have become much more aware of the potential for disturbances in postnatal function resulting from developmental exposure (see chapters in the section "Perinatal and Postnatal Functional Evaluations" in this volume). Stanton (24) has reviewed the factors important

TABLE 1. Summary of developmental lead toxicity

FUNCTIONAL SYSTEMS

| Lead exposure[a] | Growth and development | Reproduction | CNS | Immune | Spleen and Kidney (9 mo. offspring) | Other | Toxic response? |
|---|---|---|---|---|---|---|---|
| 250 ppm | No ↑ mortality. Growth retardation in maternal animals and offspring. | No effect other than delayed vaginal opening. | No neuropathology.[b] Delayed locomotor development and surface righting. T-maze task. Shuttle box avoidance. | Impaired immunologic competence | Spleen: ↑ hemosiderin and organ weight. Kidney: Impaired heme biosynthesis and mitochondrial respiration. Intranuclear inclusions. Karyomegaly and cytomegaly.[c] ↑ organ weight; ↑ body weight in males only. | No change in hematology or clinical chemistries. | Yes |
| 50 ppm | | | | | | | Yes |
| 25 ppm | | | | | | | Yes |
| 5 ppm | | | | | | | ? |
| 0.5 ppm | | | | | | | No |

[a]Lead exposure is given as the concentration in drinking water in ppm.
[b]The only evaluation was histopathology at 9 months of age.
[c]Effect observed in both sexes except in 5-ppm group; only males were affected in this group.
From Kimmel et al., (15), with permission.

in studying postnatal physiological effects of prenatal exposure to xenobiotics. All functional systems are theoretically at risk at some point in their development and maturation, and a number are relatively unexplored as yet (e.g., respiratory, cardiovascular, gastrointestinal, renal, and hepatic function).

In the few instances where these systems have been assessed, there have been indications of toxic effects. Armenti and Johnson (1) have shown that fetal exposure to excess vitamin A altered lung histology and increased neonatal mortality, possibly because of incomplete expansion of the lungs. Christian and Johnson (3) have reported alterations in gastrointestinal function (i.e., total transit time, sigmoid and rectal emptying times) following actinomycin D, hydroxyurea, or methotrexate treatment. The potential for altered renal development and function has been described by Gibson (7). Fox (6) has demonstrated that lead exposure may delay the development of temperature regulation in neonatal rats. Our laboratory is currently studying the effects of chemical agents on cardiovascular function and predisposition to hypertension (13), as suggested earlier by Grollman and Grollman (9). Another area somewhat unexplored is shortened life-span resulting from early developmental exposure (23).

Taken together, postnatal functional alterations should be viewed as important manifestations of developmental toxicity and are critical in the determination of risk estimation and extrapolation of animal data to man. This is especially true when these effects (e.g., learning impairment or metabolic alterations) occur at dose levels below those that cause the other major manifestations of developmental insult, i.e., death, malformation, or growth retardation. Once such functional alterations are linked with exposure to a particular toxicant, epidemiologic studies may be designed to evaluate such a relationship in man. This is not meant to indicate that the animal data can be expected to predict precisely an effect in man, but perhaps such data may point toward functions that have not previously been associated with developmental insult. Thus, treatment and implementation of preventive measures for functional abnormalities may become more effective once these abnormalities are identified as resulting from developmental exposure.

Another area ripe for expansion within developmental toxicology is the study of comparative pharmacokinetics. Knowledge of the disposition of chemicals and metabolites in both the mother and embryo is important for choosing the species to use in testing a particular chemical. If there is no species readily available that simulates the pharmacokinetic pattern in man, this information is still important for understanding the similarities or differences in embryotoxic outcome in the species used. The potential utility of pharmacokinetics in improving safety evaluation has been emphasized for toxicology in general (e.g., 19) and for teratology specifically (28). A few teratology studies have correlated maternal blood or embryo levels of particular chemicals with the subsequent teratogenic response (16,20,26,27,29). Rowland et al. (20) indicated differences in parent glucocorticoid levels that correlated with the differential teratogenicity of triamcinolone acetonide and cortisol in the rat. The direct correlation of pharmacokinetic parameters with embryo/fetal response has been pursued in our laboratory using sodium salicylate teratogenicity as a model system (29). In rats, fetal outcome was predictable in 74% of the litters from the pharmacokinetic profiles of the maternal animals. This study was done by obtaining individual animal pharmacokinetic patterns, a step that is essential to account for a high level of interlitter variability. It also requires fewer animals, results in a more accurate pharmacokinetic pattern, and may reveal differences in responsive versus nonresponsive individuals (28).

The third major area in which some progress has been made is the study of mechanisms of action of developmental toxicants. However, our understanding of mechanisms and subsequent developmental events is still extemely limited (see chapters by R. G. Skalko and G. L. Kimmel, *this volume*). To some extent this has been the result of technical problems involved in attempting to work with the small amounts of tissue available in embryonic and fetal organisms. More recent technology has overcome some of these barriers; however, even more serious has been the lack of interest in developmental toxicity by scientists with expertise in areas other than the morphological disciplines. This situation also is changing, and the interest of scientists in other disciplines should continue to grow as the challenges and complexities of toxicity in the developing system are recognized. Realistically, the paucity of our knowledge about mechanisms of abnormal development makes it doubtful that such information will be available in the near future for a number of agents. This fact does not negate, but rather it emphasizes the need for increased effort in this area.

## AN APPROACH TO DELINEATING A PROFILE OF DEVELOPMENTAL TOXICITY

With the pertinent information currently being gathered in specific areas of postnatal function, pharmacokinetics, and mechanisms, it should be possible to begin to define profiles of developmental toxicity. The following discussion outlines one approach that is based largely on the manner in which we have been studying salicylate teratogenesis in our laboratory (11,13,29; C. A. Kimmel, *unpublished data*) and should not be considered the only approach to collecting such data.

First, the information known about the toxicity of the agent and of structurally and pharmacologically related chemicals and possible modes of human exposure should be considered. Second, basic pharmacokinetic data should be obtained, including the time course of the agent in blood, urine, and feces of one or more species; this should then be compared with available data in man (28). Subsequent data can be gathered to determine embryo exposure levels and their relationship to maternal blood levels. Third, dose-finding studies for determining developmental toxicity endpoints should then be carried out, initially to determine the maternal maximum tolerated dose (MTD) and the viability and normality of offspring at term. Subsequent endpoints of postnatal function should be assessed if initial studies show no effects below the MTD or if a lowest effective dose is required for setting exposure limits. If the agent appears to affect embryonic development or survival, the relationship of maternal pharmacokinetics to embryonal dosimetry should then be established by collecting embryos or fetuses following treatment. Pharmacokinetic patterns and developmental toxicity endpoint evaluations should be determined in the same animals, and correlation of pharmacokinetic and developmental toxicity parameters may suggest those pharmacokinetic factors that are important in predicting developmental toxicity within and among species. These predictions should then be validated where possible (29).

The study of mechanisms may begin at any point in this sequence and should take into account the information on mechanisms that is available from other studies, e.g., carcinogenesis, mutagenesis, pharmacology. Information on pharmacokinetics and endpoints may be useful in deciding on a mechanistic approach to pursue. The study of mechanisms should include not only the interaction of an agent with a cellular or subcellular component but also the impact of this interaction on subsequent developmental events (pathogenesis) and the potential for compensation for damage resulting from the action of an agent (22). Once mechanisms of action are delineated, exposure of the target site(s) to the active agent can be more clearly defined. Information on mechanisms should also provide a clearer understanding of observed and potential manifestations of toxicity and should suggest the possibility that additional endpoints or latent effects may be predicted from early developmental alterations. Thus, the study of developmental toxicity must be an integrative one with interplay among each of the three correlates, as indicated in Fig. 2.

There are likely to be a number of effective means of gathering the necessary information for delineating a profile of developmental toxicity. In some cases, limitations in methodology may necessitate one approach versus another. However, an effort must be undertaken for a number of agents to assess the validity of this approach for more accurately predicting human hazard. Once data are available on a number of agents, approaches may be simplified and general principles established that can be used in collecting and integrating information in future studies.

## CONCLUSIONS

The importance of developmental toxicology is being realized by many in both the public and private sectors as evidenced by the proliferation of new journals and books, the number of studies in the scientific literature, and the regulatory decisions that have recently been made, e.g., concerning possible risk of exposure to DES or lead or the intake of alcohol or caffeine. In addition, the sensitivity of the developing organism has become more widely recognized in toxicology, and studies more frequently incorporate developmental exposures for assessing chemical hazards.

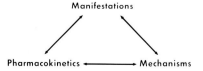

**FIG. 2.** Constant interplay among the three key correlates in the study of developmental toxicity.

The potential for advances in the future are great if we decide that developmental disabilities are of major consequence to the well-being of future generations and the quality of life. Such value judgments must be made and will most probably influence the emphasis (and thus the monetary support) that is given to the types of studies outlined in this chapter. As Campbell (2) has described for carcinogenesis, the harmfulness of a toxic event may be related to the severity and prolongation of the disease as well as to the degree of irreversibility. Within this framework, most developmental toxicities certainly would be described as very harmful. Although our current ability to accurately predict risk is limited, the benefits of an integrated approach to defining profiles of developmental toxicity would far outweigh the cost in the long run. Our ability to predict human risk would be more soundly based and provide a better means of estimating, and thus minimizing, human developmental toxicity.

## REFERENCES

1. Armenti, V. T., and Johnson, E. M. (1979): Effects of maternal hypervitaminosis A on perinatal rat lung histology. *Biol. Neonate*, 36:305–310.
2. Campbell, T. C. (1980): Chemical carcinogens and human risk assessment. *Fed. Proc.*, 39:2467–2484.
3. Christian, M. S., and Johnson, E. M. (1978): Prenatal alteration of postnatal gastrointestinal physiology. *Teratology*, 17:44A.
4. Faith, R. E., Luster, M. I., and Kimmel, C. A. (1978): Effects of chronic developmental lead exposure on cell-mediated function. *Clin. Exp. Immunol.*, 35:413–420.
5. Fowler, B. A., Kimmel, C. A., Woods, J. S., McConnell, E. E., and Grant, L. D. (1980): Chronic low-level lead toxicity in the rat. III. An integrated assessment of long-term toxicity with special reference to the kidney. *Toxicol. Appl. Pharmacol.*, 56:59–77.
6. Fox, D. A. (1979): Physiological and neurobehavioral alterations during development in lead exposed rats. *Neurobehav. Toxicol.*, 1 (Suppl.1):193–206.
7. Gibson, J. E. (1976): Perinatal nephropathies. *Environ. Health Perspect.*, 15:121–130.
8. Grant, L. D., Kimmel, C. A., West, G. L., Martinez-Vargas, C. M., and Howard, J. L. (1980): Chronic low-level lead toxicity in the rat. II. Effects on postnatal physical and behavioral development. *Toxicol. Appl. Pharmacol.*, 56:42–58.
9. Grollman, A., and Grollman, E. F. (1962): The teratogenic induction of hypertension. *J. Clin. Invest.*, 41:710–714.
10. Hicks, S. P., and D'Amato, C. J. (1966): Effects of ionizing radiations on mammalian development. In: *Advances in Teratology, Vol. 1*, edited by D. H. M. Woollam, pp. 195–250. Academic Press, New York.
11. Holson, J. F., Kimmel, C. A., and Young, J. F. (1980): The precision of pharmacokinetic parameters for predicting embryotoxicity endpoints. In: *Abstracts of Papers, Society of Toxicology, 19th Annual Meeting*, p. A24. Academic Press, New York.
12. Joffe, J. M. (1969): *Prenatal Determinants of Behavior*. Pergamon Press, New York.
13. Kimmel, C. A., and Buelke-Sam, J. (1980): Cardiovascular function following prenatal salicylate exposure to rats. *Teratology*, 21:49A.
14. Kimmel, C. A., Grant, L. D., Sloan, C. S., and Gladen, B. C. (1980): Chronic low-level lead toxicity in the rat. I. Maternal toxicity and perinatal effects. *Toxicol. Appl. Pharmacol.*, 56:28–41.
15. Kimmel, C. A., Grant, L. D., West, G. L., Martinez-Vargas, C. M., McConnell, E. E., Fowler, B. A., Woods, J. S., and Howard, J. L. (1978): Multidisciplinary approach to the assessment of developmental toxicity associated with chronic lead exposure. In: *Developmental Toxicity of Energy-Related Pollutants, DOE Symposium Series #47*, edited by D. D. Mahlum, M. R. Sikov, P. L. Hackett, and F. D. Andrew, pp. 396–409. United States Department of Energy, Washington, D.C.
16. Kimmel, C. A., Wilson J. G., and Schumacher, H. J. (1971): Studies on the metabolism and identification of the causative agent in aspirin teratogenesis in the rat. *Teratology*, 4:15–24.
17. Kretchmer, N. (1978): Perspectives in teratologic research. *Teratology*, 17:203–212.

18. Luster, M. I., Faith, R. E., and Kimmel, C. A. (1978): Humoral antibody response in rats following chronic developmental lead exposure. *J. Environ. Pathol. Toxicol.*, 1:397–402.
19. Ramsey, J. C., and Gehring, P. J. (1980): Application of pharmacokinetic principles in practice. *Fed. Proc.*, 39:60–65.
20. Rowland, J. M., Althaus, Z. R., Slikker, W., Jr., and Hendrickx, A. G. (1980): Comparative distribution of triamcinolone acetonide and cortisol in the rat embryomaternal unit. *Teratology*, 21:65A–66A.
21. Smithells, R. W. (1980): The challenge of teratology. *Teratology*, 22:77–85.
22. Snow, M. H. L., and Tam, P. P. L. (1979): Is compensatory growth a complicating factor in mouse teratology? *Nature*, 279:555–557.
23. Spyker, J. M. (1975): Assessing the impact of low level chemicals on development: Behavioral and latent effects. *Fed. Proc.*, 34:1835–1844.
24. Stanton, H. C. (1978): Factors to consider when selecting animal models for postnatal teratology studies. *J. Environ. Pathol. Toxicol.*, 2:201–210.
25. West, G. L., Kimmel, C. A., Grant, L. D., and Howard, J. L. (1981): Appetitive acquisition and performance deficits in rats with chronic low-level lead exposure. *Neurobehav. Toxicol. Terat.* *(in press)*.
26. Wilson, J. G., Ritter, E. J., Scott, W. J., and Fradkin, R. (1977): Comparative distribution and embryotoxicity of acetylsalicylic acid in pregnant rats and Rhesus monkeys. *J. Toxicol. Appl. Pharmacol.*, 41:67–78.
27. Wilson, J. G., Scott, W. J., Ritter, E. J., and Fradkin, R. (1975): Comparative distribution and embryotoxicity of hydroxyurea in pregnant rats and Rhesus monkeys. *Teratology*, 11:169–178.
28. Young, J. F., and Holson, J. F. (1978): Utility of pharmacokinetics in designing toxicological protocols and improving interspecies extrapolation. *J. Environ. Pathol. Toxicol.*, 2:169–186.
29. Young, J. F., Kimmel, C. A., and Holson, J. F. (1979): Validation of a pharmacokinetic model for rat embryonal dosimetry of salicylates during a teratogenically susceptible period. *Toxicol. Appl. Pharmacol.*, 48:A121.

# Subject Index